Mosby's PATHOLOGY *for* Massage Therapists

ELSEVIER

evolve

The Latest *Evolution* in Learning.

Evolve provides online access to free learning resources and activities designed specifically for the textbook you are using in your class. The resources will provide you with information that enhances the material covered in the book and much more.

Visit the Web address listed below to start your learning evolution today!

▶▶ *LOGIN: http://evolve.elsevier.com/Salvo/pathology/*

Evolve Learning Resources for Salvo/Anderson: *Mosby's Pathology for Massage Therapists* offer the following features:

- **Resources**
  An exciting feature that lets you link to hundreds of websites carefully chosen to supplement the content of the textbook. Resources include government agencies, researchers, and nonprofit associations, to name a few.

- **Crossword puzzles**
  Have fun reviewing pathologies and medical terminology by completing crossword puzzles!

- **Case studies**
  Read the case studies and then apply the knowledge gained from the chapters to answer the questions.

- **Client assessment section**
  To assess any pathologies, this two-part client assessment section includes a list of questions to ask the client, as well as observations and/or palpations that can be made during the intake or during treatment.

- **Pronunciation list**
  For those hard-to-read pathologies, check out the pronunciation list at your fingertips.

Think outside the book... *evolve.*

Mosby's
PATHOLOGY
for Massage
Therapists

SUSAN G. SALVO, BEd, LMT, NTS, CI, NCTMB

Co-owner, Co-director, and Instructor
Louisiana Institute of Massage Therapy
Lake Charles, Louisiana

SANDRA K. ANDERSON, BA, LMT, NCTMB

Department Head of Anatomy and Physiology
Desert Institute of the Healing Arts
Tucson, Arizona

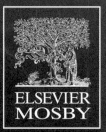

ELSEVIER
MOSBY

ELSEVIER
MOSBY

11830 Westline Industrial Drive
St. Louis, Missouri 63146

NOTICE

Massage Therapy is an ever-changing field. Standard safety precautions must be followed, but as new research and clinical experience broaden our knowledge, changes in treatment and drug therapy may become necessary or appropriate. Readers are advised to check the most current product information provided by the manufacturer of each drug to be administered to verify the recommended dose, the method and duration of administration, and contraindications. It is the responsibility of the licensed prescriber, relying on experience and knowledge of the patient, to determine dosages and the best treatment for each individual patient. Neither the publisher nor the author assumes any liability for any injury and/or damage to persons or property arising from this publication.

Library of Congress Cataloging-in-Publication Data

Salvo, Susan G.
  Mosby's pathology for massage therapists/Susan G. Salvo, Sandra Kauffman Anderson.
  p. ; cm.
Includes bibliographical references and index.
ISBN 0-323-02652-4
  1. Pathology. 2. Massage therapy. I. Title: Pathology for massage therapists. II. Anderson, Sandra Kauffman. III. Title.
[DNLM: 1. Massage—methods. 2. Diagnostic Techniques and Procedures. 3. Pathology. WB 537 S186ma 2004]
RB111.S29 2004
616.07—dc22

Publishing Director: Linda Duncan
Acquisitions Editor: Kellie White
Senior Developmental Editor: Kim Fons
Editorial Assistant: Kendra Bailey
Publishing Services Manager: Melissa Lastarria
Associate Project Manager: Bonnie Spinola
Designer: Julia Dummitt

Printed in the United States of America

Last digit is the print number: 9 8 7 6 5 4 3 2 1

The study of human pathology is as essential as bone is to muscle in the assurance of safe practice and application of massage therapy. There are so few texts available on the subject of pathology as it pertains to therapeutic massage and even fewer written in the last five decades. We who teach massage and related subjects know intimately the limitations of our available references. We have endured the painstaking task of filtering material from physical therapy and kinesiology books that make little if any mention of manual therapy. It is, therefore, with abundant pleasure that I write this foreword and congratulate Ms. Salvo for the creation of this modern resource for today's massage therapist.

In a foreword by James Little in Despard's *Textbook of Massage* from 1911, he writes, "Massage has now secured its position as a recognized therapeutic measure useful alike in medical and surgical cases . . ." He goes on to describe what he feels are the quintessential traits of massage therapists, noting that therapists should "have the physical and mental qualities necessary for its successful practice, the tact, the judicious firmness, the wise reticence, the sympathetic disposition without which success is not to be obtained." These characteristics are highly valued; even today, students who portray these qualities stand apart from the rest.

I have waited with great anticipation for books on massage published in this century. At last, they are starting to appear. This new century holds renewed promise toward the relief of human suffering through integrated healthcare. The arrival of *Mosby's Pathology for Massage Therapists* brings us one step closer to legitimacy and inclusion in the professional practice of caring for humanity.

"The physiologic research, which has been applied to the methods of massage within recent years, has clearly demonstrated the effectiveness of external manipulations as a means of influencing metabolic and other processes in the deeper parts of the organism." The above sentence, which pertains to massage research from the late 1800s and early 1900s, was written by John Harvey Kellogg in 1922. Yet, the same could be said of today's research. This text cites the latest research available and substantiates it by providing relative anatomical, physiological, and kinesthetic subject matter, manual technique, and precautions. There is no doubt that it will be an invaluable resource for the new generation of practitioners for years to come.

The chapters in the text are arranged in a logical sequence and are accompanied by hundreds of images and photographs that reinforce the recognition of pathologies. Massage therapists are often the first to notice suspicious marks on the skin or the beginning of deformities. Early detection has become vitally important as a preventive measure. The chapter on disease awareness and infection control is essential reading when so many individuals with compromised immunity are seeking relief through massage.

The journey into mainstream medicine is once again inevitable, and it is essential that we in the healing arts have a thorough knowledge of pathology. It is of equal importance that practitioners of wellness or spa massage obtain these competencies, as they too are responsible for referring clients to a doctor if and when they detect abnormalities. The authors of this book acknowledge a deep respect in regard to massage therapists' affiliation with the medical profession and accountability to the public trust. With invaluable help from her colleague Sandra K. Anderson, Ms. Salvo has brilliantly portrayed the efficacy of the oldest medicine. While most pathology texts depict the human organism at its worst, within these pages lie glimmers of hope toward some reprise of the human condition, from which no one is exempt, creating room for every kind of healing.

"It will take a society of healers to heal society."—Sherry Rosenheck, RN, LMT

Elaine Calenda
Clinical Education Director
Boulder College of Massage Therapy
2003

The study of pathology is a vital component of any massage therapy training program. The healthcare field has grown exponentially over the past few decades, and medicine has become so technologically advanced that physicians can now diagnose almost any condition by the use of scans or chemically based tests. The technology itself is amazing and has saved countless lives. However, one of the casualties of this technical revolution in medicine has been the regrettable demise of palpation. For many physicians, palpation has become a lost art replaced by these new diagnostic tests.

For massage therapists, palpation remains our primary tool of evaluation. We use it daily and are adept at recognizing the differences between the feel of healthy muscle and the taut, fibrous bands of injured tissue. Even therapists who do not know exactly what a sebaceous cyst is can tell that it feels different from a trigger point or a "knot" in a muscle. As bearers of this lost art of palpation, we are obligated to learn as much about pathology as possible. In doing so, our skills can evolve from simple touch to purposeful palpatory evaluation and informed assessment.

To achieve that end, this book has been written with two purposes in mind. First, it may be used as an initial learning tool to introduce the beginning therapist to the study of diseases. The scope of most anatomy classes and their respective textbooks does not allow the time or space for pathology to be fully developed. This book can be used as an adjunct to anatomy and physiology classes to cover the concepts of massage and disease more thoroughly. Second, it may be used for continuing education or as a desk reference for the established therapist.

The book is formatted to be reader-friendly, and it has many important and innovative features:

• **Organization** Textually, the book organizes pathologies by body system. Chapters 3 to 11 include an overview of body systems and general manifestations of the associated pathologies. Diseases and conditions are listed alphabetically. When applicable, both the technical and common pathological terms are listed. Each pathology features its Greek or Latin root derivation, a description of the disease, and any applicable massage considerations. These considerations often include suggestions for technique. Pronunciations accompany many diseases. End-of-the-chapter self-tests are included to allow the

student to check his or her understanding of the definitions.

• **Volume of Information** Covers more than 340 pathologies, almost twice that of the next best-selling pathology book on the market.

• **Tables of Medications** Various chapters include tables of commonly prescribed medications. This helps the massage therapist to understand massage considerations for medications (e.g., anticoagulants, platelet inhibitors, corticosteroids, NSAIDs, muscle relaxers, narcotic analgesics) common to the pathologies discussed, as well as possible side effects that may affect treatment. These tables include medications used to treat musculoskeletal disorders and medications used to manage mood disorders, diabetes, HIV/AIDS, cardiovascular disease, respiratory disorders, and cancer.

• **Assessment Guide** The assessment guide found in Chapter 2 is the most comprehensive on the market today. Featured assessments range from posture and gait to skin condition and range of motion. Additionally, each chapter has a brief therapeutic assessment guide applicable to the featured body system. This includes a list of questions to ask the client, as well as observations and/or palpations that can be made during the intake or during treatment.

• **Self-tests** Self-tests are included at the end of Chapters 3 to 12 to assist the student in seeing how much he or she has retained and to teach him or her how to structure study time when studying for tests. This book can also be used as a study guide to prepare for and successfully pass state and/or national examinations.

• **Cancer** A complete chapter provides an overview of cancer, its risk factors, current cancer treatments, guidelines to follow when working with cancer patients, and a special intake form to use for clients living with cancer.

• **Cardio Pulmonary Resuscitation (CPR)** CPR is featured in Chapter 1 and includes an illustration sequence to assist the reader in understanding how to apply CPR if it is ever needed. This topic is taught in most massage schools.

• **Medical Technologies** Included in numerous chapters are discussions and massage considerations for medical technologies and devices used in treatment of various acute and chronic pathologies, such as colostomies, central venous catheters, transdermal patches, pacemakers, implantable cardioverter defibrillators, and renal dialysis.

- **Additional Tables and Charts** Various chapters include statistics, tables, and charts, such as Comparative Causes of Annual Deaths in the United States, Leading Causes of Death, Tables of Joint Movements, Common Skin Lesions, Mole Changes, Comparison of Hyperglycemia to Hypoglycemia, Comparison of Type I and Type II Diabetes, Malignancies and Common Opportunistic Infections and Conditions in AIDS, Types of Hepatitis, Common Infections Transmitted by Food and Water, Risk Factors for Contracting Sexually Transmitted Diseases, and Comparison of Benign and Malignant Tumors.

- **Illustrations** This book has been lavishly illustrated to be an invaluable pictorial reference for the recognition of disease by the beginning and established therapist. The photos and drawings in this pathology book have been placed adjacent to the corresponding text.

- **Resource Lists** Each chapter provides a list of resources for further information on various diseases. Resources include government agencies, researchers, and non-profit associations along with contact information or website addresses, including the American Anorexia/Bulimia Association, the National Cancer Institute, the American Diabetes Association, and many others.

- **Quick Reference Icons** Perhaps most important for the massage therapist, this book has been designed as a quick reference text for massage-specific contraindications of all the diseases listed herein. The term *quick reference* is used because the text and illustration of each disease is presented with an icon of a traffic light. This traffic light may be green, yellow, red, or combinations of these colors.

Green denotes that massage is indicated for the given condition and that the therapist may proceed normally. For example, psoriasis, although scaly and rough, may be treated with massage. The condition represented with a green traffic light may merit lighter pressure, a shorter duration, or increased or decreased frequency of treatments.

Yellow denotes that the therapist should proceed with caution; the condition may require that massage be avoided locally in the affected area or that a physician's approval be obtained before treatment. An example of a yellow icon disease would be warts, which must be avoided locally

but do not preclude the therapist from working on the unaffected areas of the body. A yellow caution light may also represent that a condition has cycles of exacerbation and remission and that massage should be applied only when the client's condition is in remission.

Red denotes that the condition is totally contraindicated for massage and that the therapist must not perform treatment. Contagious diseases such as scabies infestation or German measles fall into this category. Red also denotes a medical emergency or a life-threatening condition, such as encephalitis or kidney failure.

By use of these icons, a therapist can quickly glance at the condition and know if he or she can proceed without caution (green), perform no massage at all (red), or if he or she needs to take the time to read further for considerations (yellow). The icon system has been designed to improve both the effectiveness and the efficiency of massage.

- **Appendixes** This text also provides five appendixes. Appendix A includes a quick reference table in which all pathologies contained in the text are listed alphabetically with the massage considerations to the right. Appendix B addresses physiological effects of massage by body system. This section also lists specific conditions in which massage has been scientifically proven to have a positive effect. Endangerment sites are covered in Appendix C. Because massage therapy also includes the use of hydrotherapy, Appendix D lists contraindications for hydrotherapy use. Appendix E includes symbols and abbreviations that are commonly used when writing treatment notes.

- **Website Support** There is an established website for both instructors and students that includes a resource section and case studies. Instructors can access an image collection, sample tests, lesson plans, and a unique forum for general questions, which are sent directly to the author. Students will enjoy crossword puzzles, pronunciations of pathologies, and a two-part client assessment section.

A few more thoughts on massage, palpation, and pathology: A large part of the success of massage lies in the fact that massage therapists spend so much time with clients; this gives them the opportunity to express health concerns, and it gives therapists the time necessary to find problem areas. Another key component of this success is the access afforded by massage. Massage therapists see and feel areas that are not commonly treated by other professions. And the frequency with which most clients schedule massages allows therapists to notice changes that may become health considerations. All of these factors, combined with superior palpatory skill and knowledge of pathology, make massage therapists an important part of the healthcare team.

Today, massage therapists are often the first healthcare practitioners to assess a possible pathology and refer the client to his or her physician for proper diagnosis and further treatment. In the spirit of this teamwork, we have gathered a prestigious group of reviewers consisting of doctors, nurses, pharmacists, and massage therapists to make sure that all pathologies have been double- and triple-checked for accuracy. But it is not enough to write a book like this. It is up to you, the therapist, to put the information to use. Each massage therapist must learn about pathology to tailor his or her massage treatments. We can ease pain and discomfort where possible, promote healing, and avoid massage when contraindicated so as to not cause harm.

Susan G. Salvo
susansalvo@hotmail.com

Sandra K. Anderson
anderkauf@msn.com

ACKNOWLEDGMENTS

We would like to acknowledge the following individuals who assisted us in writing this book:

Dr. Joseph O'Donnell
Mike Breaux
Rhiannon Roberts
Tracy Walton
Kim Fons
Dr. Maureen Oliver
Dr. Charles Woodard
Patti Phillip, RPh
Carolyn Vallery Robinson, RN

Tari Dilks, CFNP, LPC
Maggie Woosley, BA
Bonnie Spinola
Kellie White
Elaine Calenda

Susan G. Salvo, BEd, LMT, NTS, CI, NCTMB
Sandra K. Anderson, BA, LMT, NCTMB

TABLE OF CONTENTS

Mosby's PATHOLOGY for Massage Therapists

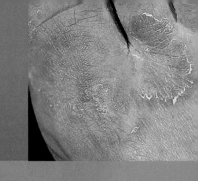

1

Disease Awareness and Infection Control

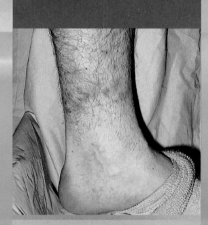

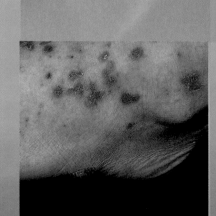

INTRODUCTION TO PATHOLOGY

As health care professionals, massage therapists seek to improve the health and well-being of their clients through massage therapy. Regardless of work setting or treatment style, the massage therapist encounters clients who have pathologies, who are under medical supervision, and/or who are taking prescription medications. The therapist needs information regarding these conditions and medications, as well as how massage can be safely administered in these situations. This information will also assist the therapist in making treatment choices such as whether to use neuromuscular therapy, manual lymphatic drainage, joint mobilizations, stretching, hydrotherapy, or other modalities and techniques that are appropriate.

To build an understanding of disease and its transmission, it is necessary to begin with a fundamental overview of pathology, also known as pathophysiology. *Pathology* is the study of biological and physical manifestation of disease. Disease occurs when there is some sort of disruption in the homeostasis of the body.

Homeostasis is a constancy within the body's internal environment. The internal environment consists of cells, tissues, organs, systems, and all the fluids associated with them. Homeostasis is a dynamic process. As conditions change in the body, the equilibrium point will change only over a narrow range. For example, blood glucose levels normally stay between 70 and 110 mg of glucose per 100 ml of blood. Blood glucose levels that stay outside this range, either above it or below it, may not be compatible with life. Every body structure, from the cells to organ systems, helps keep the internal environment within normal limits.

The body's homeostasis is constantly being challenged. The disturbances can come from the external environment, such as intense cold or lack of oxygen, or from inside the body, such as water levels in the blood that are too low. Homeostasis can also be challenged as a result of psychological stresses, such as demands from family or work. In most cases, the disturbance of homeostasis is temporary, and the body is able to quickly restore it. If the disruption is extreme, homeostasis may not be restored. In the case of uncontrolled diabetes mellitus, blood glucose levels can be far greater than 110 mg per 100 ml of blood because glucose is not entering the body cells that need it. If blood glucose levels are left uncontrolled long enough, death could occur.

Homeostasis is maintained by the interplay of regulatory processes in the body. The two major systems of the body that regulate homeostasis are the nervous system and the endocrine system. They can work together or independently to correct changes in homeostasis. The nervous system sends messages as nerve impulses to structures and organs that can counteract imbalances. The endocrine system secretes chemical messengers called hormones into the bloodstream. Nerve impulses cause rapid changes, whereas hormones usually work more slowly, but no less effectively.

The body regulates the internal environment through many feedback systems. Feedback systems are cycles of events in which conditions in the body are constantly monitored, evaluated, modified, remonitored, reevaluated, remodified, etc.

Most feedback systems of the body are negative systems. Negative feedback systems reverse a disruption in a controlled condition. For example, normal body temperature is 98.6° F, which is a controlled condition. When the external environment becomes very warm, there is a disruption in the controlled condition, and body temperature can increase as well. To maintain homeostasis, several mechanisms are activated to cool the body, including perspiring and bringing blood to the surface (the skin becomes flushed) so that excess heat can be lost from the body. These mechanisms reverse the disruption in the controlled condition.

Positive feedback systems strengthen or reinforce a change in a controlled condition. These systems continue until they are interrupted by some mechanism outside the system. An example of this kind of system is the response of the immune system when it is challenged by a disease-producing organism. When a disease-producing organism enters the body, it stimulates the proliferation of white blood cells, whose purpose is to fight off intruders. The white blood cells secrete chemicals that stimulate the formation of even more white blood cells. This cycle of increasing chemicals stimulating the formation of more white blood cells results in a continual strengthening or reinforcement of the change in the controlled environment. White blood cells proliferate until there are sufficient numbers to create an army that destroys the invading organism. This positive feedback system continues until the organism is contained, and there is no longer any need to form more white blood cells.

The body stays healthy as long as controlled conditions within the body are maintained by feedback systems. If some aspect of the body loses its ability to contribute to homeostasis, however, equilibrium in other parts of the body or the body as a whole

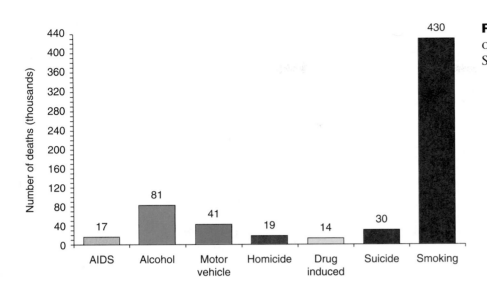

Figure 1-1. Comparative causes of annual deaths in the United States.

may be disturbed. If there is a moderate imbalance, a disorder or disease may result. If the imbalance is severe enough, death can occur.

A *disorder* is any functional abnormality; a *disease* is a more specific term that refers to any illness that is characterized by certain signs and symptoms. Signs are objective changes in the body that can be observed and measured. They include swelling, rashes, fever, high blood pressure, and paralysis. Symptoms are subjective changes in the body that only the person experiencing them is aware of. These include headaches, nausea, and anxiety. A *syndrome* is a group of signs and symptoms that occur to collectively present a pattern that defines a particular disease or abnormality. Down syndrome is a genetic disorder in which the person has delayed mental development, short stature, a round face, with a Mongoloid slant to the eyes, and possibly heart abnormalities.

A *local disease* can affect only one area of the body. An example is a foot fungus. A *systemic disease* affects many areas of the body or the entire body. An example is systemic lupus erythematosus, which is an inflammatory disease of connective tissues. Connective tissue is found everywhere in the body. *Acute diseases* have an abrupt onset of severe symptoms that run a brief course (less than 6 months) and then resolve or, in some cases, cause death (Figures 1-1 and 1-2). *Chronic diseases* develop slowly and last longer than 6 months. In some cases, chronic illness lasts a lifetime.

Diagnosing is the science and skill of distinguishing diseases or disorders from each other. It is based on signs and symptoms, physical examination, and specialized testing. Diagnoses are established only by trained health care providers. It is beyond the scope of practice for massage therapists to diagnose clients.

Types of Diseases

To understand how to reduce the likelihood of transmitting disease, it is important to look at disease itself. This section explores the types of diseases and delineates which are contagious and which are not contagious.

The types of diseases are autoimmune, cancer, deficiency, degenerative, genetic, infectious, and metabolic. There are also two important categories of disorders: congenital and traumatic.

Autoimmune Diseases

Autoimmune diseases are part of a large group of diseases marked by an inappropriate or excessive response of the body's immune functions. The immune system fails to distinguish between the body's tissue and something that is foreign to the body such as an invading organism. The immune system then attacks the tissue, which not only affects the targeted tissue but also depletes the immune system, allowing other invaders to infect the body. Examples of autoimmune diseases are rheumatoid arthritis, in which the synovial membranes of joints are attacked; systemic lupus erythematosus, in which the connective tissue of the body is attacked; and multiple sclerosis, in which the covering (myelin sheath) of nerves in the central nervous system is attacked. Autoimmune diseases are not contagious.

Cancerous Diseases

Cancer is characterized by the uncontrollable growth of abnormal cells. The excess tissue that

10 Leading Causes of Death, United States 2000, All Races, Both Sexes

Rank	<1	1-4	5-9	10-14	15-24	25-34	35-44	45-54	55-64	65+	All Ages
						Age Groups					
1	Congenital Anomalies 5,743	Unintentional Injury 1,828	Unintentional Injury 1,391	Unintentional Injury 1,588	Unintentional Injury 14,113	Unintentional Injury 11,769	Malignant Neoplasms 16,520	Malignant Neoplasms 48,034	Malignant Neoplasms 89,005	Heart Disease 593,707	Heart Disease 710,760
2	Short Gestation 4,397	Congenital Anomalies 495	Malignant Neoplasms 489	Malignant Neoplasms 525	Homicide 4,939	Suicide 4,797	Unintentional Injury 15,413	Heart Disease 35,480	Heart Disease 63,399	Malignant Neoplasms 392,386	Malignant Neoplasms 553,091
3	SIDS 2,523	Malignant Neoplasms 420	Congenital Anomalies 198	Suicide 300	Suicide 3,994	Homicide 4,164	Heart Disease 13,181	Unintentional Injury 12,278	Chronic Low. Respiratory Disease 10,739	Cerebro-vascular 148,045	Cerebro-vascular 167,661
4	Maternal Pregnancy Comp. 1,404	Homicide 358	Homicide 140	Homicide 231	Malignant Neoplasms 1,713	Malignant Neoplasms 3,916	Suicide 6,582	Live Disease 6,654	Cerebro-vascular 9,958	Chronic Low. Respiratory Disease 108,375	Chronic Low. Respiratory Disease 122,009
5	Placenta Cord Membranes 1,062	Heart Disease 181	Heart Disease 106	Congenital Anomalies 201	Heart Disease 1,031	Heart Disease 2,958	HIV 5,919	Cerebro-vascular 6,011	Diabetes Mellitus 9,186	Influenza & Pneumonia 58,557	Unintentional Injury 97,900
6	Respiratory Distress 999	Influenza & Pneumonia 103	Benign Neoplasms 62	Heart Disease 165	Congenital Anomalies 441	HIV 2,437	Liver Disease 3,371	Suicide 5,437	Unintentional Injury 7,505	Diabetes Mellitus 52,414	Diabetes Mellitus 69,301
7	Unintentional Injury 881	Septicemia 99	Chronic Low. Respiratory Disease 48	Chronic Low. Respiratory Disease 91	Chronic Low. Respiratory Disease 199	Diabetes Mellitus 623	Homicide 3,219	Diabetes Mellitus 4,954	Liver Disease 5,774	Alzheimer's Disease 43,993	Influenza & Pneumonia 65,313
8	Bacterial Sepsis 763	Perinatal Period 79	Influenza & Pneumonia 47	Influenza & Pneumonia 40	Chronic Low. Respiratory Disease 190	Cerebro-vascular 602	Cerebro-vascular 2,599	HIV 4,142	Nephritis 3,100	Nephritis 31,225	Alzheimer's Disease 49,558
9	Circulatory System Disease 663	Benign Neoplasms 53	Septicemia 38	Cerebro-vascular 51	Influenza & Pneumonia 189	Congenital Anomalies 477	Diabetes Mellitus 1,926	Chronic Low. Respiratory Disease 3,251	Suicide 2,945	Unintentional Injury 31,051	Nephritis 37,251
10	Intrauterine Hypoxia 630	Chronic Low. Respiratory Disease 51	Two Tied 25	Benign Neoplasms 37	HIV 179	Liver Disease 415	Influenza & Pneumonia 1,068	Viral Hepatitis 1,894	Septicemia 2,899	Septicemia 24,786	Septicemia 31,224

Figure 1-2. Ten leading causes of death in the United States (2000, all races, both sexes).

develops when body cells divide without control is called a *neoplasm* or tumor. The study of tumors is called oncology. The tumors can be either cancerous or harmless. A cancerous tumor is called *malignant* and will often metastasize or spread cancerous cells to other parts of the body. A *benign* tumor does not metastasize, but may become life threatening if the tumor, as it grows, puts pressure on vital areas, such as within the brain. There are many types of cancers, and they are named for the type of tissue from which they are derived. Carcinomas arise from epithelial tissue. Melanomas grow from melanocytes—skin cells that produce the pigment melanin. Sarcomas develop from muscle cells or connective tissue. Leukemia is characterized by rapid growth of abnormal white blood cells. Lymphoma is a cancer of lymphatic tissue.

Causes of cancer include carcinogens, oncogenes, and oncoviruses. *Carcinogens* are cancer-causing chemical agents or radiation. They cause permanent structural changes in the genetic material of the cell. Examples of carcinogens include cigarette tar, radon gas, and ultraviolet radiation in sunlight. *Oncogenes* are cancer-causing genes. When these genes are inappropriately activated, they transform a normal cell into a cancerous cell. It is unclear how oncogenes become activated. *Oncoviruses* cause cancer by stimulating cells to divide abnormally. For example, the human papillomavirus causes cervical cancer in women. Cancer is not contagious (Box 1-1). See Chapter 12 for more information on cancer.

Box 1-1

Leading Causes of Death in the United States (2000)	
Heart disease	710,760
Cancer	553,091
Stroke	167,661
Chronic lower respiratory disease	122,009
Accidents	97,900
Diabetes	69,301
Pneumonia/influenza	65,313
Alzheimer's disease	49,558
Nephritis, nephrotic syndrome, and nephrosis	37,251
Septicemia	31,224

From Anderson RN: National Vital Statistics Report 150(16):2002. Centers for Disease Control and Prevention (National Center for Health Statistics), Division of Vital Statistics.

Deficiency Diseases

Deficiency diseases are caused either by a lack of an essential vitamin, mineral, or nutrient in the individual's diet, or by the individual's inability to properly digest and absorb a particular nutrient. This deficiency typically interferes with the body's growth, development, and metabolism. Types of deficiency diseases are scurvy, resulting from a deficiency of ascorbic acid or vitamin C (Figure 1-3); rickets, resulting from a deficiency of vitamin D (Figure 1-4); and beriberi, resulting from a deficiency of thiamine or vitamin B_1 (Figure 1-5). Pernicious anemia is due to inadequate absorption of vitamin B_{12} because of a lack of intrinsic factor from the stomach. Deficiency diseases are not contagious.

Degenerative Diseases

Degenerative diseases refer to tissue breakdown that occurs either as a result of an overuse syndrome, or naturally as a result of the aging process (Box 1-2). Examples of degenerative diseases are osteoporosis, Alzheimer's disease, and macular degeneration. Degenerative diseases are not contagious.

Genetic Diseases

Genetic diseases are caused by an abnormality in the genetic code. Genes are the cell's hereditary units. They are arranged in single file along chromosomes, which are located in the nucleus of the cell. Each gene codes for a single protein. All the genes on the chromosomes code for all the proteins in the body, and are responsible for the physical makeup of each person. Genetic abnormalities can be passed from one generation to the next. Examples of genetic diseases are cystic fibrosis, sickle cell anemia (Figure 1-6), and hemophilia. Genetic diseases are not contagious.

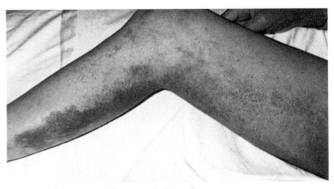

Figure 1-3. Scurvy.

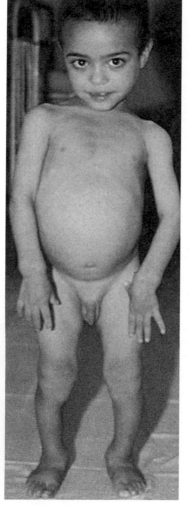

Figure 1-4.   Rickets.

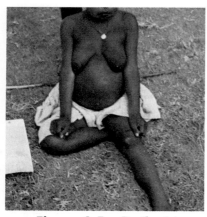

Figure 1-5.   Beriberi.

Box **1-2**

Miscellaneous Effects of Aging

As aging occurs, certain changes happen to all the body systems.

- Nerve and reflex reaction time is slower, so more time is typically needed to perform tasks such as the intake and the premassage interview.
- Because of the effect of the nervous system, there may be a loss or increased sensitivity to pain.
- There is typically a loss in hearing and vision (especially presbyopia) (i.e., nearsightedness and farsightedness) that must be taken into consideration.
- A decrease in strength and muscle tone is often noted.
- Bones are not as strong. Joints may not be as flexible and may begin to wear down. Osteoarthritis and osteoporosis are common. A mild kyphosis may be noted (dowager's hump). Joint mobilizations and stretching will need to be modified.
- The skin appears pale and wrinkled and becomes thinner, looser, and more frail. Age spots may appear on the skin as a result of blood leaking from damaged and weak capillaries. Liver spots may be seen on the skin of older people, especially those who have been exposed to excessive sun. Use adequate lubricant to prevent skin pulling.
- In the case of inactivity in some older people, circulation may not be efficient. Atherosclerosis is fairly common among older people.
- There may be an increase in incontinence resulting from loss of muscle tone in the urinary and gastrointestinal tracts.

Infectious Diseases

Infectious diseases are caused by a biologic agent such as a virus, bacterium, fungus, or parasite. Also known as communicable diseases, infectious diseases can be transmitted to a person by another person, animal, or inanimate object, called a *fomite*, either by direct or indirect contact. *Hosts* are the organisms in which the biological agents are residing. Examples of infectious disease are the common cold, strep throat, acquired immunodeficiency syndrome (AIDS), pneumonia, measles, scabies (Figure 1-7), lice (Figure 1-8), hepatitis A and hepatitis B,

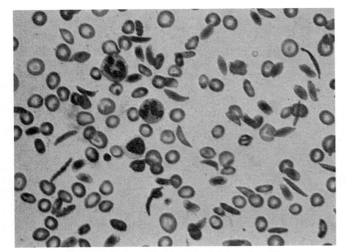

Figure 1-6. Sickled red blood cells.

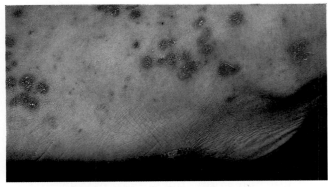

Figure 1-7. Scabies infestation.

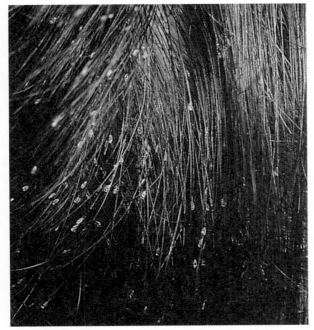

Figure 1-8. Pediculosis capitis (head lice).

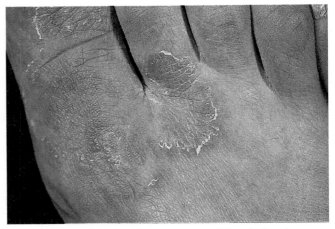

Figure 1-9. Tinea pedis (athlete's foot).

most fungal infections (Figure 1-9), and tuberculosis. Some infections, such as fungal infections (e.g., thrush, ringworm), may also be a sign of diabetes or may suggest a suppressed immune system. In these cases, general massage may be contraindicated until a physician's diagnosis and permission are obtained. All infectious diseases are contagious, some more so than others.

Metabolic Diseases

Metabolic diseases are physiologic dysfunctions that disrupt some aspect of metabolism in the body. Examples are Cushing's disease, which is an overproduction of the hormone cortisol; diabetes, which is an underproduction of the hormone insulin, or an insensitivity of body cells to insulin; cardiovascular conditions such as high blood pressure; and kidney failure, which results in the kidneys no longer being able to filter wastes from the blood. Jaundice is often a symptom of metabolic diseases of the liver. Metabolic diseases are not contagious.

Congenital Disorders

Congenital disorders are present at birth. They may result from genetic abnormalities or may be caused by a maternal diet deficient in nutrients or habits of the mother while the baby is in utero, such as use of recreational drugs, alcohol, or tobacco. Other causes of congenital abnormalities include in utero exposure of the baby to radiation, poisons, certain medications or disease-causing organisms such as rubella, or oxygen deprivation of the baby before or during birth. Examples of congenital disorders include Down syndrome (Figure 1-10), cerebral palsy, and certain heart defects. Congenital disorders are not contagious.

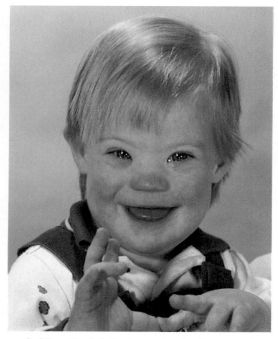

Figure 1-10. Facial features typically seen in Down syndrome.

Traumatic Disorders

Traumatic disorders are injuries that can disrupt homeostasis. Examples of traumatic disorders are open wounds, bone fractures, contusions, and concussions. Traumatic disorders are not contagious.

Infectious Diseases and the Connection to Massage Therapy

Massage therapists encounter clients with all of these types of diseases and disorders discussed previously. However, an in-depth understanding infectious disease is of paramount importance in massage therapy because of the human-to-human contact. The massage therapist, as well as the massage setting, can be sites of disease transmission, both from the therapist to the client, and vice versa. By understanding how disease transmission occurs, the massage therapist will be in a much better position to implement preventive measures to keep both the therapist and the client safe.

Agents of Disease

A *pathogen* is a living biologic agent capable of causing disease. One way to develop a disease is to be exposed to a pathogen. Effective exposure results in contamination. Contamination occurs when an infectious, or pathogenic, agent resides in or on an organism. Pathogens can be airborne, fluid-borne, or spread by direct contact.

Four basic pathogenic agents can cause disease in the body: bacteria, fungi, protozoa, and viruses (Table 1-1).

- **Bacteria:** Most bacteria are not pathogenic and do not require living tissue for survival. Some bacteria are important for plant growth, such as nitrogen-fixing bacteria in the soil. Others are used for processing certain foods such as bread, cheese, yogurt, and wine. Helpful bacteria also occur as natural flora in the body (e.g., mouth, intestines) and aid digestive processes. Harmful bacteria are transmitted directly from person to person, from animal to person, or from a fomite. Bacteria may enter the body through ingestion and lead to diseases such as botulism and salmonella. Improper food handling, such as chopping vegetables or fruits after handling raw meat, or chopping on unclean surfaces, can contaminate food. Another frequent method in which a person may obtain bacteria is by not washing hands after using the toilet and then touching the nose or mouth. Bacterial transmission can also occur by not washing hands and then touching another person; by touching the nose or mouth, and then touching another person; or by coughing or sneezing on the person. Some diseases that are caused by bacteria are boils (*Staphylococcus*), tuberculosis, strep throat, and tetanus.

- **Fungi:** Fungal agents include molds and yeast. Their growth is promoted by warm, moist environments. Only a few fungal varieties are pathogenic. When an individual has a fungal infection, it is typically superficial, tenacious, and difficult to eradicate. Generally, fungal spores are transmitted by a fomite. For example, athlete's foot fungus may be picked up from a locker room floor. Some fungal infections can infect the body internally such as thrush, which is a yeast infection of the tissues of the mouth. In a person with severely impaired immune function, fungi can become systemic and may be life threatening. Fungi can be transmitted directly from person to person. *Candida albicans* (Figure 1-11) normally grows in the mucous membranes of the mouth and vagina, can be found in the axilla and under

Table 1-1	TABLE OF RELATIONSHIPS BETWEEN THE ORGANISM/PATHOGEN, THE RESERVOIR, AND RESULTANT INFECTION/DISEASE	
ORGANISM/PATHOGEN	RESERVOIR	INFECTION/DISEASE
Bacteria		
Escherichia coli	Colon, manure	Food poisoning, diarrhea, enteritis
Staphylococcus aureus	Skin, hair, nose	Cellulitis, pneumonia, impetigo, acne, boil
Streptococcus pneumoniae	Throat, skin, lungs	Pneumonia
Streptococcus pyogenes	Throat, skin	Strep throat, scarlet fever, rheumatic fever
Mycobacterium tuberculosis	Lungs	Tuberculosis
Neisseria gonorrhoeae	Genitalia, rectum, mouth	Gonorrhea
Rickettsia rickettsii	Tick	Rocky mountain spotted fever
Borrelia burgdorferi	Tick	Lyme disease
Clostridium botulinum	Food (improperly handled)	Botulism, food poisoning, gastroenteritis
Salmonella enteritidis	Food (improperly handled)	Salmonella, food poisoning, gastroenteritis
Clostridium tetani	Intestines, feces	Tetanus
Helicobacter pylori	Duodenum, stomach, saliva	Ulcers
Chlamydia trachomatis	Urinogenital tract, eye	Chlamydia, pelvic inflammatory disease, urethritis
Fungi		
Candida albicans	Mouth, skin, genitalia, intestines	Candidiasis, thrush, dermatitis
Epidermophyton floccosum	Fomite, skin	Athlete's foot, ringworm, jock itch, onychomycosis
Protozoa		
Plasmodium falciparum	Mosquito	Malaria
Trichomonas vaginalis	Urinogenital tract	Trichomoniasis
Trypanosoma brucei rhodesiense	Tsetse fly	African sleeping sickness
Entamoeba histolytica	Water, food, feces	Amebic dysentery
Viral		
Human immunodeficiency virus	Body fluids	AIDS
Influenzavirus type A, B, C	Droplets, lung	Influenza
Paramyxovirus virus	Droplets	Measles, mumps, respiratory infections
Human papillomavirus	Skin	Warts
Rhabdovirus	Saliva, brain tissue	Rabies
Herpesvirus type 1 and 2	Mucous membrane, genitalia, rectum, blisters	Herpes simplex, genital herpes

From Salvo S: Massage therapy: principles and practice, ed 2, Philadelphia, 2003, WB Saunders.

the breast, and can be transmitted to a non-infected person through touch. Other fungal infestations are ringworm and jock itch, which manifests on the skin.

- **Protozoa:** These single-celled organisms are considered the simplest form of animal life. Pathogenic protozoa can survive only in a living subject and are commonly transmitted through contact with feces, contaminated food and water, or an insect bite or sting. Protozoa are responsible for diseases such as trichomoniasis, amebic dysentery, African sleeping sickness, and malaria.

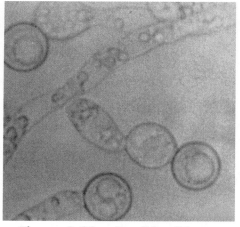

Figure 1-11. *Candida albicans.*

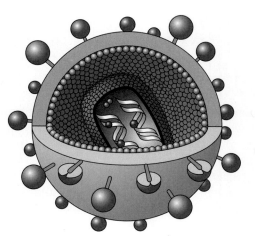

Figure 1-12. Cross-section of the human immunodeficiency virus (HIV).

- **Viruses:** Viruses are considered to be nonliving entities because they do not carry out independent metabolic activities. They can replicate themselves only within the cell of a living plant or animal. Viruses consist of a core of DNA or RNA, surrounded by a protein coat. They attach to the plasma membrane of the host cell and inject their genetic material into the cell, where it travels to the nucleus. The viral genetic material then incorporates itself into the host cell's DNA. Because DNA is a blueprint or code for proteins, the cell "reads" the code and synthesizes the corresponding protein. After the viral genetic material has become part of the host cell's DNA, the cell synthesizes viruses instead of its usual proteins. The cell will make viruses until there are so many that the cell bursts. Each virus then infects a new host cell. Viruses are difficult to treat because they easily mutate, or change, and because antibiotics are ineffective against them. Antibiotics work only on living organisms. Viruses are usually transmitted from person to person, from insect to person or from animal to person. Viral diseases include the common cold, influenza, human immunodeficiency virus (HIV) (Figure 1-12), measles, mumps, rabies, herpes simplex, viral hepatitis, and Ebola.

In addition to bacteria, fungi, protozoa, and viruses, parasites can also enter the body and cause disease. Parasites are organisms that live in or on a host organism, and rely on that host for nourishment. Examples of parasites are tapeworms, lice, and scabies.

Modes of Transmission

For infections to pass successfully from one infected agent or person to another, a mode of transmission is required. It is important to note that modes of transmission are used for noninfectious, although no less serious, toxic agents as well (animal and insect venoms, asbestos, some carcinogens). The source of infection or toxin is often referred to as a *reservoir*, which can be living or inanimate. By understanding the various modes of transmission, both massage therapists and their clients can help protect themselves from disease.

Direct Physical Contact

Pathogens and toxic agents can enter a host through contact with *mucous membranes* or *intact or broken skin*.

- **Mucous Membranes:** This category includes the touching of an infected mucous membrane to an uninfected mucous membrane, such as in the nose, mouth, and genitals, and the exchange of body fluids and secretions by oral, genital, or rectal sexual activity. This is how sexually transmitted diseases are spread. See Chapter 11 for more information on sexually transmitted diseases.
- **Intact Skin:** This method of transmission includes contact with someone or something that is infected with pathogens such as fleas (Figure 1-13), scabies (Figure 1-14), lice, ticks, other insects (Figure 1-15), and fungi. Other diseases can manifest as a result of contact with toxins such as poison oak, poison ivy, and poison sumac.

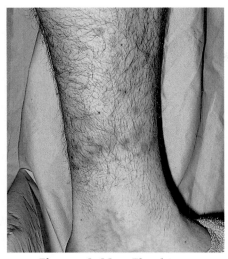

Figure 1-13. Flea bites.

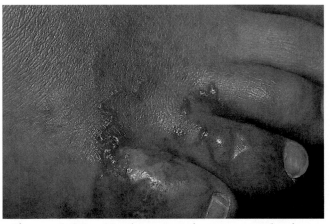

Figure 1-16. Hookworm infestation in the feet.

- **Broken Skin:** This type of transmission involves pathogen entry and toxin introduction through breaks in the skin. The skin can be broken through an accident, surgery, an animal or insect bite or sting, skin eruptions from a prior infection, a hangnail, or a self-inflicted wound such as intravenous drug use. Some parasites, such as hookworms, gain entry to the body through breaks in the skin (Figure 1-16). Malaria and rabies are two examples of diseases caused by bites or stings.

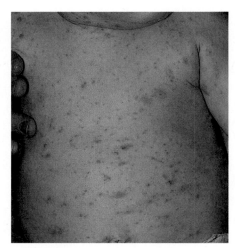

Figure 1-14. Scabies infestation.

Indirect Physical Contact

Pathogens and other disease-producing substances can enter a host by *ingestion* or *inhalation*.

- **Ingestion:** This category includes the consumption of contaminated water, undercooked meats, and food that has not been properly stored or refrigerated. Another method of ingestion of pathogens is through unwashed hands. The oral/fecal route, for example, is the mode of transmission of hepatitis A.

- **Inhalation:** This mode of transmission includes infectious agents and toxins that are inhaled and then absorbed through the lining of the lungs. Although there is no direct contact, contamination occurs after the person comes into contact with airborne droplets of fluid arising from the respiratory tract and salivary glands of the reservoir, primarily through coughing, sneezing, massaging, or talking within a 3-foot distance. Most respiratory diseases are spread by this method. Asbestos fibers, coal dust, textile fibers, and tar and particulates in

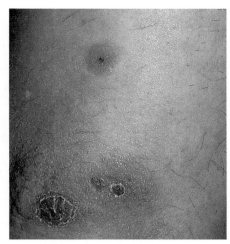

Figure 1-15. Insect bites.

cigarette smoke are toxic agents that are inhaled and can cause diseases such as emphysema and lung cancer. See Chapter 8 for more information.

Risk Factors for Disease

The susceptibility of persons to infection is dependent on risk factors such as age, genetics, nutrition, state of health, immune response, and factors that are, as yet, unknown. Risk factors, also known as *predisposing factors*, make a person or group of people more susceptible to disease. These conditions predispose an individual to certain diseases, making the onset of the disease more likely. For example, people have no control over aging or genetics, but they can make changes in regard to lifestyle, environment, and stress levels. Predisposing risk factors are described next.

Age

During different stages in the human life cycle, an individual may be more susceptible to certain diseases as a result of physiological changes that occur. For example, infants are more susceptible to some diseases such as respiratory diseases. Other diseases tend to occur between puberty and menopause in women. Older adults are more susceptible to still other diseases such as heart disease. Complications during pregnancy increase with older women.

Genetics

Genes inherited from parents may place an individual at a higher risk for one or more diseases. Coronary artery disease, high blood pressure, cancer, diabetes, and many kidney diseases are frequently genetically linked. Sickle-cell disease is another example of a condition that results from a genetic predisposition.

Lifestyle

Lifestyle factors include one's manner of living, work habits, sleep habits, dietary habits, exercise habits, and various living conditions that affect the likelihood of contracting a disease. For example, heart disease is common among those who are sedentary and have diets high in animal fat and proteins and low in fruits and vegetables. Evidence shows that smoking and high intake of saturated fats combined with a family history of certain hereditary illness compound an individual's risk of heart disease. Intravenous drug users who share needles increase their risk of contracting blood-borne diseases. Persons who have unprotected sexual intercourse with multiple partners increase their risk of sexually transmitted diseases.

Environment

Environmental factors include climate, weather, pollution, chemicals, and radiation. Water and air pollutants constitute a significant factor for cancer and respiratory disease. At this time, research is being conducted on GMOs (genetically modified organisms) and GEIs (genetically engineered ingredients) and their effect on health and disease. Other environmental factors include chemicals that are used in food and living space cleaners, preservatives, herbicides, pesticides, lead and asbestos contamination, and nuclear and other types of radiation exposure.

Stress

Stress can be categorized as physical, emotional, or even chemical challenges placed on the body. Some stress is necessary for existence, such as anger or fear responses that keep the body safe. When there is too much stress for too long a period, however, actual chemical changes occur in the way cells function, which allows diseases of various kinds to develop. Long-term stress often negatively impacts the body's immune response to disease. As the body deals with the stress, it releases hormones that interfere with healing mechanisms and decrease white blood cell production, so that the person becomes much more susceptible to infection and healing time takes longer.

Gender

Certain illnesses are more common in women, such as osteoporosis and multiple sclerosis. Likewise, some illnesses are more common in men, such as Parkinson's disease and gout.

The Host/Pathogen Relationship

The ability of the pathogen to cause disease in a person depends on various factors including the portion or number of organisms that gain access, which areas of the body are attacked, the pathogen's ability to spread and replicate itself, and its resistance to the host's defenses. Thus a weak host with a strong pathogen results in disease, whereas a strong host with a weak pathogen will overcome the introduction of disease.

The body's natural defense mechanisms against exposure to pathogens are (1) physical and chemical barriers, such as the skin, the skin's surface acidity, mucus, cilia, digestive enzymes, perspiration, and vaginal secretions; (2) inflammation to keep the infection contained; and (3) the body's immune response. Usually the first two are enough to keep pathogens from either entering the body or invading into deeper tissues. If the pathogen penetrates the physical and chemical barriers and inflammation cannot keep it contained, the immune response will go into action to destroy the pathogen. If the person's immune system is suppressed by chronic stress, malnutrition, radiation, some medications, or a preexisting illness, such as AIDS, the person is then more susceptible to diseases caused by pathogens. It is for this reason that HIV (human immunodeficiency virus) is so deadly; it weakens the host by crippling the host's immune response so that a second infection, which would normally be contained or suppressed by the immune system, can become fatal.

Signs and symptoms that demonstrate that the organism is trying to overcome a pathogen include fever, mild nausea, altered metabolism, cardiovascular changes such as an increased heart rate, anemia, an elevated white blood cell count, and a general feeling of low energy. See Chapter 7 for more information on the immune response.

The disease process includes the course of infection; the pathogen's incubation stage, the period of full-blown symptoms (exacerbation), and often a phase of partial or complete disappearance of symptoms (remission). Remission may be spontaneous or the result of therapy or, in some cases, represents a cure.

INFECTION CONTROL IN A MASSAGE PRACTICE

In general, massage therapists are exposed to no more viruses and bacteria than the average person. Because massage therapists touch an unclothed person, however, the risk of transferring pathogens from client to massage therapist, and from massage therapist to client, is greater than in the general population. Also, there is an increased risk of the massage therapist transferring pathogens from one client to another. Massage therapists who are hospital based or who work with hospice or nursing homes may be at a higher risk of transferring infections, as hospitals and hospices have a higher population of sick people.

Pathogens that the massage therapist is most likely to contract are fungi, yeasts, bacteria, and viruses. Massage therapists may not only contract the pathogens but also spread them to other parts of their client's body. Bacteria may be spread if boils are open and the massage therapist has a break in the skin of his or her hands. Viruses can spread through inhalation of infected droplets. A foot fungus on the client can be spread to other parts of the body by massage. Additionally, fungi, bacteria, and viruses can be spread through contact with linens, massage tools, and open containers of lubricant. Thus massage therapists need to learn, implement, and practice universal precautions.

In December 1991 the Occupational Safety and Health Administration (OSHA) supported and helped pass federal legislation that requires all health care providers to prescribe to a plan that helps prevent the exposure to and spreading of blood- and fluid-borne pathogens. Body fluids that can carry harmful microorganisms are mucus, sputum, respiratory droplets, semen, vaginal secretions, blood, saliva, breast milk, urine, and feces, as well as cerebrospinal, synovial, pleural, peritoneal, and pericardial fluids. From this legislation, the Centers for Disease Control and Prevention (CDC) established *universal precautions* to reduce the transmission of communicable disease. These precautions protect the client *and* the health care provider. For more information, see Box 1-3.

Universal precautions include mandatory hand washing, use of gloves, protective eyewear, nose/face masks, protective clothing, laundering linens and uniforms, cleaning or disinfecting equipment, and observing proper methods for disposing of used medical supplies and biologic material. The use of universal precautions is required when performing invasive medical procedures or when handling body fluids. Invasive medical procedures involve puncturing or penetrating body tissues or entering a body cavity.

How involved do massage therapists have to become with these medical precautions? The answer to this question varies according to the therapist's practice. Although massage therapists are not involved with surgical procedures, they do occasionally work in a body cavity such as the mouth for temporomandibular joint (TMJ) massage (in areas of the country where it is legal). A therapist who works in a medical clinic or hospital, where there is a greater population of sick people, has a greater exposure risk than the therapist who works in a private practice. In a clinical setting, the therapist may be required to perform rehabilitative therapy on patients who have pins, wires, stitches, staples, or open wounds near the treatment area; thus there is a greater risk of the massage therapist spreading contagion to the client.

Contact with body fluids seldom occurs in a private massage therapy practice; a small blemish may break, lesions or minute scabs on recently

Box **1-3**

Infection Control and Universal Precautions

Guidelines: Treat blood and body fluids as if infected and remember to use the following precautions. Not all 10 precautions will apply to a massage therapist in his or her practice setting.

1. Practice frequent and thorough hand washing.
2. Report any accidental needle sticks.
3. Wear personal protective equipment, including mask, gown, gloves, and goggles.
4. Use caution with laboratory specimens.
5. Dispose of contaminated sharps in a designated biohazard container. Caution: Do not recap or break needles.
6. Use proper linen disposal containers.
7. Use clean mouthpieces and resuscitation bags.
8. Obtain hepatitis B vaccination for occupational exposure to blood.
9. Use proper decontamination techniques.
10. Blood spills should be absorbed with paper towels, the area cleaned with soap and water, and then disinfected with a 1:10 solution of household bleach.

From Frazier M, Dryzmkowski J: Essentials of human diseases and conditions, *ed 2, Philadelphia, 2000, WB Saunders.*

shaved legs may drain, a client may cough or sneeze and expel mucus, or a nauseated client may vomit. These and similar situations must be handled according to sanitary procedures, which involves the use of methods to eliminate the presence of pathogens and are outlined next.

Sanitary Procedures for the Massage Therapist

Part of infection control is following basic guidelines of sanitation. *Sanitation* involves the application of measures to promote a healthful, disease-free environment. Like universal precautions, sanitary procedures include laundering the massage linens after each use, cleaning and disinfecting massage equipment and supplies used for the client, and following a hand washing procedure. Included in these guidelines are additional recommendations for a safe massage procedure.

In some circumstances, state law or employers require the massage therapist to be immunized against diseases such as rubella, rubeola, poliomyelitis, diphtheria, tuberculosis, and hepatitis B (the last is a recommendation under the guidelines for universal precautions). Some employers of massage therapists, such as hospitals, may highly recommend vaccinations, but not require them. If the massage therapist chooses not to get immunized, however, the therapist will be sent home in the event of an outbreak. The time spent away from work will vary with the disease in question. The following guidelines for sanitation will guide the massage therapist in ensuring the highest quality of health care possible.

Guidelines of Sanitation for Massage Therapists

1. Use an approved hand washing procedure. Wash and dry hands thoroughly before and after performing massage therapy. One example is provided in the next section of this chapter.
2. Wearing rings, bracelets, or wristwatches while performing massage therapy is not advisable because it is difficult to remove microorganisms from small cracks and crevices found in ornate jewelry. Furthermore, jewelry can also potentially injure the client or break the protective barrier of gloves.
3. Keep nails clean and short, and avoid the use of nail polish. Long nails or cracked nail polish also provides hiding places for microorganisms and is not in keeping with sanitary standards. Long nails can also injure the client or break the protective barrier of gloves. Artificial nails are a high risk for fungal infections that can be transmitted to the client.
4. Use only clean linens for each massage session and launder all massage linens—sheets, towels, bolster covers, and face rest covers—after each session. In the event of blood or tissue fluid seepage, remove the linens with gloved hands. Wash contaminated linens separately in hot water, using laundry detergent and $^1/_4$ cup chlorine bleach. Another recipe is 2 ounces or $^1/_4$ cup of chlorine bleach to 20 ounces

or $2\frac{1}{2}$ cups water. Dry linens using hot air. After contaminated linens have been removed from the massage table, use paper towels to absorb the blood spills, then clean the area with soap and water. Next, disinfect the table with a solution of water and chlorine bleach in a 10:1 solution. Finally, wash and dry your hands.

5. Wear a clean uniform each day. Do not wear massage uniforms, including lab coats, for other purposes. The uniform should not fit too loosely, as it will brush up against the client when the therapist leans over the table. The sleeves should be short to allow easy washing and use of forearms and elbows. Short sleeves are also more sanitary than long sleeves because they do not touch the client's skin. Avoid contact between contaminated linens and the uniform. Wash uniforms in hot water and detergent and dry them with hot air. If any exposure to contaminated fluids/droplets or a communicable disease is suspected, add $\frac{1}{4}$ cup chlorine bleach to the detergent and wash water while laundering. Dry using hot air.

6. *Cross-contamination* (the passing of microorganisms from one person to another) can occur if the lubricant becomes contaminated and reused. To prevent this problem, use only closed dispenser-type containers. Use of open jar containers risks cross-contamination because the therapist must remove the lubricant from the jar, place it on the client's skin, and reach back into the jar for additional lubricant. Unless a single-use container is used, the lubricant in the container is used for another massage. The therapist can use a clean spatula or tongue depressor and remove enough lubricant for single-client use, placing it on a disposable palette or in a separate sanitary container.

7. Disposable gloves should be worn anytime the therapist has a cut or open wound on the hands, when handling contaminated linens, when disposing of trash, or when cleaning massage equipment that contains body fluids. A finger cot may be used over a bandage to keep the edges smooth or instead of a glove if the area of broken skin is contained to one finger. Guidelines for protective glove use are found in the section Glove Use in Massage Therapy.

Another alternative to finger cots or gloves is a product that can be painted over a cut to seal it.

8. Do not perform massage therapy if ill or have coldlike symptoms, such as sneezing, coughing, fever, or a runny nose. In these cases, it is preferable to cancel appointments or arrange for an associate to substitute rather than to wear a surgical mask to prevent the spread of airborne pathogenic microorganisms. In some states, such as Arkansas, it is against the law for the massage therapist to work while ill.

9. Do not perform massage therapy under the influence of alcohol or recreational drugs. It is difficult to make good judgments regarding infection control while under the influence of mood-altering substances.

Safety Guidelines for Massage Therapists

The following guidelines will help ensure the safety of the massage procedure.

1. Obtain and maintain training or certification for first aid and cardiopulmonary resuscitation (Table 1-2).
2. Keep a first-aid kit on the premises in a location known by all personnel.
3. After each massage, wipe the client's feet to remove the massage lubricant. This decreases the likelihood of the client slipping. The massage therapist may wish to spray witch hazel, isopropyl alcohol, or a natural product such as pure grain alcohol, on the client's feet and wipe it off with a paper towel to more effectively remove the lubricant. However, do not use alcohol on the client's feet if the skin is broken or if athlete's foot is present.
4. Be able to identify endangerment sites and contraindications of massage therapy. Use this information in your massage therapy practice. This book will be a great resource. Be sure to review the appendices.

Glove Use in Massage Therapy

The following are guidelines for glove use during massage therapy:

1. When handling any form of blood or other body fluid or secretions, including removal of contaminated massage table linens or disposal of trash.

Table **1-2** BASIC LIFE SUPPORT FOR ADULTS AND CHILDREN

OBJECTIVES	ACTIONS		
	ADULT (OVER 8 YR)	CHILD (1 TO 8 YR)	INFANT (UNDER 1 YR)
A—Airway			
1. Assessment: Determine unresponsiveness.	Tap or gently shake shoulder. Ask, "Are you okay?"		Observe.
2. Position victim.	Turn on back as unit, supporting head and neck if necessary.		
3. Open airway.	Open airway with head-tilt/chin-lift.		
B—Breathing			
4. Assessment: Determine breathlessness.	Maintain open airway. Place ear over mouth, observing chest. Look, listen, feel for breathing (3-5 sec).		
5. Give two rescue breaths.	Seal mouth-to-mouth with barrier device or bag-valve device.		Seal mouth-to-mouth/ nose with barrier device.
	Give two rescue breaths 1$\frac{1}{2}$-2 sec each. Observe chest rise. Allow lung deflation between breaths.		
C—Circulation			
6. Assessment: Determine pulselessness.	Feel for carotid pulse (5-10 sec); maintain head-tilt.		Feel for brachial pulse; maintain head-tilt.
7. If pulseless, begin chest compressions.	Run middle finger along bottom edge of rib cage to notch at center (tip of sternum).		Imagine line drawn between nipples.

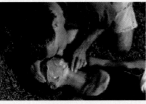

Continued

Table **1-2** **BASIC LIFE SUPPORT FOR ADULTS AND CHILDREN—CONT'D**

ACTIONS

OBJECTIVES	ADULT (OVER 8 YR)	CHILD (1 TO 8 YR)	INFANT (UNDER 1 YR)
a. Landmark check. b. Hand placement.	Place index finger to finger on notch. Place two hands next to index finger. Depress $1\frac{1}{2}$-2 inches.	Place heel of one hand next to index finger. Depress 1-$1\frac{1}{2}$ inches.	Place 2-3 fingers on sternum, 1 finger's width below line. Depress $\frac{1}{2}$-1 inch.
c. Compression rate.	Give 80-100 compressions per min.	Give 100 compressions per min.	

CPR cycles

8. Compressions to one breath.	Give two breaths every 15 compressions.	Give one breath every five compressions.	
9. Number of cycles. 10. Reassessment.	4 (52-73 sec) Feel for carotid pulse.	10 (60-87 sec)	20 (approx. 60 sec) Feel for brachial pulse.

If there is no pulse, resume CPR.

Entrance of sound rescuer.

Second rescuer should perform one-rescuer CPR when first rescuer becomes fatigued. Compression rate for two-rescuer CPR is 80-100 per min; compression ratio is five chest compressions to one breath.

Option for pulse return

If not breathing, give rescue breaths.	Give one breath every 5 sec (12 per min).	Give one breath every 3 sec (20 per min).	

From Sanders MJ: Mosby's paramedic textbook, ed 2, St Louis, 2000, Mosby. Illustrations from Stoy WA: Mosby's first responder textbook, St Louis, 1997, Mosby.

2. Anytime the therapist has a break in the skin or a skin infection on one or both hands. If the injury or infection is only on the end of the finger, a finger cot may be worn, or a suitable product painted over it.
3. When working in the oral cavity, such as for internal TMJ massage.
4. Whenever the client requests that the therapist wear gloves.

If one or several of these conditions are present, then the therapist may decide that the risk factor is high enough to warrant double gloving or rescheduling the massage until after conditions change.

If gloves must be worn during a massage, the massage therapist needs to make sure they fit his or her hands. The massage therapist should be aware that glove use may reduce palpatory abilities. Performing massage with gloved hands also creates more friction, especially in areas of thick body hair; this may be uncomfortable for the client. The two most popular glove materials used in the health care industry are latex and vinyl. Each has its assets and liabilities.

Latex gloves are very thin and very strong, and conform to the therapist's hands like second skin. They are readily available in a variety of sizes and are affordably priced. However, most massage lubricants are oil based and break down latex glove material. If latex gloves are used, a water-based lubricant is needed. Additionally, many people have latex allergies or are latex-sensitive. Symptoms can include rashes, itching or, more seriously, respiratory difficulties. If any of these occur, the massage therapist needs to remove the gloves immediately and seek medical attention.

Vinyl gloves may be used with oil-based lubricants and are fine for clients with latex allergies. Vinyl gloves are thicker and greatly reduce the tactile sensitivity of the therapist. Because they do not have the stretch capability of latex, they do not conform to the therapist's hands as readily. Vinyl gloves are also more expensive than latex gloves.

The massage therapist needs to inform the client about the use of gloves for safety and protection (e.g., open cuts). Some clients may be offended that the massage therapist is donning gloves before the massage and ask that the gloves be removed; the therapist may then refuse to perform the massage on the client if this situation occurs. Conversely, the client may refuse the massage if the client notices or suspects that the therapist has an open wound or an infection (e.g., cold or flu). Before gloving up, the massage therapist needs to wash his or her hands and dry them thoroughly. The therapist then gloves up

discreetly and quietly. If a glove is torn or damaged during a procedure, it must be removed, the hands rewashed, and a new glove replaced immediately.

Care must be taken when removing and disposing of gloves to restrict possible contamination from the glove surface. One safe method of glove removal is to peel the first glove from the cuff to fingers so that it is inside out (Figure 1-17, *A*). Then, the removed glove is placed into the palm of the other hand (Figure 1-17, *B*) so that when the second glove is peeled off, the first will be contained inside (Figure 1-17, *C*). The removed gloves need to be disposed of in a closed container (Figure 1-17, *D*). The therapist should wash hands thoroughly after removing and discarding the used gloves.

Hand Washing

The number one source of microorganism cross-contamination is by contact with human hands. It seems reasonable that the best measure to prevent the spread of infection would be hand washing. Hand washing removes or destroys pathogens from the forearms, hands, and nails. Other hand washing techniques include the use of special hand-cleaning solutions that are used without water. These high-alcohol content gels are designed for field use in sporting events and on-site chair massage appointments where hand washing may not be convenient or even possible. The massage therapist needs to be sure to follow the directions listed on the container.

Massage therapists must wash their hands before and after each massage; using gloves for massage therapy does not preclude hand washing. The following hand washing procedure is recommended for health care professionals to ensure that appropriate steps have been taken to protect them and their clients.

Hand Washing Procedure

1. Approach the sink. Turn the valves on (Figure 1-18, *A*). Adjust the hot and cold water valves until the water is a comfortable temperature and is not splashing in the sink.
2. Wet hands, forearms, and elbows, keeping hands lower than elbows. This will prevent water, soil, and microorganisms from running up the arms and onto garments (Figure 1-18, *B*). Using a nail brush or orange stick, clean underneath the nails (Figure 1-18, *C*). A single-use nail brush or orange stick is preferred. Nails must be cleaned before hands are cleaned.
3. Using soap, generate a lather in your hands, and briskly rub the soap up the forearms using a firm, circular motion. When washing,

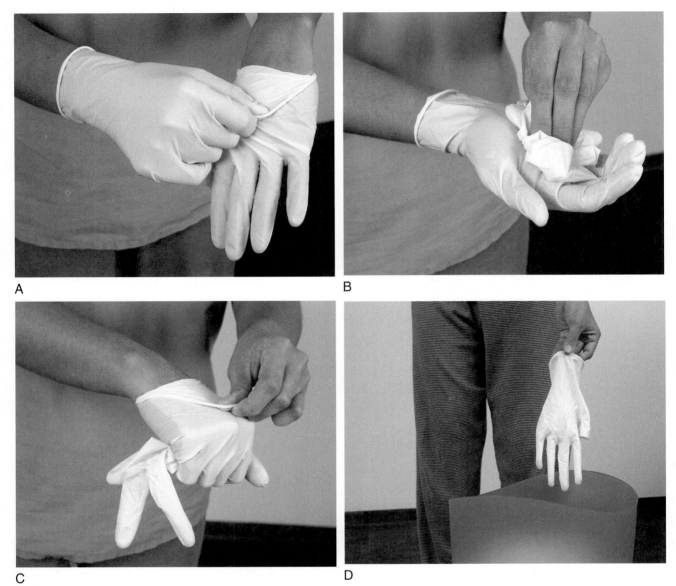

A

B

C

D

Figure 1-17. Proper removal of disposable gloves. **A,** Pulling off one glove. **B,** Putting the removed glove in the palm of the gloved hand. **C,** Removing the other glove with the first removed glove inside. **D,** Disposal of the used gloves.

include the areas between the fingers (Figure 1-18, *D*). Massage soapy hands, forearms, and elbows for 30 seconds. If there is broken skin on the fingers, hands, forearms, or elbows, or if there has been accidental emission of and contact with body fluids such as blood, *increase the hand-washing time to 2 minutes*.

a. The friction created by rubbing hands together is essential to emulsify the oils on the skin and to lift microorganisms and dirt from the skin's surface. These unwanted impurities become suspended in the lather, which will be rinsed away.

b. Liquid soap in a pump dispenser is preferred over bar soap because the soap does not become contaminated by direct contact and is therefore more sanitary. If bar soap is used, rinse the bar before and after use. Liquid dishwashing soap can be used as an alternative to liquid hand soap.

4. Rinse the hands and forearms thoroughly, using tap water until all lather is removed (Figure 1-18, *E*). Allow the water to run from the fingers to the elbows. This rinsing technique ensures that the hands will be the most sanitary area. Do not skimp on this step.

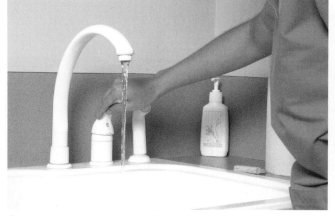

A

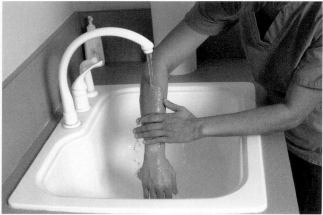

B

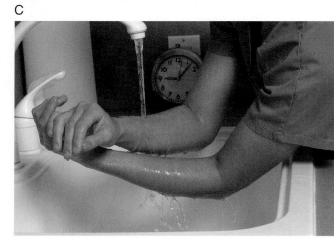

C

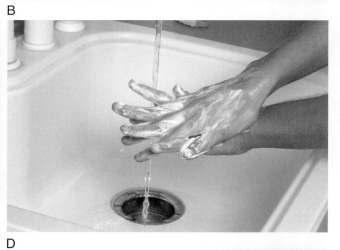

D

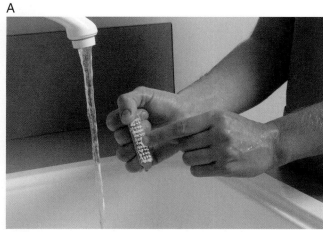

E

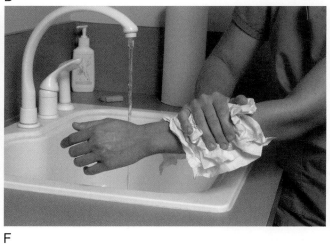

F

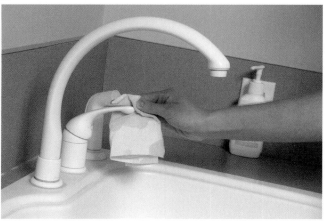

G

Figure 1-18. Hand washing. **A,** Turning on the water. **B,** Wetting hands, forearms, and elbows. **C,** Cleaning underneath fingernails. **D,** Soaping the hands. **E,** Rinsing. **F,** Drying the hands. **G,** Turning off the water.

Leaving soap residue on the skin may result in chapped or dry skin.

5. Using paper towels, dry the hands and forearms well (Figure 1-18, *F*). Using the same paper towels, turn off the water valves (Figure 1-18, *G*). Continue to use the same paper towels to open door handles until reaching the room in which the massage is performed. Discard the paper towels.

SUMMARY

Pathology is the study of disease as it is manifested biologically and physically. There are many types of diseases: autoimmune, cancer, deficiency, degenerative, genetic, infectious, and metabolic. Two significant disorders are congenital and traumatic. A living biologic agent capable of causing disease is known as a pathogen. Examples of pathogens are bacteria, fungi, protozoa, and viruses; they may be airborne, fluid-borne, or spread by direct contact. Exposure to a pathogen results in contamination. Once contaminated, the organism may or may not become infected depending on the strength of the pathogen and the resistance of the host organism.

Risk factors for disease include age, genetics, lifestyle, environment, stress, and gender. Once infection occurs, pathologies will develop that disrupt homeostasis as is evidenced by the presence of measurable signs and symptoms that deviate from the body's normal functions. Identifying the path of infection allows control of transmission.

To control infection in a massage practice, a therapist must be familiar with correct sanitary procedures including hand washing, glove use, and disinfecting of equipment. Regardless of the work setting or treatment style, the massage therapist will encounter clients who have various pathologies, who are under medical supervision, and who are taking prescription medications. Information regarding these situations will assist the therapist in making appropriate treatment choices for his or her clients.

2

Client Intake and Health Assessment

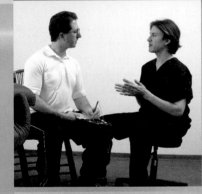

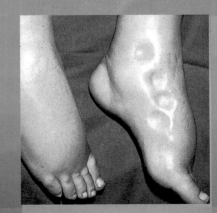

INTRODUCTION

This chapter examines the process of collecting client information, or intake information, and assessing the client. As massage therapists begin their journey into practice, they must be aware of and use all the types of communication techniques: *verbal, nonverbal,* and *written.* A prudent therapist uses patience, skill, knowledge, and a positive frame of mind. All of these affect the outcome of a massage session.

Experience is the best teacher. By palpating, questioning, listening, and treating, the massage therapist develops a sense of what is familiar, which, in turn, breeds knowledge, enhances skill, and promotes confidence. Massage therapists learn that mastery comes not only in the doing but also in the deciding. Many small decisions are made in the course of a workday. Good decisions are more easily made as the massage therapist develops professionalism. Professionalism is essential to developing and maintaining a practice.

It is the therapist's responsibility to gain and utilize the following three areas of professionalism in order to practice massage therapy safely, ethically, and successfully:

- **Personal Professionalism:** The therapist is professional in appearance and mannerism, and is knowledgeable, skilled, self-aware, focused, calm, confident, and prepared. Personal professionalism is maintained when dealing with clients, the public, or with colleagues.
- **Client Precaution Knowledge:** The therapist becomes familiar with the client and the client's needs through an assessment process that includes visual and auditory assessments, determination of client health conditions and issues via a written intake form and/or verbal questioning, and physical assessments of soft tissue through palpation. This includes documenting your findings. This process ensures proper client screening and professional competency.
- **Professional Environment:** The massage environment needs to be safe and comfortable for the client. The therapist should see to client needs such as room temperature, music selection and volume, choice of lubricant, and table dressing. The area needs to be clutter-free and devoid of barriers so clients with special needs will have access to the office, the bathroom, and treatment room.

This chapter focuses on client precaution knowledge (Figure 2-1).

ASSESSING THE CLIENT: SUBJECTIVE AND OBJECTIVE DATA

The primary assessment rule is to use an empirical process that entails using the senses: what is seen, heard, touched, and even smelled throughout the assessment. During the assessment, the massage therapist collects subjective and objective information and combines the findings to decide what type, length of time, and frequency of treatment is needed. *Subjective data* are any information that can be gained from the client; it includes all written disclosure given on the intake form and all the information gathered during the massage consultation. It is referred to as subjective because the client cannot present the information without personal bias—the client is the one experiencing symptoms. Of special note are the client's chief concern or complaint and the client explanations of various symptoms. A *symptom* may be anything the client subjectively notices as unusual or uncomfortable. While all senses are being used, listening is a vital component while gathering subjective information.

Objective data are measurable and quantitative, such as the size and shape of a mole, whether the right shoulder is higher than the left, or if the left knee is larger (swollen) than the right, and by how much. Objective data may be a comparison of range of motion in one hip joint as compared to the other. Objective data are gained through the massage therapist's assessments. The main components used for gathering objective information are observation and palpation, even though all senses participate in the process.

The choice of therapy depends on the assessments garnered through the subjective and objective data. Numerous modalities can be used to give the client maximum benefit from the session, and the modalities chosen by the massage therapist need to be based on the assessments. If a local or absolute contraindication is determined through assessment, it influences how massage will be applied, or may rule out massage therapy entirely.

DOCUMENTATION

Documentation is an important component of client care. The massage therapist needs to document important aspects of premassage assessments, and assessments made during the massage treatment. Documentation of the types of modalities

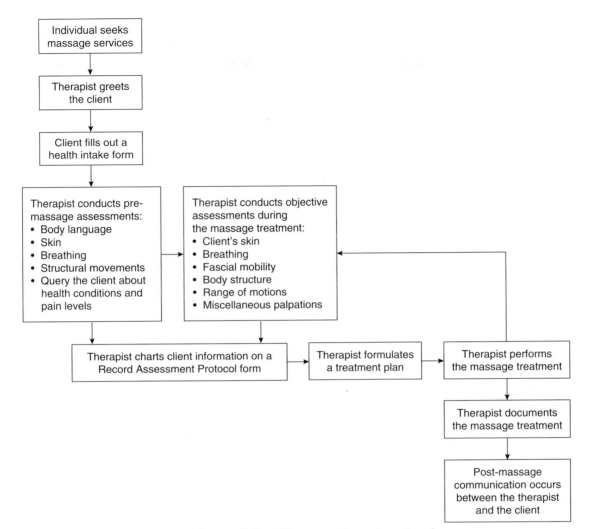

Figure 2-1.   Client treatment protocol.

used will help the therapist, and anyone else who performs massage on the client, recall what was done for the client, and if the client reports receiving benefit. Documentation protects the client by being a source of valuable information for the massage therapist and future therapists. Documentation and client records are legal evidence; this serves to protect the therapist by establishing professional accountability. It decreases liability risks by showing a history of communication with the client and a history of treatment methods. Adequate and accurate documentation also helps justify reimbursement, improve the quality of care, and demonstrates to the public that the massage therapist follows the accepted standards of care mandated by law, the profession, and the health care facility.

The therapist must keep important records for an established period of time; the National Certification Board of Therapeutic Massage and Bodywork-

ers recommends four years, but requirements may vary from state to state.

Computerized documentation is becoming more popular. Fewer errors are made because the formats are standardized, legibility is improved over handwriting, and less time and expense are required to record.

Documentation should use accepted abbreviations common to the medical profession. See Appendix E for Medical Abbreviations.

The three major ways client information is documented are through a (1) client health intake form, (2) a Record Assessment Protocol (RAP) and (3) session charting. The intake form records subjective information the client imparts. The RAP records both subjective information from the client and objective information gathered by the massage therapist. Session charting records subjective and objective information the massage therapist learns about the client throughout the massage treatment, information for future sessions, and suggestions for the client.

Designing the Health Intake Form

Information gathered and documented on a health intake form varies among questionnaires. To keep from overlooking and forgetting vital information, a well-designed health intake form is essential. The type style (font) on the intake form must be read-able, and the form must be logically organized, appropriate to massage, and ideally one to two pages long. The form should encompass a variety of information, such as the client's personal and contact information (an example is provided below), health and medical history, and client consent. The intake form needs to be "user friendly" so the client can write in, circle, or check off information quickly.

Information on the Client Intake Form can be looked at in sections:

PERSONAL AND CONTACT INFORMATION

Name _____ Date _____

Street address _____

City, state, ZIP Code _____

Social security number (if applicable) _____

Date of birth _____ Occupation _____

Contact numbers: home _____ work _____ cell _____
pager _____

Emergency contact person: name _____
relation to client _____ phone number _____

Insurance information (if applicable) _____

How were you referred to this office? _____

Health and Medical History

Health and medical history information can be solicited on the intake form in several ways. One way is with open-ended questions that allow the client to write in all the information. The following is an example:

Why are you seeking massage services?

What causes you stress, and where in your body do you feel it?

Do you have any current or recent (within the last 12 months) illnesses, injuries, accidents, or surgeries (including cosmetic surgeries)?

Have you had any serious illnesses, injuries, accidents, or surgeries before the last 12 months?

Are there any past illnesses, injuries, accidents, or surgeries that are still affecting you?

What medications, either prescribed or over-the-counter, are you currently taking? Why are you taking them?

What, if any, side effects are you experiencing from these medications?

What do you do for relaxation?

What is the name and phone number of your primary health care provider?

Another way to obtain health information on the intake form is to provide a list of conditions with a space next to each one. The client can then check off those health conditions that are relevant to the client's health history. The following is an example of some conditions that can be included:

Please check off all that apply to you:

Allergies _____	Insomnia _____	Seizure disorders _____
Anxiety _____	Leg/foot problems _____	Skin conditions _____
Arm/hand problems _____	Motor vehicle accident _____	Spinal problems _____
Asthma _____	Muscular problems _____	Stress _____
Back problems _____	Neck problems _____	Temperature sensitivity _____
Bruises _____	Numbness/tingling/ pins and needles _____	Urinary problems _____
Contact lenses _____	Paralysis _____	Varicosities _____
Depression _____	Pregnant _____	
Fatigue _____	Pressure sensitivity _____	
Gastrointestinal discomfort _____	Reduced sensations _____	
Headaches _____	Respiratory problems _____	
Heart problems _____		
High blood pressure _____		

Please explain any of the above conditions that you have checked.

The information given by the client in the health and medical history section of the intake form is not designed to be all encompassing. Rather, its purpose is to give the massage therapist an overall view of the client's health. During the massage consultation, discussed later in this chapter, the massage therapist can ask for more specific information on anything the client has written down or checked off.

Informed Consent

Informed consent is a client's authorization for professional services based on information provided by the massage therapist. Essentially, it is permission for treatment. The contents include the therapist's credentials, the modalities used, expectations and potential benefits, possible undesirable effects, and professional and ethical responsibility. This information can help the client make an educated decision about participating in the care. The consent may be on a separate document or combined on the health intake form.

Ideally, the contents of the document are discussed with the client during the massage consultation so that the client has a chance to ask questions and receive answers before signing the document. If the therapy is provided to a minor, a parent or guardian needs to sign the consent. The consent may also be acquired verbally, but it is better to obtain consent in writing, as this proves the document was presented to the client.

The following are samples of items to include in the client consent. Any or all can be used.

The therapist's credentials are _____. (This is a list that includes the massage school the massage therapist attended, the year of graduation, any postgraduate training and certifications held, any college diplomas held, and professional affiliations. If the massage therapist works in an office where all therapists share the client intake forms and consent documents, this information needs to be verbalized to the client.)

OR: The therapist has told me of his or her credentials.

The information attained on the intake form is true to the best of my knowledge.

I freely give my permission to receive massage therapy treatment.

I understand that massage is contraindicated for some medical conditions and that it may be necessary to obtain a physician's clearance, release, or prescription before beginning treatment.

The primary modalities used will be _____. Secondary modalities will be _____. (What is placed in these blanks will depend on the massage therapist's education, skills, and abilities, and will vary between therapists.)

Using these modalities, the client can expect _____. These are the potential benefits of massage.

Potential undesirable effects of massage are _____. (These are mainly soreness and a mild inflammatory response. The massage therapist can suggest the use of ice and increasing water intake, which will greatly reduce these side effects.)

I agree to inform the therapist of any experience of pain during the initial and subsequent sessions.

I understand that I have the right to refuse any treatment or ask that it be modified in regard to pressure or modality.

I understand that I will be draped during treatment in accordance with state laws and that I may request additional draping if desired.

During future sessions, I agree to update the therapist on changes in my health status and medical history and understand that there shall be no liability on the therapist's part if I should neglect to do so.

I understand that massage therapy should not be construed as a substitute for medical examination, diagnosis, and treatment, and that I should see a medical physician, chiropractic physician, or other health care specialist to address concerns that are outside the scope of a massage therapist's practice.

Patient signature _____

Therapist signature _____

Date of signature _____

Record Assessment Protocol

A Record Assessment Protocol (RAP sheet) such as the one presented here ensures consistency in assessment. This list is derived from observable and palpable data, as well as direct client inquiry; thus it includes both subjective and objective data. This protocol is a checklist of assessment criteria that will help prevent errors of omission. Each item on this checklist is discussed in more detail in the sections titled Pre-Massage Assessments and Assessments Made During the Massage Treatment.

The massage therapist can fill out the RAP sheet during the client interview and assessment and/or after the massage treatment, as some items will be noted during treatment. It is not necessary for the massage therapist to waste time and space charting normal conditions. Only deviations from the norm need to be charted.

```
RECORD ASSESSMENT PROTOCOL

☐ Gait Assessment
☐ Structural (Postural) Assessment
☐ Skin Color
☐ Skin Temperature
☐ Skin Condition
☐ Skin Pigmentation
☐ Nail Condition
☐ Breathing
☐ Swollen Lymph Nodes
☐ Anomalies (masses, lipomas)
☐ Pain Assessment (if applicable)
☐ Fascial Assessment
☐ Muscle Assessment
☐ Range of Motion Assessment
```

Session Charting

Session charting records important information about the treatment. Charting helps the massage therapist evaluate the effectiveness, problems, or concerns of the session, and reach a posttreatment conclusion. It includes:

- Information regarding whether the client needed assistance
- Use of support/bolstering devices that are out of the ordinary
- Techniques used by the therapist during the treatment
- Relevant communication from the client about pressure and effectiveness of techniques
- Outcomes of specific techniques and of the massage treatment as a whole
- Progress toward short- or long-term treatment goals
- Any revisions to the massage treatment plan
- Recommendations made by the therapist for future massage treatments for the client
- Recommendations for "homework" and self-care for the client such as specific stretches or stress reduction techniques
- Use of any adjunctive therapies such as aromatherapy or hydrotherapy

CLIENT TREATMENT PROTOCOL

From the moment a client enters the massage therapist's office until the client leaves, the massage experience is literally and figuratively in the massage therapist's hands. Whether the client has a good or bad experience greatly depends on the therapist's personal professionalism, communication skills, critical thinking skills, and hands-on skills. When the massage therapist has mastered all of the facets of these skills, the therapist is regarded not only as a professional but also as a master of his craft.

There are steps the massage therapist follows to make the massage treatment the best experience possible for the client. These start with greeting the client, having him fill out an intake form, conducting premassage assessments (include the premassage interview), conducting assessments during the massage treatment, formulating a treatment plan, performing appropriate massage techniques, and communicating with the client after the treatment.

Greeting the Client

The massage therapist should greet the client warmly and introduce herself by name. She should make direct eye contact and offer to shake hands.

Filling out the Health Intake Form

After greeting the client, the massage therapist should escort the client to a quiet area with adequate lighting for reading and writing. The client is given a writing utensil and the health intake form on a clipboard to fill out. The massage therapist needs to point out the informed consent document and ask the client to read it. The therapist should tell the client that they will go over it together before the client signs the form.

If this is a returning client, the therapist should update the previously filled-out intake form. If a physician requested massage services, important forms such as a prescription or a referral form can be obtained from the client at this time.

While the client is filling out the form, the massage therapist should be available for questions. If the client is unable or unwilling to fill out the form, data may be obtained by the therapist asking questions and writing down the client's responses on the intake form. Ask the client to review the form once it is filled out by the therapist.

Premassage Assessments

The premassage interview should take place in a comfortable environment that is free of distractions

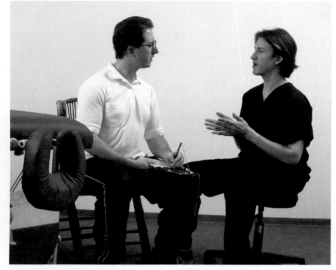

Figure 2-2. Therapist and client during massage consultation.

such as beepers, phones, television, pets, and other people. During the interview, the massage therapist sits facing the client at the client's eye level (Figure 2-2). For example, if the client is sitting in a chair across from the therapist, the massage therapist should sit next to the client so that eye contact is easily made and conversation flows freely. This, along with a nod of the head while the client is speaking, lets the client know that the client is worth listening to and that the therapist is interested in helping the client.

After the client fills out the intake form, the massage therapist needs to ask the client to hand it to the therapist. The massage therapist looks it over and makes sure that all relevant information is complete and that it is dated and signed. If there are blank lines, the therapist asks the client for the information requested and writes it in. Next, the massage therapist goes over the checklist and discusses any condition to which the client responded "yes." If a checklist was not used on the intake, the massage therapist discusses any health conditions the client wrote in. Last, the massage therapist reads aloud each item in the informed consent document. The therapist answers any questions the client has about the informed consent, then obtains the client's signature on it.

The premassage interview builds rapport between the therapist and the client. It also gives the therapist greater insight into the client's overall health and any conditions the client may have. The therapist can ask for specific information and necessary details during the consultation. This will help the therapist screen for contraindications or realize the need for adaptive measures during treatment.

During the premassage interview, the massage therapist is receiving information from the client in several ways: (1) through body language, (2) through questioning the client, and (3) through objective assessment.

Body Language

While being interviewed, the client may use nonverbal communication when speaking. Nonverbal communication, known as body language, includes body gestures, facial expression, changes in posture, and signs indicating discomfort and change in emotions. The therapist observes the client's body language to gain clues about the client's feelings. The therapist should note whether the client is focused and attentive or distracted and fatigued during the client consultation. If the client is focused and attentive, that can indicate health and vigor. Stress, illness, pain, and anxiety can all be projected through body language and can be manifested as distraction.

Nonverbal communication is a reciprocal process, so the massage therapist needs to be aware of own body language. The massage therapist should project a genuine caring professional image. This strengthens the weight carried by the therapist's words. Generally, the strongest message the listener will receive and remember is the unspoken message. The massage therapist should not, however, rely solely on body language as an indicator of client health conditions.

Questioning the Client

The questions the massage therapist asks the client need to be relevant to the massage treatment. The therapist uses these questions to gain more information on health conditions the client has, how massage may affect his health, and whether any special adaptations need to be made for the client during the treatment. The massage therapist can start with general questions, then ask questions that are more specific to certain conditions. The following is a list massage therapists can use to develop their interviewing skills. Along with these questions are suggestions for the massage therapist to help develop critical thinking skills.

- *What were the client's impressions of the previous session (if applicable)? Was any relief experienced? If so, for how long? Did the client experience any adverse effects, such as soreness or bruising?* Document this important information. Repeat what has worked for

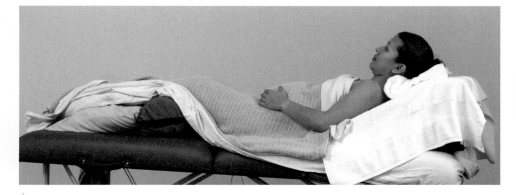

Figure 2-3. Modified supine position with leg and foot elevations.

the client and modify or avoid what did not work. If soreness or bruising was experienced, reduce pressure and length of time on the sore or bruised area.

- *What is the client's current chief complaint? What does the client hope to gain from today's and future sessions?* This will help formulate the treatment plan.
- *What sleeping positions does the client find most comfortable?* Answers to this question can help the therapist decide how best to position the client during the massage. Positional supports such as pillows and bolsters can be used to enhance client comfort. The modified supine position (semireclining) (Figure 2-3), side-lying position, or seated position may also need to be used.
- *Does the client currently receive frequent injections? If there is a regular injection site, how often is it used? Are alternate sites used? Where are they and when were they last used?* The massage therapist can ask to see injection sites. *Does the injection site appear inflamed or irritated? Does the tissue surrounding the site feel loose and fragile or dense and fibrous? Is there any discoloring such as bruising or rash near the site? Does the site look excessively moist or dry?* It is best to avoid the area for at least 10 days after the injection. Massage over a recent injection site increases the absorption rate of the medication. Avoid heat application over the injection site for at least 10 days. Avoid ice over the site for at least 3 days. Older injection sites are often adhered and fibrotic. Gentle to moderate pressure can be used initially, then pressure can gradually be increased until the massage stroke has achieved its therapeutic impact. The massage

therapist should ask the client to monitor the site for several days after the massage for any unfavorable reactions such as redness, heat, swelling, soreness to the touch, or bruising (Figure 2-4).

- *If the client has had previous surgery, was a surgical mesh implanted?* These are often used to repair or prevent hernias and to strengthen the abdominal wall. Use only gentle pressure over the mesh site, especially during the first 3 months after implantation, as moderate or deep pressure may disrupt the tissue-mesh relationship and cause damage. Most surgical meshes are placed in the anterior abdominopelvic wall, so the therapist will not be able to perform abdominal massage to increase intestinal peristalsis or go through the abdominal wall to massage the iliopsoas.
- *Does the client use implanted devices?* If so, massage should not be performed within a 4- to 6-inch radius. Heat or ice should not be used over the device.
- *Does the client use transdermal patches?* If so, massage should not be performed within a 4- to 6-inch radius. Massage near or on the skin patch increases the absorption rate of the medication. See Chapter 3 for more information on transdermal patches.
- *Does the client have any diagnosed conditions?* The client may not consider himself or herself to be under the care of a health care provider. If the client has a diagnosed condition, the massage therapist needs to encourage the client to check in with his or her health care provider as symptoms arise.
- *If the client has any known allergies, does she know what her triggers are?* The massage therapist needs to be prepared to make adjustments to the massage environment.

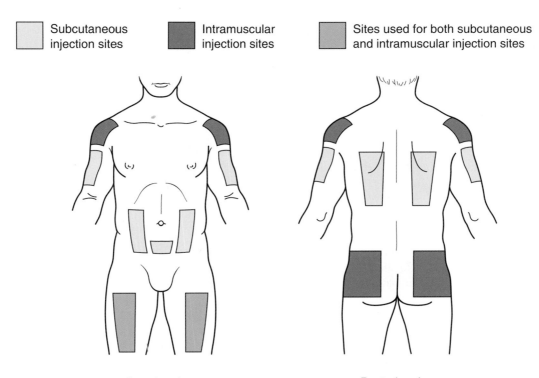

Subcutaneous injection sites

Intramuscular injection sites

Sites used for both subcutaneous and intramuscular injection sites

Anterior view   Posterior view

Figure 2-4.   Common subcutaneous (subcu) and intramuscular (IM) injection sites.

See Chapter 8 for more information on allergies.

- *Does the client bruise easily?* If so, the massage therapist should use deep pressure cautiously or avoid it altogether. The length of time spent on sensitive areas may need to be reduced as well.
- *Does the client have any cardiovascular disorders? If so, is it being managed by medication?* If medications are being used, it should be nearby if needed. Chapter 7 has more information on cardiovascular pathologies and cardiovascular medications.
- *Does the client wear contact lenses? If so, is the client using them now?* The massage therapist should be prepared to adjust the prone pillow to enhance client comfort (Figure 2-5) or use a side-lying position.
- *Does the client have diabetes? If so, when was the last dose of medication? When was the last meal eaten? When was the last glucose check? Was it within normal limits? How does this condition affect the client? Does the client have any sugar in case it is needed?* The therapist may need to make accommodations for client's medication administration or food

intake. Chapter 6 has more information on diabetes and diabetic medications.

- *Does the client have any seizure disorders? If so, what do the seizures look like and what should be done during the seizure? How often do seizures occur? When was the last seizure? What are the client's triggers?* Chapter 5 has more information on seizure disorders.
- *Does the client have feelings of fatigue, depression, insomnia, or anxiety?* Any of these are possible symptoms of a mental/ emotional condition, an endocrine dysfunction, a cardiovascular disease, or medication side effects. The massage therapist needs to ascertain from the client the causes of these symptoms, and adjust the massage to the cause. Furthermore, if the client has a short attention span, labored or uneven breathing or breathing with lots of sighs, or her eyes glaze over during the premassage interview, these can be indicators that the client is fatigued or depressed or is suffering from anxiety or lack of sleep. If so, a gentle, slower massage of shorter duration is indicated so as not to further fatigue or "stress out" the client. It is

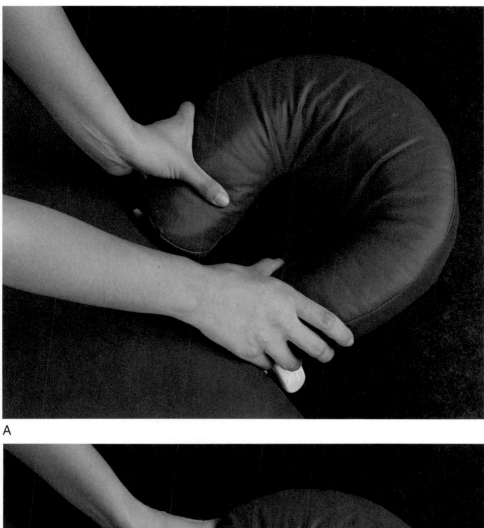

A

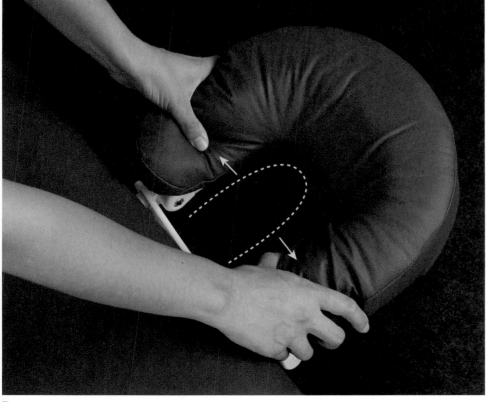

B

Figure 2-5. **A,** Adjusting the face cushion for contact lens user. **B,** Cushion once it's moved laterally.

better to "underdo" than to "overdo" treatment.

- *Does the client have gastrointestinal discomfort? What body positions make it better? Which make it worse?* The massage therapist needs to be prepared to use pillows or bolsters to increase client comfort. Chapter 9 has more information on gastrointestinal pathologies.

- *Does the client have frequent or persistent headaches?* They may be due to stress or tension, or to other disorders. Chapters 4 and 5 have more information on headaches.

- *Does the client have numbness/tingling/pins and needles sensations? Are there any reduced sensory disabilities? Is there any paralysis? Are there any involuntary movements?* These may indicate neurological problems, a diabetes symptom, or the aftermath of an injury. Chapters 5 and 6 have more information.

- *Is the client pregnant?* Chapter 11 has more information on pregnancy massage.

- *Does the client have asthma or any other respiratory problems? If so, does the client know what his or her triggers are? Does the client use an inhaler?* The massage therapist needs to be prepared to make adjustments to the massage environment. If the client uses an inhaler, it needs to be handy during treatment. Chapter 8 has more information on respiratory pathologies.

- *Does the client have sleep apnea? If so, in what positions is the client most comfortable?* The massage therapist needs to be prepared to use pillows or bolsters to increase client comfort. Chapter 8 has more information on respiratory pathologies.

- *Does the client have sensitivity to cold, heat, or pressure?* The massage therapist needs to be prepared to accommodate the client.

- *Does the client have stress (as from divorce, finances, teenagers, work)? What stress management techniques does the client use?* The massage therapist needs to be prepared to add stress reduction techniques to the treatment plan and to instruct the client in these methods. They can include receiving massage on a regular basis, frequent deep breathing, maintaining an exercise routine, healthy eating, enjoying a hobby, etc.

- *Does the client have frequent or painful urination, urine discoloration, or blood in the urine?* Any of these symptoms may be linked to a urinary infection. A kidney stone or bladder infection may produce blood in the urine. Chapter 10 has more information on urinary pathologies.

- *Has the client recently experienced a physical trauma or motor vehicle accident (MVA)? When did the physical trauma occur? Is there liability that involves a third party?* There are two main considerations for trauma or MVAs: acuteness of the injury and legal liability. If the physical trauma is less than 72 hours old, massage should be avoided because there will be pain and inflammation. Pressure from massage will only cause more pain and worsen the inflammation. Ice, however, may be applied. In regard to legal liability, the massage therapist needs to find out how the case is being handled. *Is it an on-the-job injury that will involve worker's compensation? If it is an MVA, whose fault was it and will insurance be paying? Is an attorney involved?* The answers to these questions will better enable the massage therapist to be informed about payment for services.

Assessing Pain Levels

Pain can be assessed using the following guidelines: (1) location, (2) onset and duration, (3) intensity, (4) quality, and (5) what makes it better or worse. Pain can be properly assessed with the following questions.

- *Is the client experiencing any pain? Where is it? Is it generalized or confined to a localized area? Does pressure on the painful area produce or refer sensations elsewhere? If so, where does it refer? Describe the sensation felt.* These areas often need to be addressed during treatment.

- *When did the client's pain start? Is it constant or periodic (does it come and go)?* If the pain is due to injury or other trauma, the client needs to consult his or her health care provider. Continuous or severe pain requires a medical diagnosis, and clearance for massage must be obtained from the client's health care provider before therapy can be performed.

- *On a scale from 1-5, how intense is the client's pain?* (0-1 = none to minimal, 2-3 = moderate, 4-5 = severe.) Figure 2-6 has a pain scale illustration.

The Pain Scale

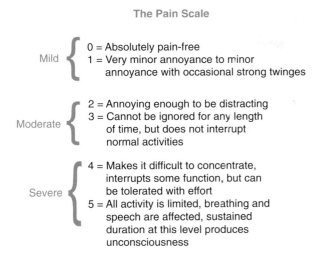

Mild {
0 = Absolutely pain-free
1 = Very minor annoyance to minor annoyance with occasional strong twinges
}

Moderate {
2 = Annoying enough to be distracting
3 = Cannot be ignored for any length of time, but does not interrupt normal activities
}

Severe {
4 = Makes it difficult to concentrate, interrupts some function, but can be tolerated with effort
5 = All activity is limited, breathing and speech are affected, sustained duration at this level produces unconsciousness
}

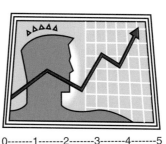

Figure 2-6.   The pain scale.

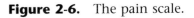
0-------1-------2-------3-------4-------5

- *Can the client describe how the pain feels? Is it sharp or dull? Does it burn, itch, or ache? Does the area go numb? Does the pain feel like tingling, shooting, or like electricity?* These signs indicate nerve entrapment, nerve compression, or severe neurologic disorders. Ascertain the cause of these sensations. Avoid areas that are numb.

- *What makes the client's pain better? Does anything make it worse?* This can be anything from a specific movement, to rest, to activity/exercise. If the client exercises and pain is exacerbated, the exercise should be modified or stopped immediately. On the flip side, if the client has been inactive, this will often give rise to pain. Moderate activity is recommended.

- *Does the client engage in any self-treatments? If so, what are the results?* Take these into consideration when adding self-care regiments.

- *Does the pain interfere with activities of daily living (ADLs)?* Document your findings. Document, also, if massage therapy increases or decreases the pain associated with ADLs.

- *Has the client seen other health care professionals or therapists? If so, what were the results?* Find out if the client is doing any exercises assigned by another healthcare provider. If so, do not add any other activities.

- *Does the client consume caffeine or sugar daily? How much or how often?* If the client is currently using these or other neurostimulants, pain perception may be increased. Reduced usage of these substances is recommended.

- *Is the client currently experiencing any lower abdominal, groin, or low back pain?* These, along with other symptoms, may be linked to a urogenital infection. Chapters 10 and 11 have more information on these pathologies.

Objective Assessments
Objective assessments begin as the client is greeted. The attentive massage therapist notices how the client stands, walks, and sits, and notes any abnormalities. The therapist notes the client's facial expression, skin color, skin condition, general stature, gait and movement patterns, any physical deformity, and limb size and shape. The therapist looks for swelling or signs of trauma. The therapist may begin to draw conclusions; a high right shoulder may be from carrying a heavy purse, or a chronic ankle and knee pain may be from a pronated gait pattern caused by fallen arches.

The following are assessments in specific areas of the client's body. The therapist can observe and palpate these during the premassage interview as well as during the actual massage treatment. Along with these assessments are suggestions for the massage therapist to help develop critical thinking skills.

Skin Assessment
Skin Color

- *Is the color normal for client's race, skin texture, and tone?* If not, conduct further assessments.
- *Is it ashen, gray, or pale (ischemic or low blood flow to areas)* (Figure 2-7)? *Is it bluish or cyanotic (low oxygen levels in the blood or tissues)* (Figure 2-8)? *Is it yellowish (jaundiced)? Is it pinkish or reddish (inflamed, burned)? Is it dark and raised (necrotic)* (Figure 2-9)? *Is the skin mottled?* Mottled skin will appear as pink, purple, or white patches from poor circulation most often found in the lower extremities or hands (Figure 2-10).

Any of these are indicators for the massage therapist to ask the client for more information on health conditions or areas to avoid on the client's body during the massage treatment.

Skin Condition

- *Is the skin moist or dry?* Overly moist skin suggests endocrine pathologies. Dryness suggests hyperactivity of the sympathetic nervous system.
- *Does the skin look stretched and shiny? Or do the areas feel swollen, "doughy," and congested?* These signs may suggest edema. Pitting edema is the prolonged existence of pits produced by applying pressure (Figure 2-11). The best places to check for pitting edema are the extremities. If prolonged pressure to the skin leaves a dent, this indicates edema (Figure 2-12). If edema is present, caution is advised. The massage therapist needs to ascertain the cause of the edema from the client and clearance may need to be

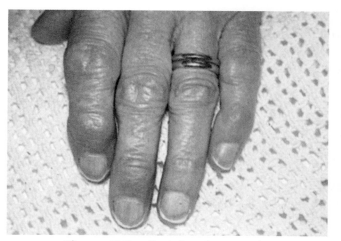

Figure 2-8.   Peripheral cyanosis.

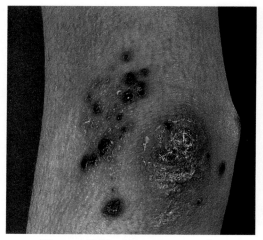

Figure 2-9.   Tissue necrosis.

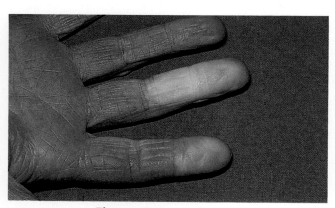

Figure 2-7.   Ischemia.

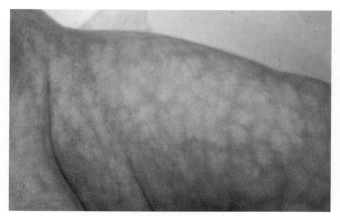

Figure 2-10.   Skin mottling.

obtained from the client's physician. If the edema is not due to a serious condition such as congestive heart failure or renal failure, massage can be performed. The massage therapist should elevate the affected area during treatment to promote drainage.

- *Are skin pigmentations present?* Box 3-2 in Chapter 3 has more information.
- *Are there any skin lesions? Are they healing properly?* If the client does not heal reasonably fast, this may indicate diabetes or immune suppression. Query the client. Box 3-2 in Chapter 3 has more information.
- *Are all birthmarks and moles normal?* Box 3-3 in Chapter 3 has more information on birthmarks and mole changes.
- *Are all scars properly healed and accounted for on the client intake form?* Document all findings.
- *Are there any bruises?* Document all findings.
- *Are there any varicosities or petechiae?* These are often visibly apparent to the therapist.

Varicosities look like blue or purple streaks and are the result of blood pooling in veins with incompetent valves (Figure 2-13). Petechiae appears as small reddish or purple spots on the skin from capillary hemorrhage.

Skin Pigmentation

- *Are skin pigmentations present?* Massage can be performed on individuals with skin pigmentations. Bronzing skin may indicate endocrine pathologies such as Addison's disease. Chapter 3 has more information on skin pigmentations. Chapter 6 has more information on endocrine pathologies.

Nail Condition

- *Are the client's nail bed color and shape in good condition?* Bluish (cyanotic) nail beds or fingernail clubbing (Figure 2-14) can indicate a respiratory disorder in which the client is not getting enough oxygen. Spooning nails

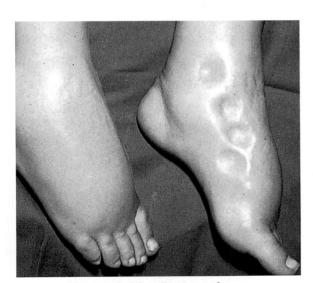

Figure 2-11. Pitting edema.

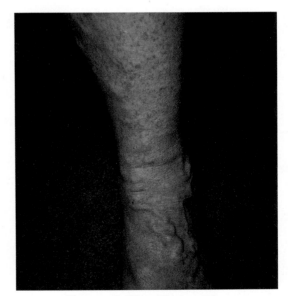

Figure 2-13. Varicosities.

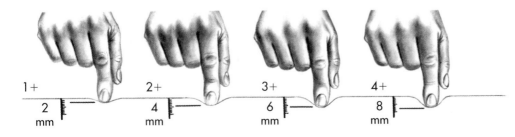

Figure 2-12. Assessing for pitting edema.

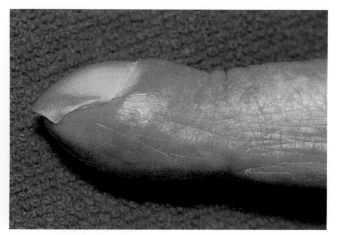

Figure 2-14. Fingernail clubbing.

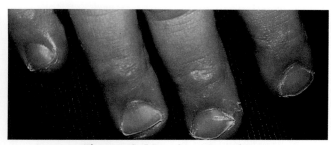

Figure 2-15. Spoon nails.

(Figure 2-15) are associated with iron deficiency anemia, syphilis, hypothyroidism, or a fungal infection.

Breathing Assessment

- *What is the client's respiration rate?* Normal adult respiration is about 16 breaths (1 inhale and 1 exhale) per minute. Every 15 seconds, there should be about 4 complete breaths. Increased respiration rate may be due to respiratory distress. However, the sympathetic nervous system does increase respiration, so fear and anxiety will result in more rapid breaths.
- *What areas of the client's body move during respiration? Does the client do diaphragmatic (abdominal) or costal (shallow) breathing? Are there any postural deviations that affect breathing (e.g., barrel chest, kyphosis, forward head posture)?* Unless massage is contraindicated, these movements or postures will help the massage therapist decide on which muscles to focus treatment.

- *During respiration, are there any respiratory-related sounds?* The massage therapist should listen for high-pitched sounds, wheezing, rattling or crackling, and deep or harsh sounds. Wheezing indicates a narrowing of respiratory passageways, perhaps resulting from illness such as asthma, hay fever, common cold or flu, or more serious illness such as tuberculosis. Crackling or rattling may indicate that the respiratory passageways contain mucus. These sounds can be heard with a stethoscope and with the human ear.
- *What are the client's breathing patterns? Are there signs of shortness of breath? Is the client a nose breather? A mouth breather?* Shortness of breath can indicate anything from rushing to make the massage appointment to anxiety to a respiratory disorder. Mouth breathing can indicate constrictions or blockages in the air passageways.

Structural (Postural) Assessment

Posture is the position of the body in space, such as standing, sitting, and lying down. Standing is considered the baseline measure of balance and alignment because standing posture is maintained through strength and tone of the muscles against gravitational forces. Structural misalignment is often the source of chronic pain. Disruption in the normal balance of the vertebrae can lead to degenerative disk disease, chronic myofascial pain, and further misalignment and compensation. Forward head posture creates excessive strain on neck muscles, throwing the whole body out of alignment in an attempt to compensate. Posterior neck muscles that could be affected are upper trapezius, splenius capitis and cervicis, and levator scapula. Anterior neck muscles that could be affected are longus colli and sternocleidomastoid. Lung capacity may be affected because of compressive forces in the chest cavity as a result of a flexed or abnormal posture. Chronic diseases of the lung, abnormal shape of the ribcage, or a barrel chest may rotate the shoulders forward as well. Fascial network, regarded as an intricate component of structure, may become restricted as a result of structural abnormalities and compensation. Long leg/short leg syndrome often produces knee and low back discomfort, and even temporomandibular joint dysfunction. The following areas should be noted when assessing structure.

Body Structure

- *Are there any spinal curve deviations (e.g., lordosis (Figure 2-16), kyphosis (Figure 2-17), dowager's hump (Figure 2-18), and scoliosis (Figure 2-19)? Chapter 4 has more information on these spinal deviations.* These conditions may require additional bolstering to increase client comfort while on the massage table.

- *Does the client's bone structure appear symmetrical bilaterally in the horizontal, midsagittal, and frontal planes when assessed while standing (Figure 2-20)?* Through training, the massage therapist's eyes can evaluate the structure by taking a baseline measurement in these body planes to locate deviations. Ways to assess the clients structure are to use the following anterior, posterior, and vertical landmarks (Figure 2-21):

Lordosis

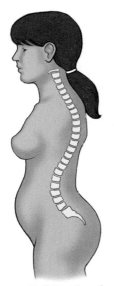

Figure 2-16. Lordosis.

Kyphosis

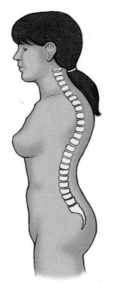

Figure 2-17. Kyphosis.

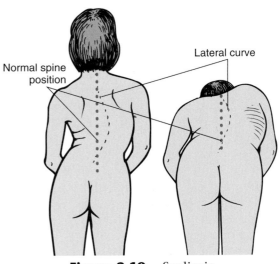

Figure 2-18. Dowager's hump.

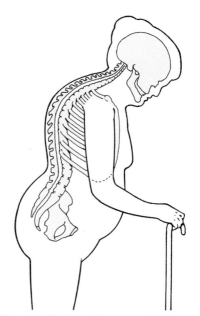

Figure 2-19. Scoliosis.

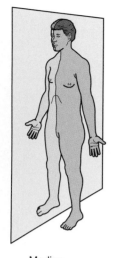
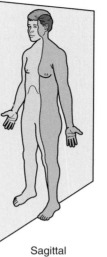

Median
(midsagittal)
plane

Sagittal
plane

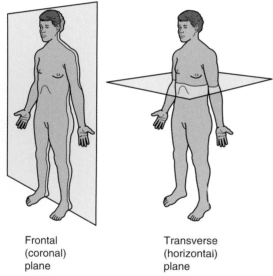

Frontal
(coronal)
plane

Transverse
(horizontal)
plane

Figure 2-20. Planes of the body.

- Anterior landmarks in the horizontal/ transverse plane: the following should be symmetric on both sides of the body and equidistant from the ground in the horizontal plane.
  - Ears
  - Eyes
  - Top of the acromioclavicular joints
  - Anterior superior iliac spines
  - Top of the greater trochanters
  - Top of the patellas
  - Top of the fibular heads
  - Top of the medial malleoli

- Posterior landmarks in the horizontal/ transverse plane should be symmetrical:
  - Ears
  - Occiput
  - Scapulas
  - Posterior superior iliac spines
  - Top of the greater trochanters
  - Calcaneus
- Vertical landmarks in the midsagittal plane should be in a straight line:
  - Nasal septum
  - Manubrium
  - Umbilicus
  - Pubic symphysis
- Vertical landmarks in the frontal plane should be in a straight line:
  - External auditory meatus
  - Humeral head
  - Femoral head
  - Lateral epicondyle of femur
  - Lateral malleolus

Movement Assessments: Gait

- *Does the client move with grace and balance?* If not, suspect problems with nerves, muscles, or the skeletal system. In an efficient gait pattern, the body is erect and the eyes are looking forward.
- *Does the client list or lean?* If so, the massage therapist needs to ask if it is due to pain, muscle weakness, structural abnormalities, brain disorders, or use of prosthesis. The low back, ankle, and foot are common problem areas.
- *How fast or slow does the client walk?* A slow gait may be pain related, age related, or an indication of a neurological disorder. The massage therapist needs to find out from the client the cause of his or her slow gait.
- *Is the client using a normal cross-pattern gait?* During a normal cross-pattern gait, the arms hang freely at the sides and swing alternately in opposition to the legs.
- *Does the client use short, shuffling steps?* This may be the result of weak quadriceps or a neurological disorder such as Parkinson's disease. The massage therapist needs to find out from the client the cause of the short, shuffling steps.
- *Are both arms swinging freely at the client's side?* Tight shoulder girdle or neck muscles prevent arm movement while walking.
- *Are one or both arms crossing the midline during stride?* If so, this indicates torquing or

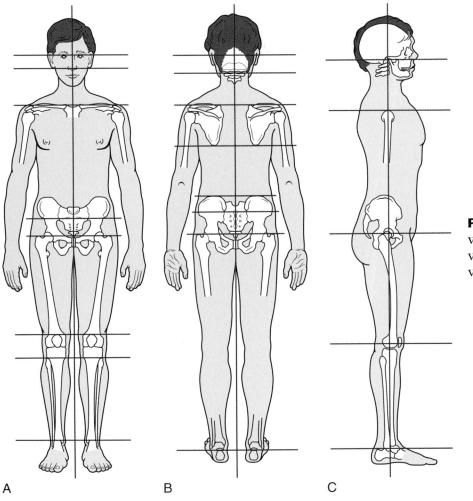

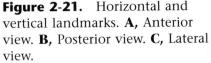

Figure 2-21. Horizontal and vertical landmarks. **A,** Anterior view. **B,** Posterior view. **C,** Lateral view.

A   B   C

listing movements in the torso. See next bullet for additional information.

- *Are both feet pointing forward?* If not, this indicates torquing or listing movements in the torso. This may also be due to pain in the low back, hip, knee, ankle, generalized leg pain, or tightness in the hip rotators. The massage therapist needs to ask the client where any pain and/or muscle tightness is felt.
- *Do the client's feet drag?* This is called foot-drop and can be an indicator of weakness in the ankle dorsiflexors. This may suggest a neurological disorder. The massage therapist needs to find out from the client the cause of the foot-drop.
- *Does the client's gait pattern waddle?* This may be the result of complaints of pain in the

lower back, hip, knees, ankle, or generalized leg pain, or improper use of prosthesis, orthotics, or pregnancy. Furthermore, a waddling gait pattern can contribute to lumbar disk deterioration. The massage therapist needs to ask the client where any pain and/or muscle tightness is felt.

- *Is the client limping or compensating?* This may be from a muscle cramp, bone spur, recent injury, neurological disorder, sacroiliac joint dysfunction, or a chronic condition such as sciatica. The massage therapist needs to ask the client the reason for limping or compensating.
- *While walking, does the client's facial expression indicate discomfort?* Ascertain the cause of the discomfort.

Considerations When Progressing from Premassage Assessment to Treatment

Once the premassage assessments are complete, the massage therapist may decide that the client requires services that are out of the therapist's scope of practice. If this occurs, the therapist needs to refer the client to the proper health care provider for further evaluation and treatment.

In another scenario, massage could be beneficial to the client, but only after clearance for massage has been obtained from the client's health care provider. The massage therapist needs to explain to the client the necessity of contacting the client's health care provider, and obtaining a signed release form. See Figure 2-22 for a sample release form.

If the premassage assessments indicate that massage therapy is appropriate, the massage therapist will then conduct assessments during the massage treatment itself. These will complete the "overall picture" the massage therapist has of the client and the particular massage needs. Based on all information gathered, the massage therapist will form a treatment plan and discuss it with the client. The treatment plan outlines the best possible approach both the therapist and client can use to address his or her needs.

Assessments Made During the Massage Treatment

The two primary methods of conducting assessments during the massage are palpation (touch assessment) and observation (visual assessment). Most of the time these are done simultaneously.

Palpation is defined as assessment through touching with purpose and intent. Palpatory assessment begins as the therapist runs the fingers over the client's main areas of complaint to note tissue health and abnormalities. The hands need to be thoroughly washed when conducting palpatory assessments. Examination is easier when a small amount of lubricant is used to reduce surface friction, allowing for easier recognition of tissues below the skin. When palpating, gentle to moderate pressure is best. Gloves may be worn if either the client or the therapist has broken skin, but the glove

---

Release of Information

Client name: _____ Medical record no: _____

Address: _____

Phone: (___)_____ DOB: _____

City, state, ZIP code: _____

Releasing facility: _____

Address: _____

City, state, ZIP code: _____

Fax: (___)_____ Phone: (___)_____

Send or fax information to:

Receiving facility: _____

Address: _____

City, state, ZIP code: _____

Fax: (___)_____ Phone: (___)_____

I hereby grant permission to release health information regarding my care for the dates:

_____ to _____. This release expires on _____ .

_____   _____
(Patient signature)   (Date)

Figure 2-22. Sample release form.

material may reduce palpatory effectiveness until the therapist becomes skilled at palpating while using them.

The following are assessments of specific areas of the client's body. As stated previously, the therapist can observe these during the premassage interview as well as during the actual massage treatment. Along with these areas are suggestions for the massage therapist to help develop critical thinking skills.

When the client is on the massage table, the massage therapist can quickly check areas not addressed during the consultation, such as skin assessments, breathing assessments, and structural assessments. These areas and others are described in the next sections.

Skin Temperature and Skin Condition
- *Is skin temperature consistent? Is the skin warm (normal) or hot (inflamed) or cool (ischemic)?* The presence of fever denotes a systemic infection. Local heat suggests local inflammation such as phlebitis or cellulitis; these are local contraindications for massage. The massage therapist takes into account outdoor and room temperature or if his or her own hands have been cooled as a result of hand washing.
- *Does the client appear to be dehydrated? Does the skin leave an elevation when pinched?* The massage therapist can check for lack of turgor (the normal resiliency of the skin caused by the outward pressure) (Figure 2-23). The massage therapist may want to moderately pinch the skin. If prolonged pressure produces a tent, this suggests that the client is most likely dehydrated. The best place to check for tenting is on the sternum or back of the hand (Figure 2-24).

Nail Condition
- *Is the client's nail bed color and shape in good condition?* To check circulation in the nail beds, the massage therapist can conduct a blanch test: press the nail firmly and release; normal color should return in less than 5 seconds. Nail condition is discussed in the previous section.

Structural (Postural) Assessment
Fascial Mobility
- *Does the skin glide easily when moved over underlying structures, or is it difficult to move?* The latter indicates restrictions or adhesions

of superficial fascia. Myofascial release techniques such as deep gliding, pin and glide, torquing, and skin rolling may be used to address these restrictions.
Body Structure
- *Does the client appear to have one leg shorter/longer than the other when assessed while lying down?* If so, the massage therapist needs to ask the client if it is structural (unilateral bone length discrepancy) or functional (muscular imbalance that torques the pelvis, creating a shorter leg). A functional short leg can be addressed through a pelvic stabilization routine or a targeted stretching of pelvic girdle and hip muscles.

Muscle and Movement Assessments
Structure relates to function. Any deviation in structure (e.g., spinal curvatures, high/low hip, long/short leg, forward head posture) produces distortions in body function and movement. Two areas to assess are muscles and movement (joint range of motion). Muscles can be assessed by palpation. The massage therapist should note local tenderness and spasms, trigger points and the local twitch response they often produce, increased tone, fibrosis, and even flaccidity and atrophy.
Muscle Assessment
- *During palpation, are there areas of generalized tension and excessive tone indicated by the client wincing, jumping, or verbalizing on application of pressure?* Other signs to look for are changes in facial expression and breathing patterns; feet, head, or knees leaving the bolster; fist tightening; and change in emotions. These indicate pain or discomfort. Pain assessment is covered in a previous section in this chapter. The massage therapist needs to ask the client if the pain or discomfort is due to therapist pressure or client injury and make a determination if the pressure should be modified. If the pain is due to injury or condition, ask the origin.
- *During palpation, is there referred pain?* It may be due to trigger points. Trigger points are hypersensitive points within a muscle, fascia, ligaments, and other structures. Trigger points can be treated using ischemic compression. Trigger points refer pain distally 73% of the time; 27% of the time, pain is produced locally.
- *During palpation, does the muscle twitch involuntarily?* This is called a local twitch

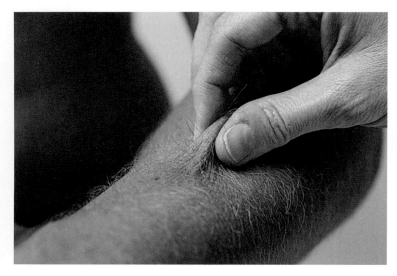

Figure 2-23.   Testing for skin turgor.

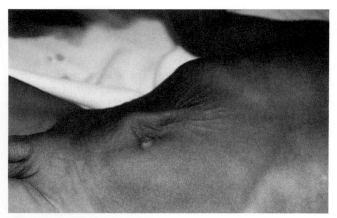

Figure 2-24.   Poor skin turgor resulting from dehydration.

response (an involuntary firing or twitching in a muscle in response to the sensory stimulation on a trigger point). The trigger point that produces the twitch response should be treated with ischemic compression until the twitching stops.

• *During palpation, is the client experiencing rebound tenderness?* This is discomfort felt as the fingertips are lifted off the abdomen instead of felt during the application of pressure. Rebound tenderness can indicate conditions such as peritonitis or appendicitis, which would require that the client receive immediate medical attention.

• *During palpation, are there areas that lack tone or feel flaccid?* This is generally due to lack of neural stimulation or lack of use. The latter can be helped by vibration, percussion and, more important, exercise.

Movement Assessments: Range of Motion The next part is to assess movement by evaluating joint range of motion (ROM). ROM can be assessed just before, during, and after the massage. In this way, a clearer picture emerges of the client's improvement. In charting treatment, the massage therapist notes which joint and what particular movement have improved (Figure 2-25). Table 2-1 lists major joints and their movements. The name of the joint (e.g., glenohumeral, iliofemoral) and the name of the action the joint were tested for (i.e., flexion, extension) need to be charted (Figure 2-26). The type of test performed on the joint also needs to be listed, such as active, active assisted, active resisted, or passive.

Pain or restriction of movement during active, active assisted, and active resisted testing, but not during passive testing, indicates a muscular or other soft tissue issue such as tight muscles or adhesions. Pain and/or restricted movement during both active and passive testing indicates a joint problem such as arthritis. Pain may be indicated by facial grimaces, muscle guarding, apprehension, or the use of accessory muscles. Any crepitus (sounds originating within the body) during joint movement should also be charted. Joint crepitations are sounds such as grating, clicking, or cracking during movement and are not necessarily a contraindication for massage.

The massage therapist needs to explain to the client that these tests will give information about the condition of the joint and the surrounding muscles.

Active ROM

• The massage therapist demonstrates the movement so that the client will know what

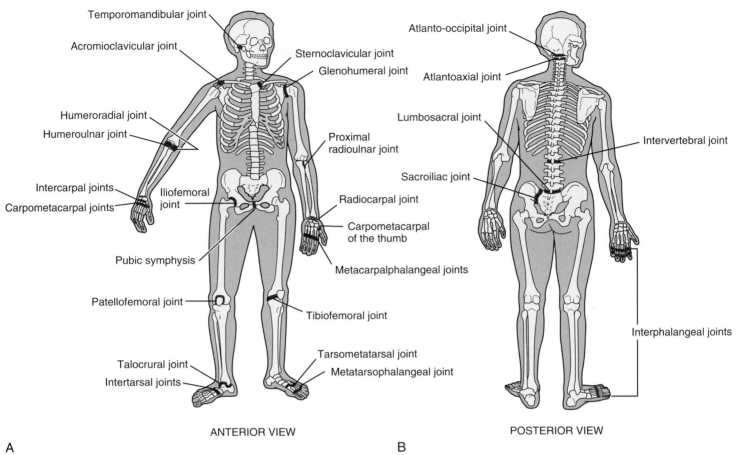

Figure 2-25. Synovial joints of the body. **A,** Anterior view. **B,** Posterior view.

movement to perform. The client first moves the unaffected side (if there is one) to establish a baseline for the client's "normal" range. The client would then move the affected side, stopping at the point of discomfort. The massage therapist should emphasize to the client not to move the joint if there is excessive discomfort when initiating movement.

- The therapist should confirm a contraction of the muscle with palpation to identify very weak muscles or if the client is using accessory muscles to perform the movement.

Active Assisted ROM

- The therapist assists the client in performing the movement correctly as long as this does not elicit excessive discomfort.
- The therapist should confirm a contraction of the muscle with palpation to identify very weak muscles or if the client is using accessory muscles to perform the movement.

Active Resisted ROM

- The client performs the movement of the joint while the massage therapist applies resistance to the movement.
- The therapist should confirm a contraction of the muscle with palpation to identify very weak muscles or if the client is using accessory muscles to perform the movement.

Passive ROM

- The massage therapist takes the client's joint through the movements without any assistance from the client

What to Note During ROM

The following observations made during the ROM assessments and accompanying suggestions can help the massage therapist develop critical thinking skills.

- *During active joint mobilizations, does the client guard movement?* The massage therapist should note any comments or reactions made by the client.

Table **2-1**   **JOINT MOVEMENTS**

Scapular Movements

ELEVATION	DEPRESSION	UPWARD ROTATION	DOWNWARD ROTATION	PROTRACTION	RETRACTION
Trapezius (upper fibers)	Trapezius (lower fibers)	Trapezius (upper fibers)	Levator scapulae	Serratus anterior	Trapezius (middle fibers)
Levator scapulae	Pectoralis minor	Serratus anterior	Rhomboids	Pectoralis minor	Rhomboids

Shoulder Joint Movements

FLEXION	EXTENSION	MEDIAL ROTATION	LATERAL ROTATION	ABDUCTION	ADDUCTION
Deltoids (anterior fibers)	Latissimus dorsi	Latissimus dorsi	Infraspinatus	Supraspinatus	Latissimus dorsi
Pectoralis major	Teres major	Teres major	Teres minor	Deltoids (middle fibers)	Teres major
Coracobrachialis	Deltoids (posterior fibers)	Subscapularis	Deltoids (posterior fibers)		Teres minor
Biceps brachii	Pectoralis major (sternal/costal portion)	Deltoids (anterior fibers)			Pectoralis major
	Triceps brachii	Pectoralis major			Coracobrachialis

Elbow Movements

FLEXION	EXTENSION
Biceps brachii	Triceps brachii
Brachialis	Anconeus
Brachioradialis	
Pronator teres	

Forearm, Wrist, and Hand Movements

FLEXION	EXTENSION	ABDUCTION	ADDUCTION	PRONATION	SUPINATION
Flexor carpi radialis	Extensor carpi radialis longus	Flexor carpi radialis	Flexor carpi ulnaris	Pronator teres	Supinator
Flexor carpi ulnaris					
Palmaris longus	Extensor carpi radialis brevis	Extensor carpi radialis longus	Extensor carpi ulnaris	Pronator quadratus	Biceps brachii
Flexor digitorum superficialis	Extensor carpi ulnaris	Extensor carpi radialis brevis			
	Extensor digitorum				

Hip Joint Movements

FLEXION	EXTENSION	MEDIAL ROTATION	LATERAL ROTATION	ABDUCTION	ADDUCTION
Psoas major	Gluteus maximus	Gluteus medius	Psoas major	Piriformis	Gluteus maximus
Iliacus	Semimembranosus	Gluteus minimus	Iliacus	Gluteus medius	Gracilis
Tensor fascia lata	Semitendinosus	Tensor fascia lata	Piriformis	Gluteus minimus	Adductor magnus
Rectus femoris	Biceps femoris	Semimembranosus	Gemellus superior	Tensor fascia lata	Adductor longus
Sartorius	Adductor magnus	Semitendinosus	Gemellus inferior	Sartorius	Adductor brevis
Gracilis			Obturator externus		Pectineus
Adductor magnus			Obturator internus		
Pectineus			Quadratus femoris		
			Gluteus maximus		
			Sartorius		
			Biceps femoris		

Table **2-1** **JOINT MOVEMENTS—CONT'D**

Knee Joint Movements

FLEXION	EXTENSION	MEDIAL ROTATION	LATERAL ROTATION
Semimembranosus	Rectus femoris	Sartorius	Sartorius
Semitendinosus	Vastus intermedius	Semimembranosus	Biceps femoris
Biceps femoris	Vastus lateralis	Semitendinosus	
Gracilis	Vastus medialis	Gracilis	
Gastrocnemius		Popliteus	
Plantaris			
Popliteus			

Ankle and Foot Movements

PLANTAR FLEXION	DORSIFLEXION	INVERSION	EVERSION
Gastrocnemius	Tibialis anterior	Tibialis anterior	Peroneus longus
Plantaris	Extensor digitorum longus	Tibialis posterior	Peroneus brevis
Soleus	Extensor hallucis longus		
Peroneus longus			
Peroneus brevis			
Tibialis posterior			
Flexor digitorum longus			
Flexor hallicis longus			

Mandible Movements

ELEVATION	DEPRESSION	PROTRACTION	RETRACTION	LATERAL MOVEMENTS
Temporalis	Platysma	Masseter	Temporalis	Pterygoid lateralis
Masseter	Pterygoid lateralis	Pterygoid lateralis		Pterygoid medialis
Pterygoid medialis		Pterygoid medialis		

Head and Neck Movements

FLEXION	EXTENSION	LATERAL FLEXION	ROTATION
Longus capitis	Splenius capitis	Longus colli	Trapezius
Longus colli	Splenius cervicis	Sternocleidomastoid	Longus capitis
Sternocleidomastoid	Rectus capitis posterior major	Scalenus anterior	Longus colli
	Rectus capitis posterior minor	Scalenus medius	Sternocleidomastoid
	Oblique capitis superior	Scalenus posterior	Scalenus anterior
	Trapezius	Splenius capitis	Scalenus medius
	Spinalis	Splenius cervicis	Scalenus posterior
			Splenius capitis
			Splenius cervicis
	Longissimus	Trapezius	Rectus capitis posterior major
		Levator scapulae	Oblique capitis superior
			Oblique capitis inferior

Vertebral Column Movements

FLEXION	EXTENSION	LATERAL FLEXION	ROTATION
Psoas major	Quadratus lumborum	External obliques	External obliques
Rectus abdominis	Semispinalis	Internal obliques	Internal obliques
External obliques	Rotatores	Quadratus lumborum	Semispinalis
Internal obliques	Multifidus	Spinalis	Rotatores
	Spinalis	Longissimus	Multifidus
	Longissimus	Iliocostalis	
	Iliocostalis		

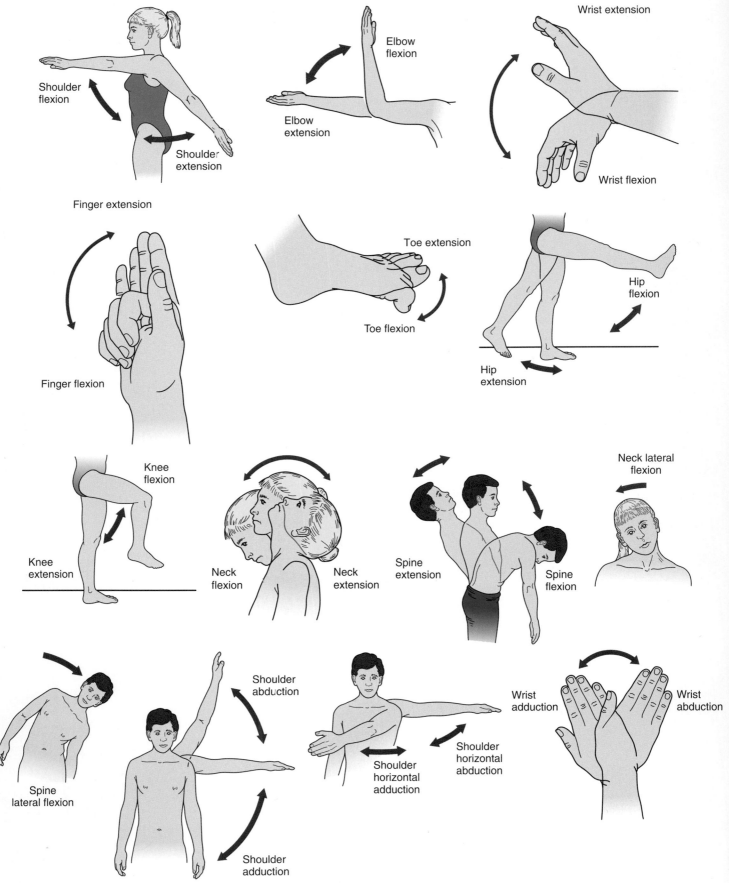

Figure 2-26. Joint movements.

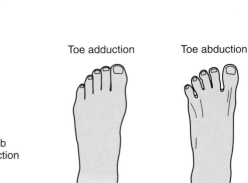
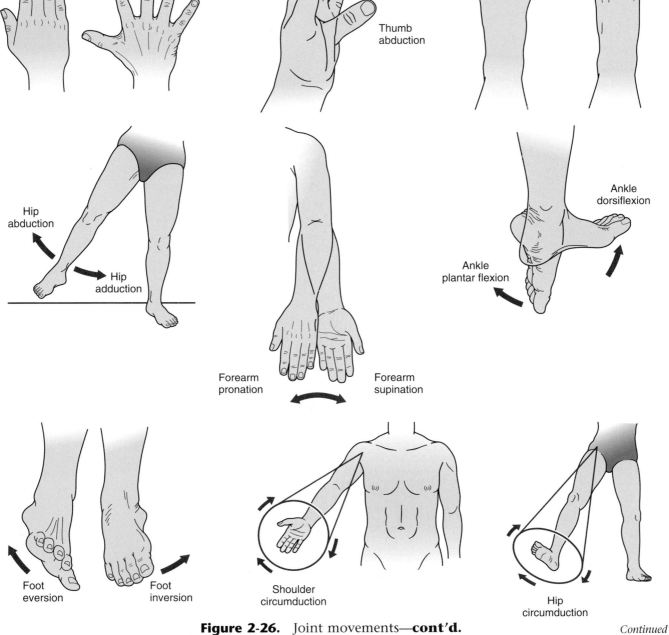

Figure 2-26. Joint movements—**cont'd.**   *Continued*

- *At the end of passive joint movements, is the endfeel hard or soft?* Endfeel is what is felt at the end of a passive ROM. Hard endfeel has an abrupt stop of motion such as felt at the end of elbow and knee extension. Soft endfeel has a springy, spongy feel, such as

the end of finger, shoulder, and hip movement. If a hard endfeel is felt at a joint that normally has a soft endfeel, this may indicate the presence of abnormal muscle contraction such as a contracture.

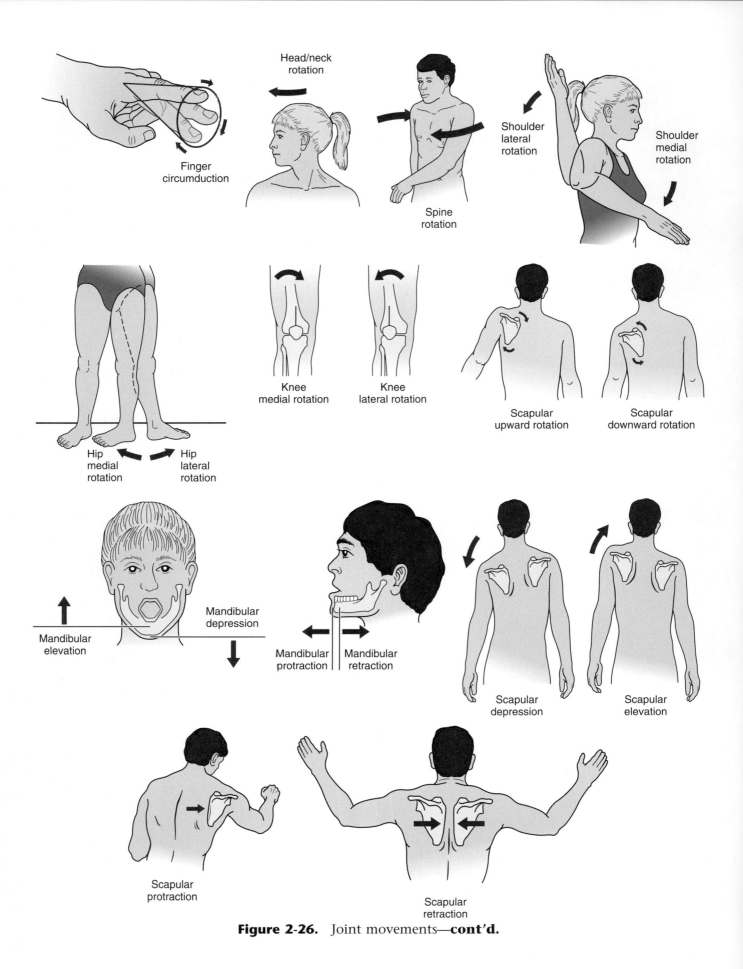

Finger circumduction

Head/neck rotation

Spine rotation

Shoulder lateral rotation

Shoulder medial rotation

Hip medial rotation

Hip lateral rotation

Knee medial rotation

Knee lateral rotation

Scapular upward rotation

Scapular downward rotation

Mandibular elevation

Mandibular depression

Mandibular protraction

Mandibular retraction

Scapular depression

Scapular elevation

Scapular protraction

Scapular retraction

Figure 2-26. Joint movements—**cont'd.**

- *Are there any sounds of crepitation?* This may indicate irregularities on articulating surfaces such as deterioration of cartilage.

Miscellaneous Palpatory Assessments

- *Can swollen lymph nodes be palpated?* The presence of swollen lymph nodes denotes possible local or systemic infection or a cancerous enlargement (Figures 2-27 through 2-31). Massage may be contraindicated if the client has an infection.
- *Are there any superficial and deep masses such as lipomas (Figure 2-32) or other anomalies?* If found during the massage treatment, avoid the area in question and refer the client to the client's health care provider for evaluation.
- *During palpation, are any hard masses felt in the abdomen?* If found during the massage treatment, avoid the area in question and refer the client to the client's health care provider for evaluation. However, formed or partially formed stools often feel hard. If a mass is felt in the region of the descending or sigmoid colon, it may be assumed that it is a stool. In either case, the massage may proceed while avoiding the abdominal region.

Formulating a Treatment Plan

A treatment plan is the approach the massage therapist will use to address a client's massage therapy needs. It is based on all the information the massage therapist has gathered: the client's health intake form, the premassage interview, premassage assessments, soft tissue palpation, and any joint ROM assessments. After integrating all this information, the massage therapist uses critical thinking skills, knowledge of anatomy and physiology, massage therapy skills, and awareness of the effectiveness of techniques to determine what will work best for the

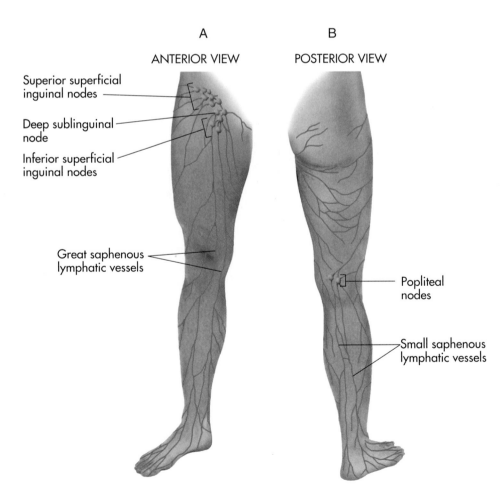

A
ANTERIOR VIEW

B
POSTERIOR VIEW

Superior superficial inguinal nodes

Deep sublinguinal node

Inferior superficial inguinal nodes

Great saphenous lymphatic vessels

Popliteal nodes

Small saphenous lymphatic vessels

Figure 2-27. Inguinal lymph nodes and lymphatics of lower extremities. **A,** Anterior view. **B,** Posterior view.

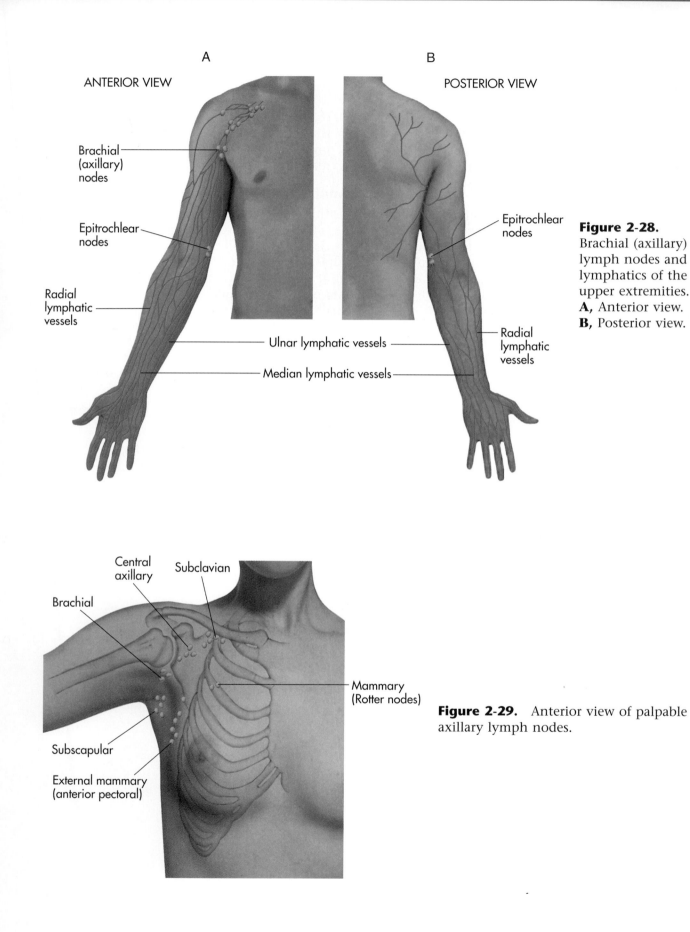

A

ANTERIOR VIEW

Brachial (axillary) nodes

Epitrochlear nodes

Radial lymphatic vessels

Ulnar lymphatic vessels

Median lymphatic vessels

B

POSTERIOR VIEW

Epitrochlear nodes

Radial lymphatic vessels

Figure 2-28. Brachial (axillary) lymph nodes and lymphatics of the upper extremities. **A,** Anterior view. **B,** Posterior view.

Central axillary

Subclavian

Brachial

Mammary (Rotter nodes)

Subscapular

External mammary (anterior pectoral)

Figure 2-29. Anterior view of palpable axillary lymph nodes.

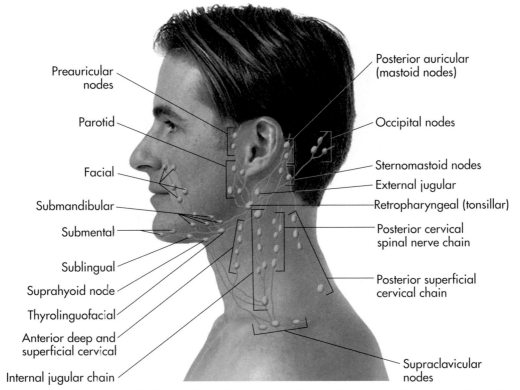

Figure 2-30. Lateral view of lymph nodes and lymphatics of the face and neck.

Preauricular nodes

Parotid

Facial

Submandibular

Submental

Sublingual

Suprahyoid node

Thyrolinguofacial

Anterior deep and superficial cervical

Internal jugular chain

Posterior auricular (mastoid nodes)

Occipital nodes

Sternomastoid nodes

External jugular

Retropharyngeal (tonsillar)

Posterior cervical spinal nerve chain

Posterior superficial cervical chain

Supraclavicular nodes

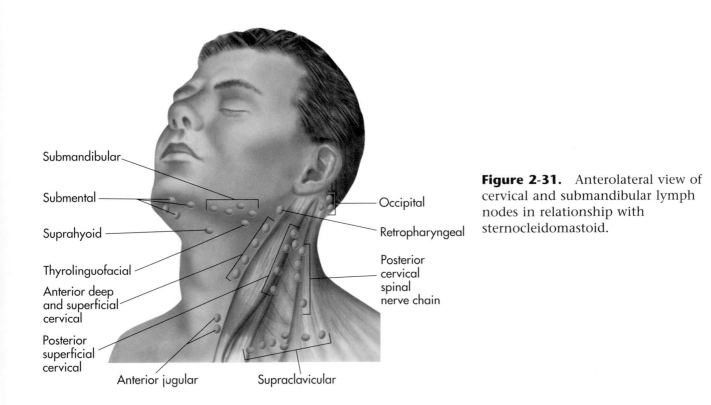

Submandibular

Submental

Suprahyoid

Thyrolinguofacial

Anterior deep and superficial cervical

Posterior superficial cervical

Anterior jugular

Supraclavicular

Occipital

Retropharyngeal

Posterior cervical spinal nerve chain

Figure 2-31. Anterolateral view of cervical and submandibular lymph nodes in relationship with sternocleidomastoid.

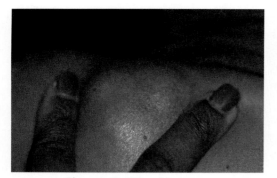

Figure 2-32.   Lipoma.

client. (See Appendix B for the physiological effects of massage.)

Short- and long-term goals are then determined. Short-term goals involve using specific modalities to decrease discomfort in a specific area by the end of a session. The short-term goal for a session may be reducing pain and discomfort by applying ischemic compression to active trigger points in the client's right shoulder. Subsequent treatments may focus on deeper musculature, passive ROM, and finally active ROM. Each of these short-term goals represents increments of progress that assists in reaching a long-term goal. Long-term goals focus on restoration of normal function; the goal is generally to return to the same level or close to the same level of health enjoyed before an accident. For example, a muscle spasm that is relieved in a session is a short-term goal; the ability to return to work, pain free, without the use of a brace is a long-term goal. Both short- and long-term goals should be simple and realistic.

The massage therapist and the client would then discuss the massage therapist's findings to develop a workable treatment plan.

Aspects of a treatment plan can include, but are not limited to, the following:

- Short-term massage goals
- Long-term massage goals
- Specific areas of the client's body to be treated during massage
- Any special testing (such as joint ROM) to be done before, during, or after massage treatments
- How often the client would need massage to address areas of complaint
- Specific techniques to be used during treatment
- Whether any adjunctive therapies, such as aromatherapy or hydrotherapy, will be used

- Self-care activities that support short- and long-term goals

The treatment plan is a malleable instrument. That is, it changes as the client's needs change. The treatment plan, and any modifications to it, is recorded during charting.

Performing the Massage Techniques

After determining the massage needs of the client, the client's overall health, and specifics of any disorders the client may have, the massage therapist performs a client-centered treatment with appropriate massage techniques.

Postmassage Communication

The end of each massage session includes evaluation by the client of the effectiveness of the techniques used and modifications to the treatment plan. If the client is not experiencing success with the massage treatments, the therapist needs to reevaluate the treatment plan. Client education and various homework assignments for the client can also be discussed when appropriate. Client education empowers the client to take control of his or her own health. The client needs to understand all the factors that can play a part in the healing process.

Areas of education include specifics about a disorder the client may have, ergonomics, musculoskeletal self-care activities, exercises, and postural adjustments. Health-related information for specific conditions such as arthritis and fibromyalgia can be kept on hand and given to the client. If handout literature includes exercises or stretches, the massage therapist needs to demonstrate them before giving the information to the client. Or the massage therapist can ask the client to mirror the exercise so that the client will do it properly and not cause injury. If stretches or joint mobilizations are to be performed bilaterally, ask the client to perform the movement on both the left and right sides.

Homework assignments can be joint mobilizations and stretches the client can do alone. Again, the massage therapist needs to demonstrate them to the client, and ask the client to mirror them to make sure the client is doing them properly. Strength-building exercises can also be demonstrated. However, if a health care provider or physical therapist is assigning and working with exercise with the client, it would be inappropriate for the massage therapist to add more or different activities.

Suggestions for lifestyle modifications can assist the client in reaching personal goals. For instance, if a client needs to lose weight, the massage therapist can support this by approaching weight loss as a health care issue. The therapist can mention the benefits to the body of weight loss, such as increased stamina, increased flexibility, and increased ROM. The massage therapist can point out, for instance, that the pain of arthritis decreases with weight loss because the joints are less stressed.

If the client needs help with stress management, the massage therapist can suggest ways for the client to acquire stress management tools, such as mild exercise (as simple as going for a walk around the block), decreasing sugar and caffeine intake, and taking time out for personal needs. Again, the massage therapist can approach stress management as a health care issue by pointing out all the benefits the body receives from lowered stress levels—increased stamina, more efficient metabolism, and longer attention span.

If the client is not an avid water drinker, the massage therapist can help the client design creative ways to increase water consumption. The therapist can explain the benefits of water, how water intake improves the body's metabolism, how it slows the aging process, and how it helps metabolize fat. The therapist can give the client relevant articles on water intake and a schedule on how to "sneak" water into the diet.

The client needs continued success to maintain motivation and healthy habits. The massage therapist needs to find ways to support and encourage the client. Teaching a client a health-building skill is an important part of the treatment plan.

The massage therapist, in working with clients, needs to realize that a 100% return of function and complete freedom from pain are not possible in all cases. Sometimes 50% improvement is tremendous progress. The purpose of the massage treatments is to benefit the client and to meet the client's needs, not the needs and goals of the massage therapist. A massage therapist who is mindful of this purpose is truly a professional.

SUMMARY

One of the most valuable skills a therapist can use is to be an effective listener and communicator. To accomplish this goal, a therapist must become familiar with three areas of professionalism: personal professionalism, client precaution knowledge, and professional environment. These skills are vital for practicing massage safely, ethically, and successfully.

Most of the subjective data on a client will be gathered by a written health intake form and oral premassage interview. A well-written intake form should contain the client's personal information, health and medical history, and an informed consent to agree to massage therapy treatment. The consultation should also assess client pain levels.

Objective data will be gathered through therapist observations of the skin, breathing, posture, movement patterns, measurements of range of motion, and palpation of the soft tissues for condition and anomalies. These observations are made during the premassage interview and during the massage treatment itself.

All relevant information needs to be documented. Documentation includes the client health intake form, a Record Assessment Protocol, and charting.

Postmassage communication is important in evaluating the effectiveness of the massage treatment and in supporting the client to meet his goals.

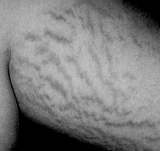

3

Dermatological Pathologies

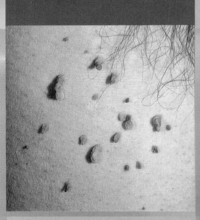

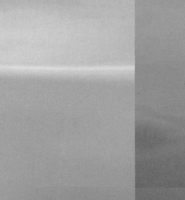

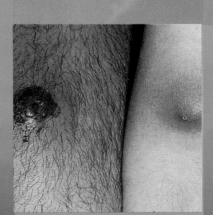

INTEGUMENTARY SYSTEM OVERVIEW

The integumentary system is an essential system for massage therapists to study and understand. The skin presents the first opportunity for the massage therapist to assess a client. Many disorders, whether or not they are dermatological, manifest themselves on the skin. Other disorders include symptoms that show on the skin. Additionally, the skin is the first body structure contacted directly during massage. By palpating the skin and underlying muscles, tendons, and other structures, the massage therapist is able to further evaluate client needs.

The skin (integument) and its accessory structures make up the integumentary system. The accessory structures include hair, nails, various glands, muscles, and nerves. The skin is divided into two distinct regions: the *epidermis* and the *dermis*. The epidermis, the most superficial layer, contains melanocytes (which contribute to skin color), nails, and pores to allow passage for hair and specialized glands (Figure 3-1).

The dermis is located beneath the epidermis and contains numerous blood vessels and many sensory nerve receptors. It also has pores for hair follicles and associated oil (sebaceous) glands, sweat (sudoriferous) glands, and cerumen or ear wax (ceruminous) glands. Mammary glands, which are modified sudoriferous glands, are often regarded as part of the integumentary system.

Collagen, the main component of connective tissue, is an insoluble, fibrous protein that constitutes about 70% of the dermis and offers support to the nerves, blood vessels, hair follicles, and glands. Within the dermis are elastin fibers, which give the skin its elasticity and resilience. Underneath the dermis is a layer of tissue known as the *subcutaneous layer*. It is also called *superficial fascia* or *hypodermis*. The subcutaneous layer is not part of the skin. Rather, it anchors the skin to underlying tissues and organs. It consists of loose connective tissue and adipose tissue, serves as a storage depot for fat, and contains blood vessels that supply the skin.

One of the functions of the skin is protection. It protects by acting as a physical barrier, biological barrier, and a chemical barrier. As a *physical barrier*, the skin is essential for protecting the underlying tissues from abrasion. The skin also provides waterproofing through a protein called keratin

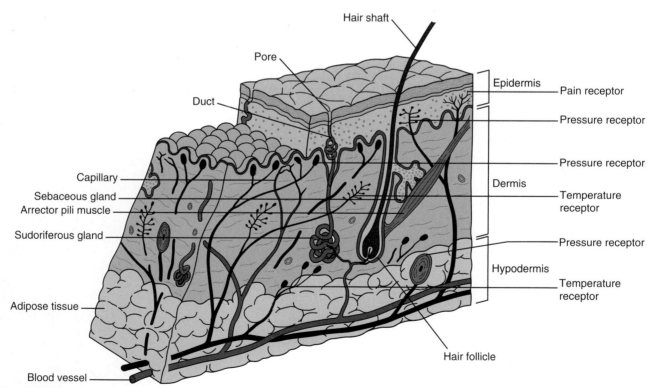

Figure 3-1. Cross section of the skin.

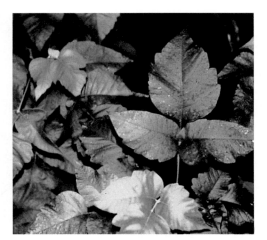

Figure 3-2. Poison ivy.

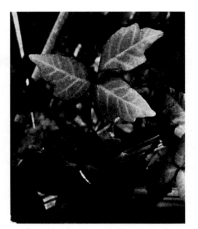

Figure 3-3. Poison oak.

and limited protection from ultraviolet radiation through a pigment called melanin produced by the melanocytes.

Intact skin functions as a *biological barrier*, and is extremely effective against many foreign agents, such as bacteria and viruses. Because the cells of the skin are tightly packed, it is difficult for pathogens to work their way through the skin into deeper tissues unless there is a break in the skin. The surface acidity provides skin with a *chemical barrier*. Sebum, the oil secreted by sebaceous glands, forms an acidic film over skin that inhibits the growth of many pathogens.

The skin also has limited properties of absorption. Examples of absorbable substances are gases such as oxygen and carbon dioxide; the fat-soluble vitamins A, D, E, and K; steroids; resins of certain plants such as poison ivy (Figure 3-2) and poison oak (Figure 3-3); organic solvents such as paint thinner, which can cause brain and kidney damage; and salts of heavy metals such as lead, mercury, and nickel. The use of medicated transdermal patches is based on the absorptive properties of the skin (Box 3-1).

Skin has many sensory receptors. Sensory receptors are specialized nerve endings that receive stimuli such as pressure, pain, and temperature from the external environment. The application of massage techniques stimulates these sensory receptors.

Skin also has a regulatory role in body temperature by changing blood flow to the skin. As the blood moves toward the body's surface and the blood vessels dilate, internal heat is released. Heat can also be dissipated through the evaporation of perspiration produced by the sudoriferous glands. Wastes are

---

Box 3-1

Transdermal Patches

The massage therapist should not work within a 4- to 6-inch radius of the patch. The client should never be asked to remove the patch so that massage can be performed under the area. Doing so could put the client at risk for medically related issues. Massage near the skin patch has the ability to alter the absorption rate of the medication. Additionally, asking a client to remove a transdermal patch is typically outside the massage therapist's scope of practice. These patches are often used to administer nitroglycerin, birth control, antinausea medication, and medication used to stop smoking or to reduce pain (lidocaine).

also removed through perspiration. Hence, the skin also functions as a miniexcretory system.

Located in the skin are precursor molecules that are converted to vitamin D with the help of sunlight. Vitamin D is important because it stimulates the absorption of calcium and phosphorus from food.

Hairs, or *pili*, are found throughout the skin except the palms, palmar surfaces of the fingers, soles, and plantar surfaces of the feet. Hair follicles are the structures in the skin from which hair grows. Hair protects the scalp from injury and ultraviolet radiation. Eyebrows and eyelashes guard the eyes from foreign particles; hair in the nostrils and external ear canal protect the nose and ears, respectively. Hairs

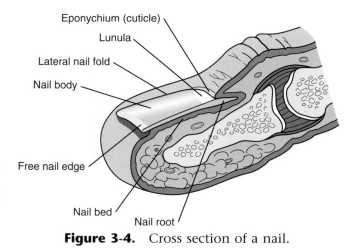

Figure 3-4. Cross section of a nail.

also function in light touch because touch receptors that are associated with them are activated whenever the hairs move. Muscles called *arrector pili* raise hairs during cold or fright. In areas where there is not much hair, goose bumps result from the contraction of the arrector pili muscles.

Nails are plates of tightly packed cells derived from the epidermis. Figure 3-4 includes main parts of a nail. They help in grasping and manipulating small objects, protect the ends of the fingers and toes from trauma, and enable scratching to remove irritating substances.

THERAPEUTIC ASSESSMENT OF THE SKIN

During the premassage interview, the massage therapist should conduct a general survey of the skin by observing any areas not covered with clothing. When the client is on the massage table, the areas not checked during the consultation can be quickly scanned and palpated. The massage therapist should inspect the skin for color, condition, and temperature. Below is a list of pertinent questions to serve as a review of how to evaluate the integumentary system. Findings need to be documented.

The client should be asked the following questions in the premassage interview:

- *Does the client intake or consultation indicate the presence of skin pathologies?* See Table 3-1 for more information.
- *Does the client have any anomalies such as superficial and deep masses?* These include lipomas and other irregularities and are a local contraindication.
- *Are all scars listed on the intake form properly healed and accounted for?* Avoid any unhealed scars.

Table 3-1 SKIN INFECTIONS		
BACTERIAL	**FUNGAL**	**VIRAL**
Acne vulgaris	Athlete's foot	Chickenpox
Cellulitis	Jock itch	German
Folliculitis	Onychomycosis	measles
Furuncle/	Ringworm	Herpes
carbuncle	Thrush	simplex
Impetigo		Measles
Onychomycosis		Shingles
Paronychia		Warts

- *Does the client have any bruises?* As with any other irregularities, document your findings.

The massage therapist should make the following observations and palpations during the premassage interview and massage treatment.

Skin Color

- *Is the color normal for the client's race, skin texture, and tone?* If not, conduct further assessments.
- *Is the skin ashen, gray, or pale indicating ischemia (low blood flow to areas)? Is it bluish or cyanotic (low oxygen levels in the blood or tissues)? Is it yellowish (jaundiced)? Is it pinkish or reddish (inflamed, burned)?* Any of these are indicators for the massage therapist to ask the client for more information on health conditions or areas to avoid on the client's body during the massage treatment.

Skin Condition

- *Is the skin moist or dry?* Dryness suggests hyperactivity of the sympathetic nervous system.
- *Does the skin look stretched and shiny? Or does the area feel swollen, "doughy," and congested?* These signs may suggest edema. Pitting edema is the prolonged existence of pits produced by applying pressure. The best place to check for pitting edema is the extremities. Prolonged pressure to the skin that leaves a dent suggests edema. If edema is present, caution is advised. The massage therapist needs to ascertain the cause of the edema from the client, and clearance may need to be obtained from the client's physician before massage therapy can be performed. If the edema is not due to a serious condition such as congestive heart failure or renal failure, massage can be performed. If

massage can be performed, the massage therapist should elevate the affected area during treatment to promote drainage.

- *Does the skin leave an elevation when pinched?* Tenting is the prolonged existence of a tent produced by pinching an area. The best place to check for tenting is the back of the palm or the sternum. If the skin tents, this suggests dehydration.
- *Are skin pigmentations present?* Massage can be performed on individuals with skin pigmentations. Bronzing skin may indicate endocrine pathologies, such as Addison's disease.
- *Are there skin lesions?* See Box 3-2 for more information. If the client does not heal reasonably fast, this may indicate diabetes or immune suppression. Query the client.
- *Are all birthmarks, moles, nails, and body hair normal?* See Box 3-3 for more information.
- *Are there any anomalies the client did not mention on the client intake form or during the premassage interview?* If so, the massage therapist needs to bring them to the attention of the client and discuss them to see if the massage should be performed.
- *Does the skin glide easily or with difficulty when moved over the underlying structures?* The latter indicates adhesions to superficial fascia. Myofascial release techniques can be used to address these restrictions.
- *Can swollen lymph nodes be palpated?* The presence of swollen lymph nodes denotes possible local or systemic infection, or a cancerous enlargement. The massage therapist needs to bring these to the attention of the client and discuss them to see if the massage should be performed.

Skin Temperature

- *Is temperature consistent throughout the client's body?* If not, conduct further assessments.
- *Is the skin warm or hot, indicating inflammation, or cool, indicating ischemia?* The presence of fever may implicate a systemic infection. Local heat suggests inflammation. This is a local contraindication.

GENERAL MANIFESTATIONS OF DERMATOLOGICAL DISEASE

If a client has any of the following, the massage therapist needs to refer the client to the client's health care provider for diagnosis and treatment.

- Lesions or eruptions
- Lumps, nodules, or masses
- Pain
- Inflammation
- Persistent itching
- Areas of redness, cyanosis, or jaundice
- Cold or overly warm skin
- Signs of edema or dehydration
- Unhealed wounds
- Excessive bruising
- Hives or rashes of unknown origin
- Swollen lymph nodes
- Any suspicious-looking moles
- Any suspicious-looking lesions

SPECIFIC DERMATOLOGICAL PATHOLOGIES

In general, most skin pathologies are treated as a local contraindication; do not apply massage on the area in question. For clients with normal pigmentation, massage can be performed. For clients with abnormal pigmentation, massage may be performed as long as the pigmentation is not cancerous.

Acne Vulgaris (Acne) (ak´·nee vuhl·gar´·uhs)

Gr. Point; Common or Ordinary

Description—Acne is a bacterial infection of the hair follicles and associated sebaceous glands (i.e., pilosebaceous unit). Acne causes inflammation and pus formation. It usually begins at puberty and may continue throughout adolescence. Whiteheads are accumulations of dead bacteria, cell debris, and dead white blood cells (Figure 3-5). Blackheads are accumulations of dried sebum and bacteria in the gland and its duct. The black appearance is due to oxidation of the sebum. Acne is most commonly found on the face, but can also

Text continued on p. 69

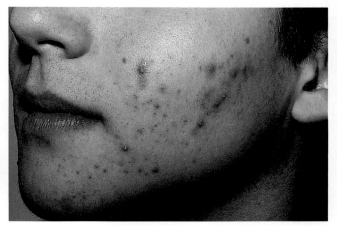

Figure 3-5. Acne.

Box **3-2**

Common Skin Lesions

Since lesions are defined as any deviation from the norm, they include pigmentations as well as pathologies. Therefore, the massage therapist should evaluate each skin lesion for the appropriateness of massage. For instance, some pathologies, such as ulcers, are always local contraindications. Pigmentations, such as freckles, are not contraindicated. Pigmentations, such as moles, and pathologies, such as scars, may sometimes be indicated and other times be contraindicated, depending on their condition. The following chart will aid the therapist in making these determinations.

Description	Examples		
Macule A flat, circumscribed area that is a change in the color of the skin; less than 1 cm in diameter	Freckles, flat moles (nevi), petechiae, measles, scarlet fever	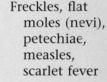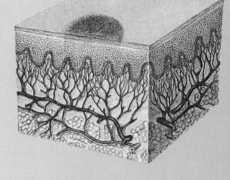	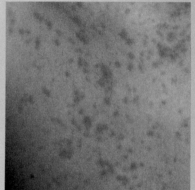Measles. (From Habif, 1996.)
Papule An elevated, firm, circumscribed area; less than 1 cm in diameter	Wart (verruca), elevated moles, lichen planus	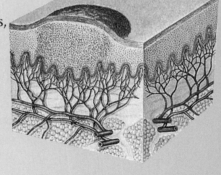	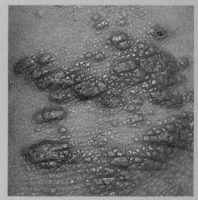Lichen planus. (From Weston, Lane, Morelli, 1996.)
Patch A flat, nonpalpable, irregular-shaped macule greater than 1 cm in diameter	Vitiligo, port-wine stains, Mongolian spots, cafe au lait patch	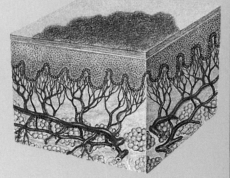	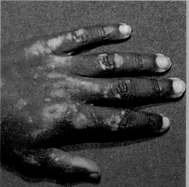Vitiligo. (From Weston, Lane, Morelli, 1991.)

Box **3-2**

Description	Examples

Plaque

Elevated, firm, and rough lesion with flat top surface greater than 1 cm in diameter

Psoriasis, seborrheic and actinic keratoses

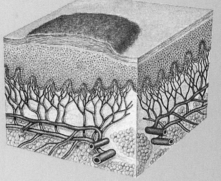

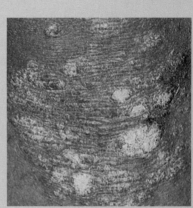

Plaque. (From Habif, 1996.)

Wheal

Elevated, irregular-shaped area of cutaneous edema; solid, transient, variable diameter

Insect bites, urticaria, allergic reaction

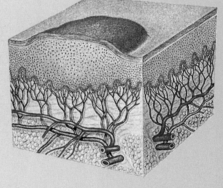

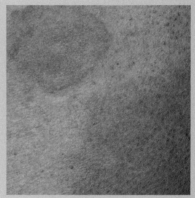

Wheal. (From Farrar et al., 1992.)

Nodule

Elevated, firm, circumscribed lesion; deeper in dermis than a papule; 1 to 2 cm in diameter

Hypertrophic nodule, lipomas

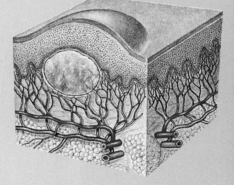

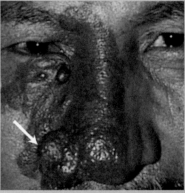

Hypertrophic nodule. (From Goldman, Fitzpatrick, 1994.)

Continued

Box **3-2**

Common Skin Lesions—cont'd

Description	**Examples**		

Tumor

Elevated and solid lesion; may or may not be clearly demarcated; deeper in dermis; greater than 2 cm in diameter

Neoplasms, benign tumor, lipoma, hemangioma

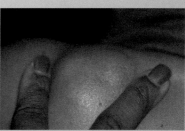

Lipoma. (From Lemmi, Lemmi, 2000.)

Vesicle

Elevated circumscribed, superficial, not into dermis; filled with serous fluid; less than 1 cm in diameter

Varicella (chickenpox), herpes zoster (shingles)

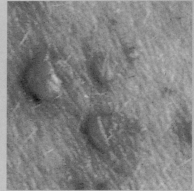

Vesicles caused by varicella. (From Farrar et al., 1992.)

Bulla

Vesicle greater than 1 cm in diameter

Blister

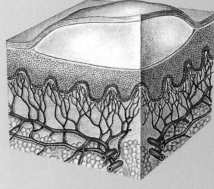
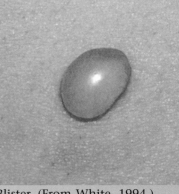

Blister. (From White, 1994.)

Box **3-2**

Common Skin Lesions—cont'd

Description	Examples		

Pustule

Elevated, superficial lesion; similar to a vesicle but filled with purulent fluid

Impetigo, acne

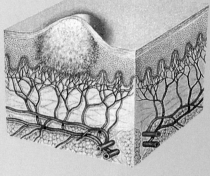

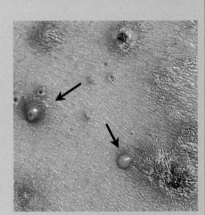

Acne. (From Weston, Lane, Morelli, 1996.)

Cyst

Elevated, circumscribed, encapsulated lesion; in dermis or subcutaneous layer; filled with liquid or semi-solid material

Sebaceous cyst, cystic acne

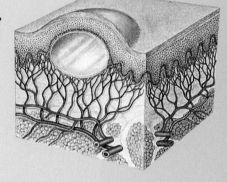

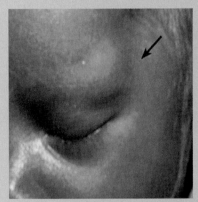

Sebaceous cyst. (From Weston, Lane, Morelli, 1996.)

Telangiectasia

Fine, irregular, red lines produced by capillary dilation

Telangiectasia in rosacea

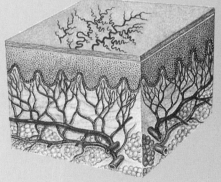

Telangiectasia. (From Lemmi, Lemmi, 2000.)

Continued

Box **3-2**

Common Skin Lesions—cont'd

Description	Examples

Scale

Heaped-up, keratinized cells; flaky skin; irregular; thick or thin; dry or oily; variation in size

Flaking of skin with seborrheic dermatitis following scarlet fever, or flaking of skin follow- ing a drug reaction; dry skin

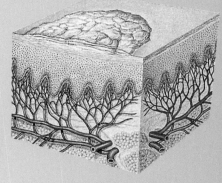

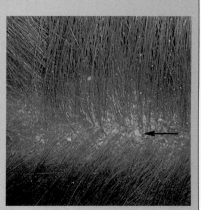

Fine scaling. (From Baran, Dawher, Levene, 1991.)

Lichenification

Rough, thickened epidermis secondary to persistent rubbing, itching, or skin irritation; often involves flexor surface of extremity

Chronic dermatitis

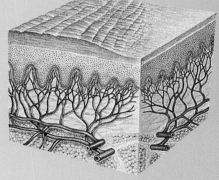

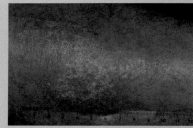

Lichenification. (From Lemmi, Lemmi, 2000.)

Keloid

Irregular-shaped, elevated, progressively enlarging scar; grows beyond the boundaries of the wound; caused by excessive collagen formation during healing

Keloid formation following surgery

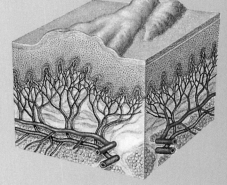

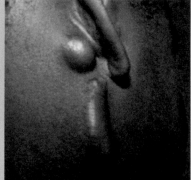

Keloid. (From Weston, Lane, Morelli, 1996.)

Box **3-2**

Common Skin Lesions—cont'd

Description	Examples		
Scar			
Thin to thick fibrous tissue that replaces normal skin following injury or laceration to the dermis	Healed wound or surgical incision	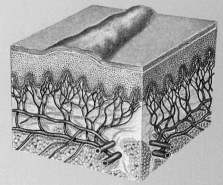	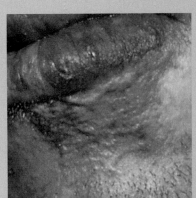 Hypertrophic scar. (From Goldman, Fitzpatrick, 1994.)
Excoriation			
Loss of the epidermis; linear hollowed-out, crusted area	Abrasion or scratch, scabies	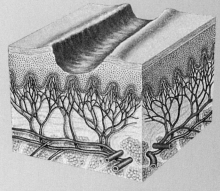	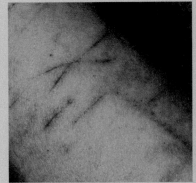 Abrasion from tree branch. (From Goldman, Fitzpatrick, 1994.)
Fissure			
Linear crack or break from the epidermis to the dermis; may be moist or dry	Athlete's foot, cracks at the corner of the mouth	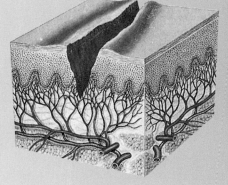	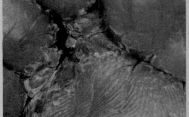 Scaling and fissures of athlete's foot. (From Lemmi, Lemmi, 2000.)

Continued

Box **3-2**

Description	**Examples**		

Erosion

Loss of part of the epidermis; depressed, moist, glistening; follows rupture of a vesicle or bulla

Varicella, variola after rupture

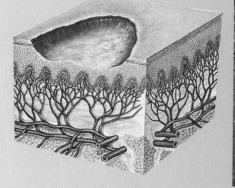

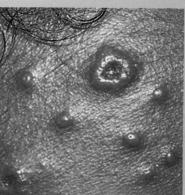

Erosion. (From Cohen, 1993.)

Ulcer

Loss of epidermis and dermis; concave; varies in size

Decubiti, stasis ulcers

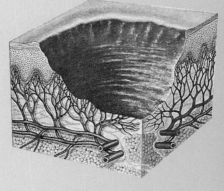

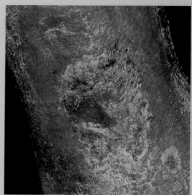

Stasis ulcer. (From Habif, 1996.)

Crust

Dried serum, blood, or purulent exudates; slightly elevated; size varies; brown, red, black, tan, or straw-colored

Scab on abrasion, eczema

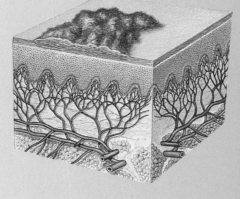

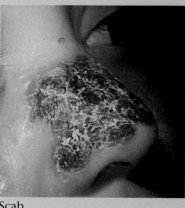

Scab.

Box **3-2**

Common Skin Lesions—cont'd

Description	**Examples**	
Atrophy		
Thinning of skin surface and loss of skin markings; skin translucent and paperlike	Striae; aged skin	

Striae.

appear on the chest, neck, shoulders, and back. Drainage of acne pustules (i.e., extracting) is beyond the scope of practice for most massage therapists. Check with your state board for more information.

Massage Consideration/s—Massage over the infected area is contraindicated if there is extensive inflammation because pressure of the massage will cause pain and also worsen the inflammation. The client with mild acne may prefer facial massage without oil. It is important that the massage therapist wash the hands thoroughly before and after massaging areas with acne so as not to spread the infection.

Athlete's Foot (Tinea Pedis) (ti·nee´·uh pee´·dis)

L. Worm; Foot

Description—Athlete's foot is a contagious superficial fungal infection of the foot characterized by discoloration of the skin and a ridge of red tissue. The skin may also break, bleed, or ooze clear fluid (Figures 3-6 through 3-8). The infected foot often has an unpleasant odor.

Massage Consideration/s—Local massage is contraindicated because this fungal infection is contagious and spreads easily.

Bruise (Contusion, Ecchymosis) (e`·ki·moh´·suhs)

O.Fr. To Break

Description—A bruise is an injury that does not break the skin. It is caused by mechanical trauma such as a blow and is

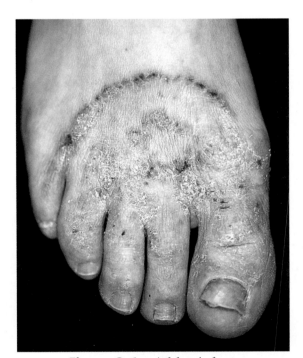

Figure 3-6. Athlete's foot.

characterized by swelling, discoloration, and pain. The color of a bruise is caused by blood from ruptured vessels that have leaked into the interstitial spaces.

Massage Consideration/s—Local massage is contraindicated until the bruise begins to turn yellowish. Massage over the bruise before this stage

Box **3-3**

Mole Changes

Observing any changes and reporting those changes to the client are an added service in massage therapy. Because the profession uses the skin as the primary organ of contact, the massage therapist has the unique opportunity to notice any changes in the skin surface. These changes are noted by both observation and palpation.

Mole changes may occur more frequently in people who are exposed to natural and artificial ultraviolet light. Mole changes may also be associated with friction or irritation from clothing (particularly bra straps), elastic waistbands, eyeglasses, or hard hats. Changes in moles can also be an indication of melanoma. Common moles and melanomas do not look alike. Using the ABCDEF method of mole assessment listed below, the massage therapist will be able to detect changing moles as they occur. The massage therapist needs to point out these moles to the client and ask the client to continue checking the moles at home. A mirror can be used for hard-to-see places on the body. A referral may be made to a health care provider for diagnosis and possible treatment.

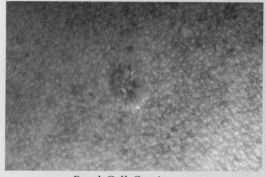

Basal Cell Carcinoma

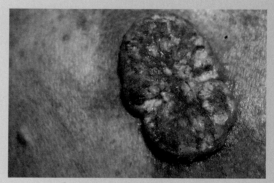

Squamous Cell Carcinoma

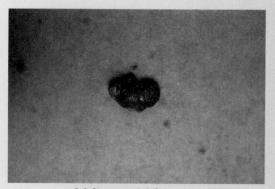

Malignant Melanoma

Asymmetry. Asymmetry means that if a line is drawn down the middle of the mole, it does not create two equal halves. Common moles are symmetrical and round. Malignant moles are asymmetrical.

Border. The edges or borders of atypical moles and malignant melanomas are irregular, scalloped, or notched.

Color. Different shades of brown or black are often the first sign of a problem. Common moles are evenly shaded brown. A health care provider should check moles that are darker than the other moles.

Diameter. Benign moles are usually less than 6 mm, the size of a pencil eraser. Early melanomas tend to be larger than benign moles.

Elevated. Benign moles are usually flat to the skin, whereas malignant moles may be elevated from the skin.

Fast-growing. Benign moles do not grow fast, if at all. Malignant moles change their size rapidly.

Sores that do not heal properly may indicate skin cancer (e.g., basal and squamous cell carcinomas and malignant melanomas) or other disorders. In these cases, the massage therapist should refer the client to the client's health care provider.

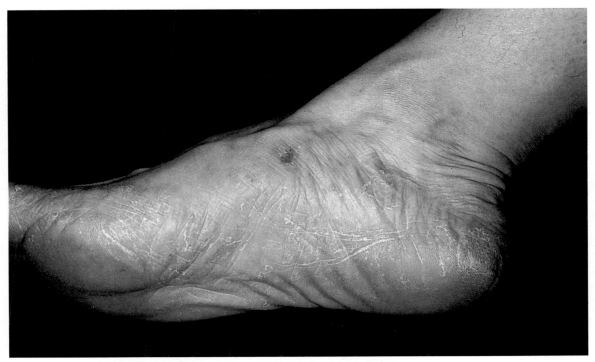

Figure 3-7. Athlete's foot, medial aspect.

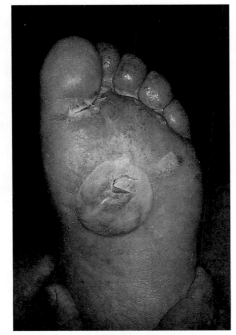

Figure 3-8. Athlete's foot, plantar aspect.

would be painful, possibly dislodge a blood clot, and may do further damage to the injured tissue. Massage around the bruise while it is bluish/purple may help facilitate its healing by increasing circulation and nutrition to and removal of wastes from the area.

Burns

A.S. To Burn

Description—When heat, radiation, electricity, or chemical agents damage the skin, cells perish. The damage that results is called a burn. A formula is used for estimating the amount of body surface covered by burns. This is called the rule of nines and it assigns 9% (or multiples of 9) to specific body areas. This formula is modified for infants and children because of the different body proportions (Figure 3-9). Burns can be classified into three categories, depending on the depth of damage to the tissues and the area of involvement.

A *first-degree burn* damages the epidermis. Symptoms are redness and mild pain. An example of a first-degree burn is a mild sunburn, which typically heals in 2 to 3 days (Figure 3-10).

A *second-degree burn* damages the epidermis and the upper layers of the dermis. Some symptoms associated with second-degree burns are swelling, blistering, and pain. Hair follicles and sweat glands usually remain functional. Healing time can be from 7 days to 4 weeks. Once the burn heals, a mild scar may remain (Figure 3-11).

A *third-degree burn* destroys the epidermis, dermis, hair follicles, and associated glands (Figure 3-12). Because of the damage to the glands and follicles, the functions of the skin are reduced or nonexistent. Because of injury of the lymphatics and

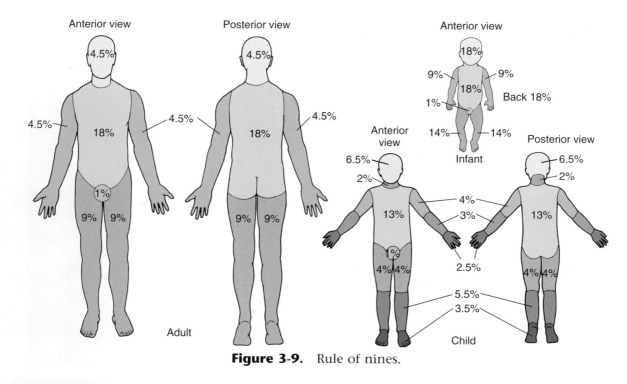

Figure 3-9. Rule of nines.

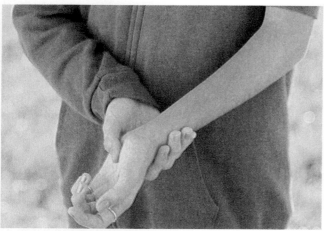

Figure 3-10. First-degree burn.

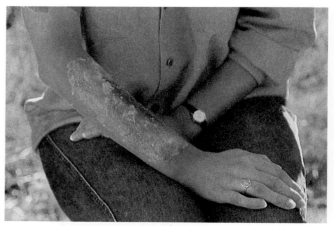

Figure 3-12. Third-degree burn.

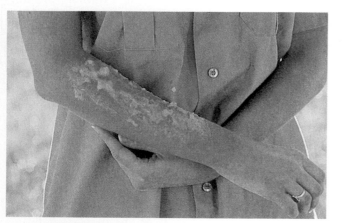

Figure 3-11. Second-degree burn.

nerve endings, there is little swelling and pain. A client with third-degree burns may experience limited mobility because of the restrictive effect of scar tissue. Almost all third-degree burns require skin grafting.

Massage Consideration/s—For clients with recent burns, the massage therapist needs to obtain clearance for massage from the client's health care provider. Massage should be performed only when tissue is fully healed and can withstand pressure. Unhealed skin is pink, thin, and delicate and should not be massaged because of the risk of the massage damaging the healing tissues. Once healing is complete and the client is cleared for massage, gentle massage is indicated, and no movements should be forced. Friction, skin rolling, and cross-fiber friction over healed and scarred tissue may help break up adhesions. Gentle stretching and joint mobilizations can help to increase mobility. The intent of massage for clients with healed skin grafts should be to soften and loosen the graft and improve circulation. The area over the graft can be massaged only after complete healing. A good-quality lubricant, preferably one with cocoa butter, aloe vera, and vitamin E, can be used. Hot packs and all forms of thermotherapy are contraindicated for all burns because they will further damage the tissues. Cold packs and all forms of cryotherapy are contraindicated for third-degree burns because of local nerve damage; the client will not be able to give accurate feedback on temperature, and thus there is an increased risk of tissue damage.

Cellulitis (sel`·yuh·lai´·tuhs)

L. Little Cell; Inflammation

Description—Cellulitis is an acute infection of the subcutaneous tissues caused by staphylococci or streptococci. It is characterized by localized swelling, redness, abscess formation, and warm and tender skin (Figure 3-13). Bacteria often enter the skin by a wound and spread to surrounding tissues.

Massage Consideration/s—If the cellulitis is in a small area, local massage is contraindicated to prevent spreading of the infection. If a larger area is involved, massage is contraindicated because of the pain, swelling, and risk of spreading the infection.

Chickenpox (Varicella) (vahr`·uh·se´·luh)

Description—Chickenpox is a highly contagious disease caused by varicella-zoster virus. The virus is transmitted by direct contact or contact with respiratory droplets. Chickenpox appears as vesicles become pustules and then crust over (Figure 3-14). Itching occurs 10 to 14 days after exposure. People are infectious from about 48 hours before the rash appears until all vesicles are crusted. Healing of the lesions occurs about a week after they appear.

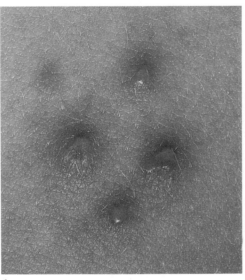

A

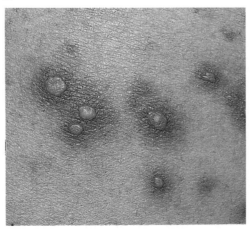

B

Figure 3-14. **A,** Chickenpox lesions. **B,** Close-ups of vesicles.

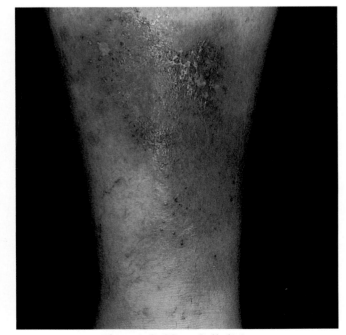

Figure 3-13. Cellulitis.

Massage Consideration/s—Massage is contraindicated until the client is completely recovered because this is a contagious disease. Also, because this is a systemic infection, massage will only make the client feel worse.

Contact Dermatitis (Allergic Dermatitis, Irritant Dermatitis)

L. Skin; Gr. Inflammation

Description—Contact dermatitis is often due to allergic reactions of the skin when the skin comes into "contact" with various substances, creating an inflammatory response (Figures 3-15 through 3-18).

Massage Consideration/s—The massage therapist needs to ask the client where the contact dermatitis is located and how widespread the area. Massage is contraindicated if there is a widespread area involved, such as with poison ivy, because it will make the dermatitis worse. If a small area is involved, local massage is contraindicated, but general massage could be performed. The massage therapist needs to make sure lubricants do not contain substances to which the client is allergic.

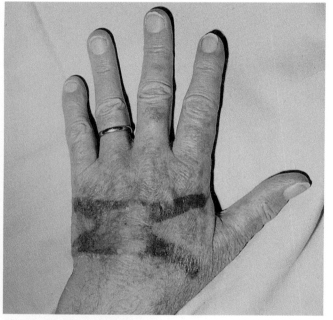

Figure 3-15. Contact dermatitis resulting from adhesive tape.

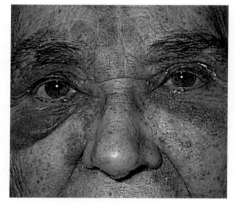

Figure 3-16. Contact dermatitis resulting from use of eye drops.

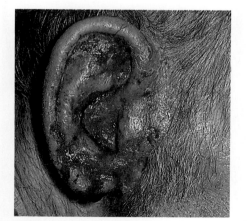

Figure 3-17. Contact dermatitis due to eardrops.

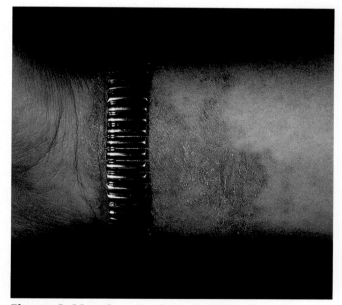

Figure 3-18. Contact dermatitis resulting from a nickel wristband.

Corn/Callus (Clavus) (ka´·luhs)

L. Horn. L. Hardened Skin

🚦 **Description**—A corn or callus is thickened, cone-shaped skin involving the uppermost layer of epidermis. It forms because of repeated friction or pressure, and occurs primarily over toe joints and between the toes (Figure 3-19).

Massage Consideration/s—The massage therapist needs to ask the client how sensitive the area is. If it is sensitive, the area should be avoided, or only gentle pressure within the client's tolerance should be used. Lemon or peppermint essential oils may help reduce the size of corns.

Decubitus Ulcer (Bed Sore, Pressure Sore) (duh·kyoo´·buh·tuhs ul´·ser)

L. A Lying Down; A Sore

🚦 **Description**—Decubitus ulcers are caused by local ischemia of tissues that have been subjected to prolonged pressure. This restriction of the normal blood supply to the skin results in cell necrosis (death). The weight of the body puts pressure on the skin (especially over bony projections). As cells die, ulcers form (Figure 3-20). Decubitus ulcers occur in bedridden patients who are not turned regularly and in people who use wheelchairs, braces, or have casts. If decubitus ulcers are not treated immediately, they can be life threatening.

Massage Consideration/s—Local massage is contraindicated because pressure from the massage would damage the tissues further. Gentle massage, using gliding strokes, in a wide area encircling the ulcer may be beneficial to increase blood flow to an area that has been deprived. Gentle active and passive joint mobilizations will help bedridden clients regain or maintain joint mobility. The client's caregiver should be advised of any redness, blistering, or ulcers noticed by the massage therapist.

Eczema (Atopic Dermatitis) (eg´·zuh·muh)

L. To Boil Out

🚦 **Description**—Eczema is an acute or chronic inflammatory disorder of the skin characterized by redness, watery discharge, crusting, scaling, itching, and burning. This disorder has no known cause and may be hereditary. Eczema is not contagious (Figures 3-21 and 3-22).

Massage Consideration/s—Massage can be performed on clients with eczema. The massage therapist needs to ask the client how sensitive the areas are, and how much pressure can be used on them. Massage over affected areas is contraindicated if there are openings in the skin and watery discharge. The massage therapist should use a high-quality

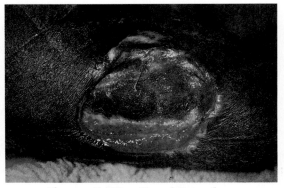

Figure 3-20. Decubitus ulcer.

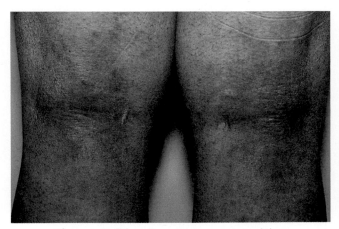

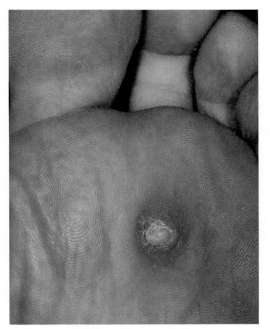

Figure 3-19. Close-up of a corn.

Figure 3-21. Eczema on extremities.

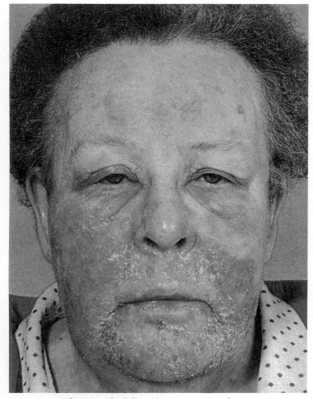

Figure 3-22. Eczema on face.

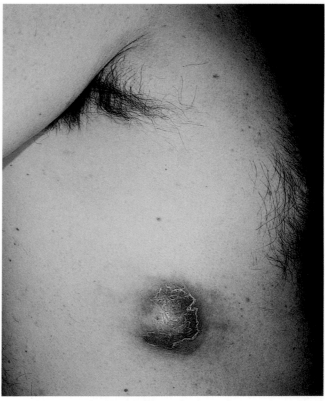

Figure 3-24. Carbuncle.

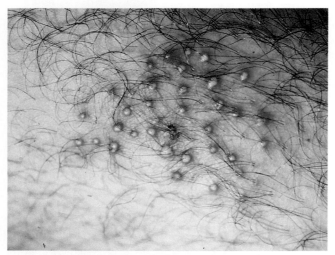

Figure 3-23. Close-up of folliculitis.

lubricant, preferably one that is highly emollient and highly nutritive.

Folliculitis (fuh·li`·kyuh·lai´·tuhs)
L. Little Bag or Sac; Gr. Inflammation

Description—When hair follicles become inflamed, it is referred to as folliculitis. This condition is often due to *Staphylococcus aureus*

(Figure 3-23). A form of folliculitis, folliculitis barbae, can develop on the bearded areas of male clients.

Massage Consideration/s—Local massage is contraindicated because massage will make the inflammation worse, and the pressure of massage could be painful. General massage can be performed.

Furuncle/Carbuncle (Boil)
(fyur´·uhng· kuhl) (kahr´·buhn·kuhl)

L. A Boil

Description—Carbuncles are clusters of furuncles connected by many drainage canals or a single, large furuncle (Figure 3-24). A furuncle is a boil or an abscess caused by the staphylococcal bacteria in the dermis or hair follicle. It is characterized by pain, redness, and swelling (Figure 3-25). Necrosis results in a core of dead tissue that may extrude.

Massage Consideration/s—Local massage is contraindicated because massage will make the inflammation worse, and the pressure of massage would be painful. Lymph nodes near the area may be enlarged and painful, so massage over them should be avoided.

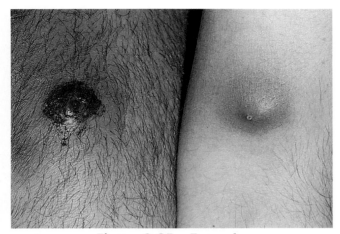

Figure 3-25. Furuncle.

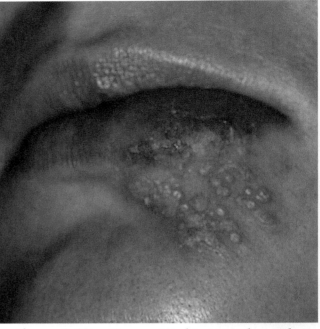

Figure 3-27. Herpes simplex around mouth.

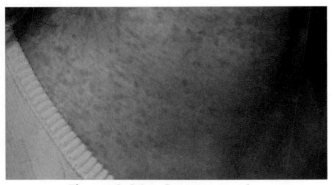

Figure 3-26. German measles.

German Measles (Rubella) (roo·be´·luh)

ME. Skin Spots; L. Reddish

Description—German measles are caused by the rubella virus. It is very contagious and is transmitted by airborne droplets from an infected person. Symptoms are mild. Some people develop a rash (Figure 3-26). Joint pain and enlarged lymph nodes may be present. The incubation period is 16 to 18 days. The infected person may spread the virus for up to 8 days after the onset of symptoms. If a pregnant woman is exposed to the virus, her fetus can develop severe abnormalities.

Massage Consideration/s—Massage is contraindicated until the client is completely recovered because this is a contagious disease.

Herpes Simplex (Cold Sores, Fever Blisters) (her´·pees sim´·pleks)

Gr. Creeping Skin Disease; L. Uncomplicated

Description—Herpes simplex is a highly contagious viral infection that has the ability to remain dormant within the dorsal nerve root ganglion corresponding to the site of infection for extended periods without expressing any signs or symptoms of disease. Flare-ups are characterized by cold sores on the skin and mucous membranes (Figure 3-27). The appearance of cold sores can be triggered by stimuli such as ultraviolet radiation from the sun, hormonal changes that occur during menstruation and pregnancy, or emotional upset.

Massage Consideration/s—Local massage is contraindicated because herpes is very contagious. General massage may be performed. If the massage therapist accidentally brushes over the cold sore, the therapist must immediately wash the area of skin that came into contact with the cold sore. The client's sheets need to be treated as infectious (see Chapter 1).

Hives (Urticaria) (uhr·tuh·kar´·ee·uh)

L. Nettle

Description—Hives are an inflammatory disorder consisting of localized edema, with development of wheals (Figure 3-28). The presence of hives is often due to an allergic reaction to food, insect bites or stings, or medications. Hives may be either acute and transient, or chronic; the former evolves over a few hours and last less than 24 hours and the latter is continuous or persists episodically for 6 weeks or more.

Massage Consideration/s—During the acute phase, general massage is contraindicated because massage will make the inflammation worse. Local massage is contraindicated, but general massage may be performed when the wheals are still visible, but not inflamed.

Ichthyosis Vulgaris (ik·thee·oh´·sis vuhl·ga´·ris)

Gr. Fish; Condition

Description—Ichthyosis vulgaris is a noncontagious group of skin disorders characterized by increased thickening of the skin, resulting in skin scaling (Figure 3-29); most are noninflammatory. Many ichthyoses are hereditary, but some may be acquired and develop in conjunction with various systemic diseases or may be a prominent feature in certain syndromes (Figure 3-30).

Massage Consideration/s—Massage may be performed and may help reduce the dryness caused by ichthyosis vulgaris. The massage therapist needs to ask the client about pressure sensitivity over the affected areas, and if there are any inflamed areas. Inflamed areas should be avoided because massage will make the inflammation worse.

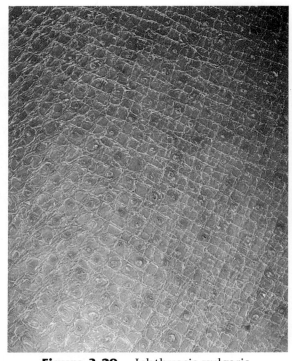

Figure 3-29. Ichthyosis vulgaris.

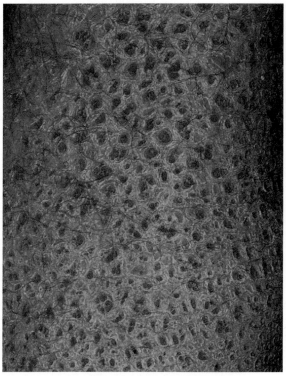

Figure 3-30. Genetically linked ichthyosis.

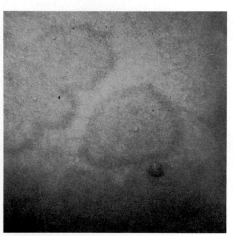

Figure 3-28. Hives (urticaria).

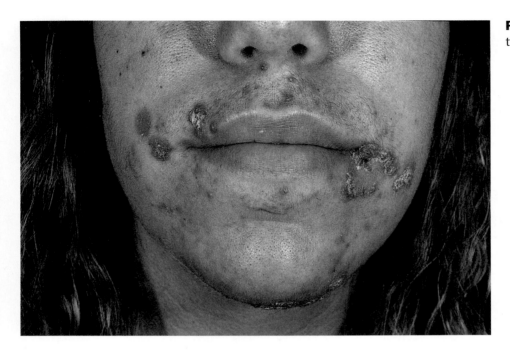

Figure 3-31. Impetigo on the face.

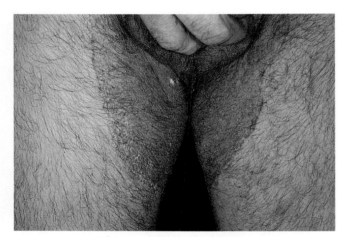

Figure 3-32. Jock itch.

Impetigo (im`·puh·tee´·goh)

L. To Attack

Description—Impetigo is an inflammatory skin infection caused by staphylococci or streptococci. It is characterized by raised, fluid-filled sores that itch or burn (Figure 3-31). This condition is most common in children, and it occurs mainly around the mouth, nose, and hands. Impetigo is highly contagious and can be spread by hand contact and handling contaminated objects such as linens, doorknobs, and toothbrushes.

Massage Consideration/s—Local massage is contraindicated because this is a highly contagious disease.

Jock Itch (Tinea Cruris) (ti·nee´·uh krur´·uhs)

L. Worm; Leg or Thigh

Description—Tinea cruris, or jock itch, is a fungal infection in the groin or perineal area, sometimes spreading to nearby areas. It is generally seen in males and is characterized by an itchy, dry, scaly area with a raised, red border (Figure 3-32).

Massage Consideration/s—As massage therapists do not massage the genitals, general massage can be performed on clients with jock itch. Since the infection may spread to the medial thigh area, the massage therapist needs to ask the client how widespread the fungal infection is. All infected areas should be avoided.

Lice (Pediculosis Capitis, Pediculosis Corpus, Pediculosis Palpebrarum, and Pediculosis Pubis) (pi·di`·kyuh·loh´·sis ka´·pi·tis) (pi·di`·kyuh·loh´·sis pyoo´·bis)

L. a Louse; Infestation; Head and L. a Louse; Infestation; Body, Eyelid; Grown Up

Description—The body louse is a parasitic insect that is highly contagious (Figures 3-33 and 3-34). Lice present on pubic hair are commonly called "crabs" (Figures 3-35 and 3-36). Lice are typically found in hair and are diagnosed with the presence of egg sacs, called nits, on the hair shaft (Figure 3-37).

Massage Consideration/s—Massage is contraindicated because lice are very contagious. Also, because lice are an infestation, massage may spread the lice on the client.

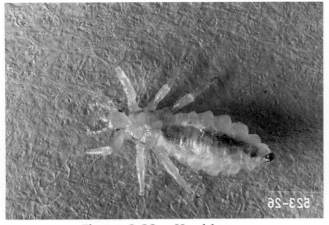

Figure 3-33.   Head louse.

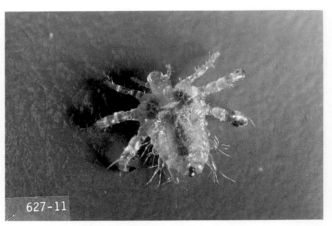

Figure 3-35.   Pubic louse.

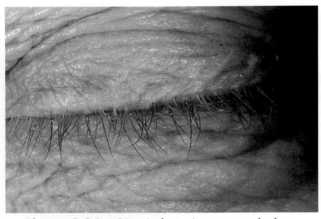

Figure 3-34.   Lice infestation on eyelashes.

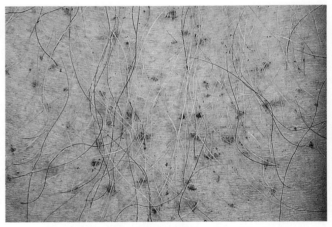

Figure 3-36.   Infestation of pubic lice.

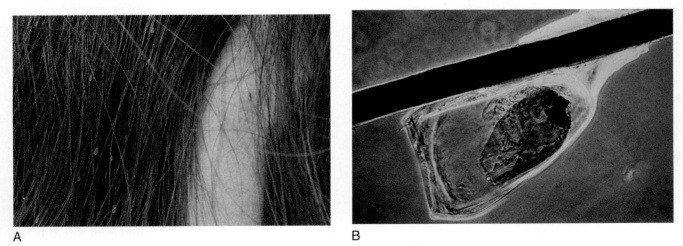

A   B

Figure 3-37.   **A,** Nits. **B,** Close-up of louse egg sac.

Measles

ME. Skin Spots

Description—Measles is caused by the measles virus, which is spread by airborne and droplet contact. Fever, coughing, watery eyes, and nasal congestion develop 2 to 3 days before the rash appears (Figure 3-38). The rash appears as small reddish spots over the face, head, arms, trunk, and back. The spots clump together in large reddish areas.

Massage Consideration/s—Massage is contraindicated until the client has completely recovered because this is a contagious disease.

Onychomycosis (Tinea Unguium)

(ah`·nee·koh·mai·koh´·sis) (ti·nee´·uh un´·gwee·uhm)

Gr. Nail; Fungus; Condition; L. Worm; Nail

Description—Onychomycosis is an infection involving the nails, usually caused by a combination of bacteria and fungi, particularly *Candida*. It is usually first seen as white patches or pits on or around the nail surface or its edges, followed by establishment of infection beneath the nail plate (Figure 3-39).

Massage Consideration/s—Local massage is contraindicated because onychomycosis is contagious. Also, massage will only worsen the symptoms.

Open Wounds

Description—Open wounds are injuries to a limited area of skin that disrupts the skin's normal continuity, resulting in a lesion. Soft tissues underneath may also be involved. These wounds can range from an abrasion, to an avulsion, laceration, incisions, puncture, or ulcer (Figure 3-40).

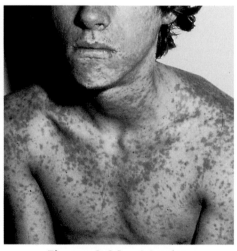

Figure 3-38. Measles.

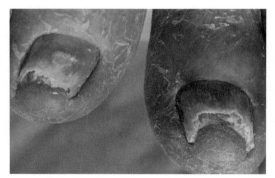

Figure 3-39. Onychomycosis.

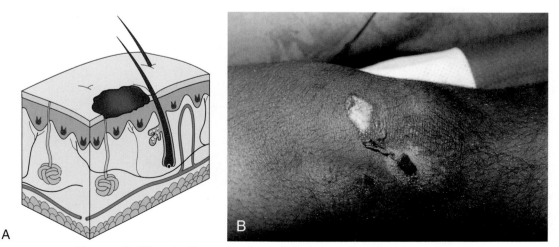

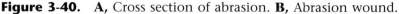

Figure 3-40. **A,** Cross section of abrasion. **B,** Abrasion wound.

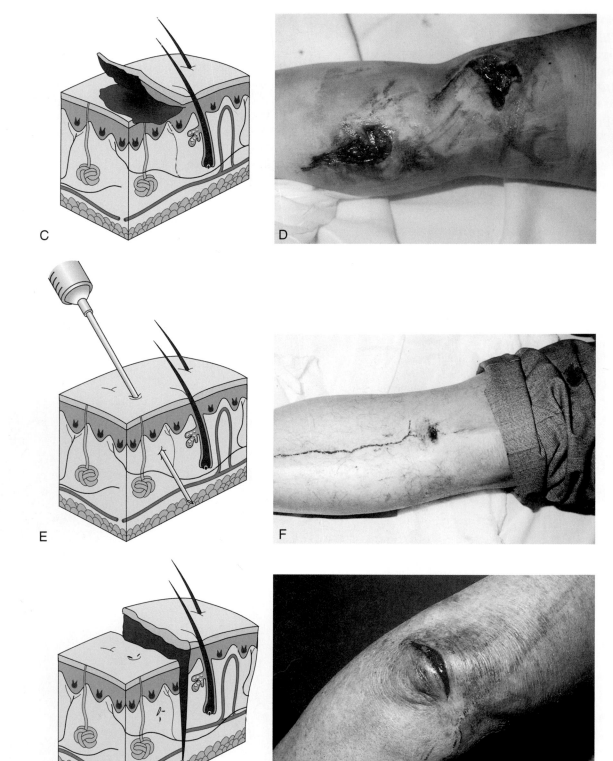

Figure 3-40, cont'd. C, Cross section of an avulsion. **D,** Avulsion wound. **E,** Cross section of a puncture. **F,** Puncture wound. **G,** Cross section of a laceration. **H,** Laceration wound.

Massage Consideration/s—Local massage is contraindicated because of the risk of massage introducing pathogens into the client's body, and the pressure of massage would cause pain and damage the tissues further. Gentle massage of the surrounding tissues may help the healing process by increasing circulation and nutrition to, and removal of wastes from, the area.

Paronychia (pa`·ruh·ni´·kee·uh)

Gr. Near; Nail

Description—Inflammation and infection of the tissue surrounding the nail caused by staphylococci is called paronychia.

Massage Consideration/s—Local massage is contraindicated because paronychia is contagious. Also, massage will only worsen the symptoms.

Petechiae (puh·tee´·kee·ay)

It. Flea Bite

Description—Petechiae are tiny red to purple spots on the skin resulting from minute hemorrhages within the dermal or submucosal tissue layers (Figure 3-41). Petechiae range from pinpoint to pinhead size and are flush with the surface.

Massage Consideration/s—Local massage is contraindicated because this condition results from bleeding under the skin and massage may make it worse.

Psoriasis (suh·rai´·uh·sis)

Gr. Itching

Description—Psoriasis is characterized by red, flaky skin elevations covered by thick, dry, silvery scales (Figure 3-42). A chronic form of dermatitis, it is characterized by periods of remission and exacerbation. In severe forms, psoriasis is a disabling and disfiguring disorder and can involve the scalp, elbows, knees, back, and buttocks. Often, it is genetic. This disorder has no known cause and is not contagious. Stress can exacerbate the condition.

Massage Consideration/s—Massage can be performed on clients with psoriasis. The massage therapist needs to ask the client how sensitive the areas are, and how much pressure can be used on them. Some of the scales may dislodge during treatment.

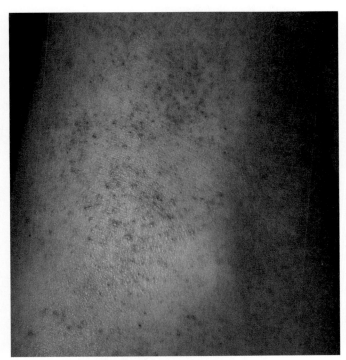

Figure 3-41. Petechiae.

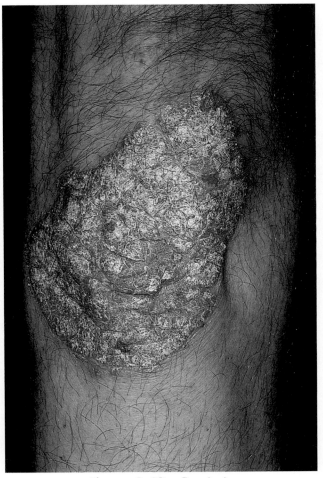

Figure 3-42. Psoriasis.

Ringworm (Tinea Corporis) (ti·nee´·uh kohr´·puh·ris)

L. Worm; Body

🚦 **Description**—Ringworm is not a worm at all, but a group of contagious fungal diseases characterized by itching, scaling, and sometimes painful lesions manifested as a raised red-ringed patch (Figure 3-43).

Massage Consideration/s—Massage is contraindicated until the client has completely recovered because ringworm is contagious.

Rosacea (roh·zay´·shuh)

L. Rosy

🚦 **Description**—A chronic inflammatory disorder affecting the blood vessels and hair follicles of the face, rosacea is characterized by persistent redness and swelling. Usually, only the middle third of the face is involved (Figure 3-44).

Massage Consideration/s—Massage can be performed on clients with rosacea. The massage therapist needs to ask the client how sensitive the areas are. Only gentle pressure, within the client's tolerance, should be used so as to not damage the inflamed blood vessels. Avoid hot immersion baths, as they may increase the redness and swelling.

Scabies

L. Itch

🚦 **Description**—Scabies is a highly contagious infestation caused by parasitic mites (Figure 3-45) that burrow and crawl under the skin's surface. The mites cannot be seen by the naked eye (Figure 3-46). The female mite excretes a material that causes intense itching (typically at night) (Figure 3-47).

Massage Consideration/s—Massage is contraindicated because scabies is highly contagious. Also, because scabies is an infestation, massage may spread the scabies on the client.

Scars

Gr. Scab Caused By A Burn

🚦 **Description**—Scar tissue is the result of the healing process. A cicatrix is a scar with substantial constriction because of the natural

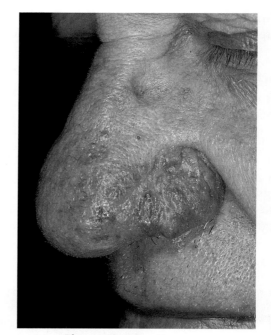

Figure 3-44.   Rosacea.

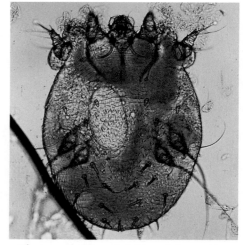

Figure 3-45.   Adult scabies mite.

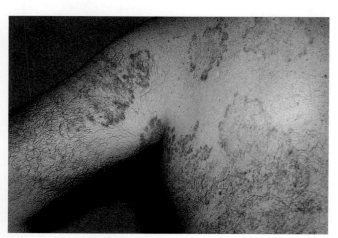

Figure 3-43.   Ringworm.

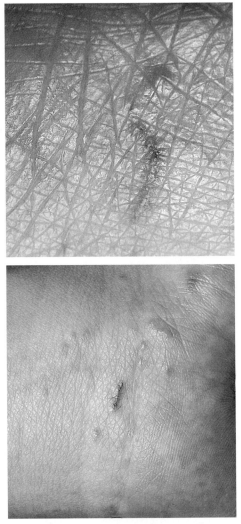

Figure 3-46. Scabies trail.

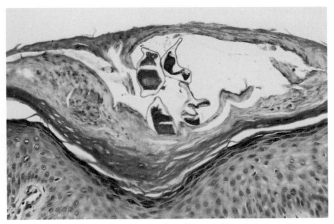

Figure 3-47. Microscopic view of scabies mite under the skin.

healing process, as in a burn, or by the way it was sutured. A keloid is a large, elevated scar that grows beyond the boundaries of the wound and that may be pink because of the presence of blood vessels (Figure 3-48). Scar tissue often creates pain and discomfort, stiffness, weakness, and loss of function.

Massage Consideration/s—The massage therapist needs to obtain clearance for massage from the client's health care provider before treating a recent but fully healed scar. Hypoallergenic lotions are recommended for sensitive skin. Cross-fiber friction or chucking friction can be applied directly to the scar. Myofascial release techniques, including skin rolling, can be used on adhesions. Gliding strokes, kneading, and deep friction can be used on muscles in the area to increase muscle tone and strength, and to alleviate muscle spasms and tense spots, working within the client's tolerance. The goals of massage treatment are to increase tissue flexibility, increase joint mobility, and counteract muscle weakness. The massage therapist needs to communicate with the client about pressure and effectiveness of techniques.

Scleroderma (Systemic Sclerosis)

(skler`·uh·der´·muh)

Gr. Hardening; Skin

Description—Scleroderma is an autoimmune disorder affecting blood vessels and connective tissue. It is characterized by excessive collagen production of the connective tissue of the skin, lungs, and internal organs. The skin tightens and becomes fixed to underlying tissues (Figure 3-49). Scleroderma is most common in middle-aged women. Death may occur because of cardiac, renal, pulmonary, or intestinal involvement. There may be localized forms with just small patches of the skin involved. Scleroderma is not contagious.

Massage Consideration/s—Massage is contraindicated for the severe forms of scleroderma because of the risk of causing further damage to the skin and underlying organs. In less severe forms, massage can be beneficial. The massage therapist needs to obtain clearance for massage from the client's health care provider. Friction and cross-fiber friction may help reduce adhesions. Deep strokes can increase local circulation and improve nutrition and drainage for tissues. Passive and active stretches and joint mobilization can help retain joint mobility. The massage therapist needs to communicate with the client about pressure and effectiveness of techniques.

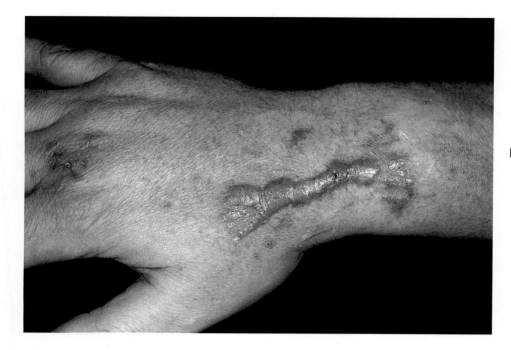

Figure 3-48.   Scar on hand.

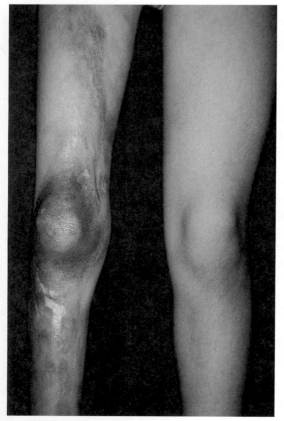

Figure 3-49.   Skin of individual with scleroderma.

Sebaceous Cyst (Epidermal Cyst, Epidermoid Cyst) (suh·bay´·shuhs sist´) (e·puh·der´·muhl sist´, e·puh·der´·moid sist´)

L. Tallow; Gr. To Flow; Gr. Bag

Description—A sebaceous cyst is a common, benign swelling beneath the skin lined by keratinizing epithelium and filled with material composed of sebum and epithelial debris (Figures 3-50 and 3-51). These cysts are mobile but attached to the skin by the remains of a sebaceous gland duct. Sebaceous cysts frequently become infected. Treatment is surgical excision.

Massage Consideration/s—Local massage is contraindicated because the pressure of massage can cause inflammation or make existing inflammation worse. New therapists are cautioned about confusing cysts with muscle knots or trigger points. If in doubt, don't.

Seborrheic Dermatitis (Dandruff and Cradle Cap) (se·buh·ree´·ik der·muh·tai´·tis)

L. Tallow; Gr. To Flow; L. Skin; Gr. Inflammation

Description—Seborrhea is dry scaly material from the scalp or any excessive scaly material from the skin (Figure 3-52) that may or may not be associated with disease (Figure 3-53). Seborrheic dermatis has no known cause (Figure 3-54).

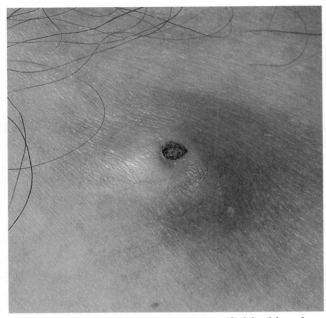

Figure 3-50.   Sebaceous cyst with blackhead.

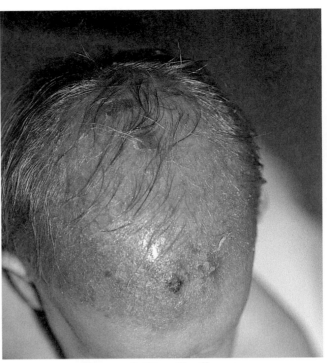

Figure 3-52.   Cradle cap.

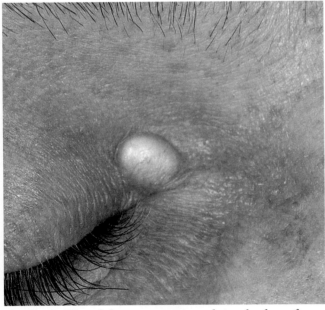

Figure 3-51.   Sebaceous cyst on lateral edge of eyelid.

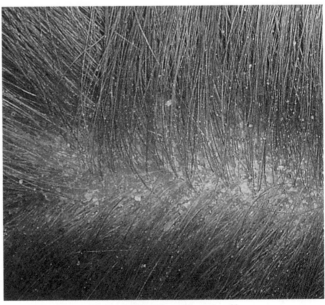

Figure 3-53.   Dandruff.

Massage Consideration/s—The massage therapist needs to ask the client if the seborrheic dermatitis is due to disease, and if so, what disease. Depending on the disease, local and possibly general massage may be contraindicated. If the dermatitis is not due to disease, massage can be performed.

Seborrheic Keratosis (se`·buh·ree´·ik ka`·ruh·toh´·sis)

L. Tallow; Gr. To Flow; Gr. Horn; Condition

Description—Seborrheic keratosis is a benign growth of epidermal cells (Figure 3-55). Usually occurring in middle life, seborrheic keratosis begins as a pink, raised patch that gradually turns tan-brown and greasy, having the appearance of being pasted on. These patches are most often located on the face, trunk, and extremities. Seborrheic keratosis has no known cause.

Massage Consideration/s—Local massage is contraindicated because the pressure of massage may cause pain and may damage the tissues.

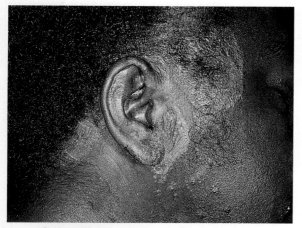

Figure 3-54. Seborrheic dermatitis.

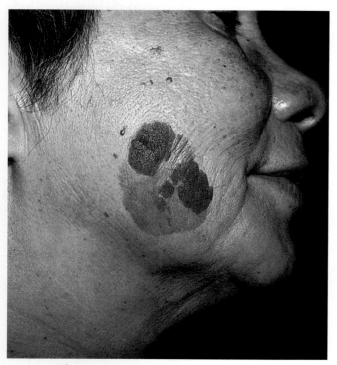

Figure 3-55. Seborrheic keratosis.

Shingles (Herpes Zoster)

Gr. Creeping Skin Disease; a Girdle

Description—Shingles occurs as a result of reactivation of the herpes zoster virus, the virus that also causes chickenpox. After a person recovers from chickenpox, the virus retreats to a posterior root ganglion. The immune system usually keeps the virus from spreading if the virus reactivates. If the immune system becomes weakened, however, the reactivated virus leaves the posterior root ganglion and travels down sensory neurons. Dermatomes are the areas of the skin that send sensory information into the central nervous system via a pair of spinal nerves, or cranial nerve V. The posterior root ganglion into which the herpes virus had retreated determines which dermatome (and area of skin) the shingles will appear (Figure 3-56). Affecting mainly adults, shingles presents itself as painful groups of vesicles (blisters) in a striplike pattern along the affected nerves of the dermatome (Figure 3-57). Scarring may result. The distribution of the blisters is usually unilateral, typically affecting the thoracic area and sometimes the face, although both sides of the body may be involved. The skin in the area of the blisters is hypersensitive.

Massage Consideration/s—Local massage is contraindicated because the pressure of massage will cause pain and worsen the inflammation. If the client feels up to it, general massage may be performed. The blisters resulting from shingles contain the varicella-zoster virus. The therapist who has not had chickenpox should not massage the client, as the virus is contagious.

Skin Tags (Acrochordon) (a·kroh·kohrʹ·duhn)

Gr. Extremity; Cord

Description—Skin tags are tiny little flaps of skin (Figure 3-58). They are most common in middle-aged men and women and are typically located around the neck, upper chest, armpit, and groin. Some are genetic; others are a result of friction such as occurs from clothes rubbing on skin.

Massage Consideration/s—Massage can be performed. The massage therapist should ask the client if the client is sensitive in the area of the skin tags, and adjust the pressure of the massage accordingly. The massage therapist should take care not to pull skin tags during the massage or when performing joint mobilizations.

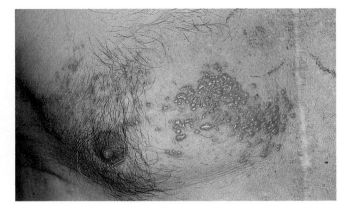

Figure 3-56. Shingles.

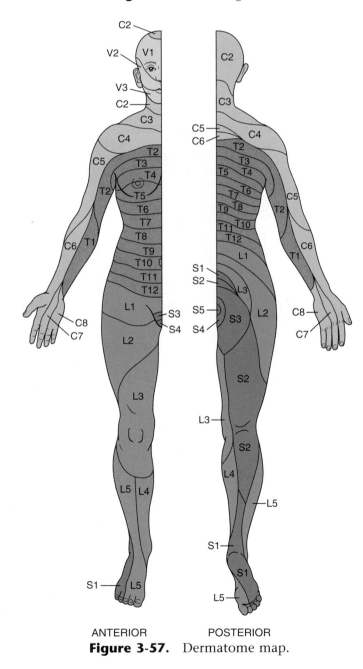

ANTERIOR   POSTERIOR
Figure 3-57. Dermatome map.

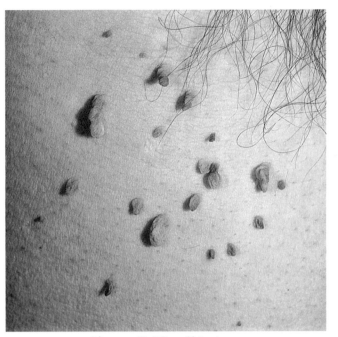

Figure 3-58. Skin tags.

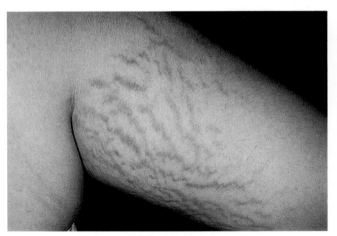

Figure 3-59. Stretch marks.

Stretch Marks (Striae) (stri´·e)

L. Channel

Description—Stretch marks are tearing, thinning, or overstretching of skin that actually reduces its thickness. They begin as red to pink streaks that eventually fade to silvery white (Figure 3-59). These streaks often result from extreme stretching of the skin such as occurs from pregnancy, body building, sudden weight gain, or severe swelling resulting from accident or surgical complications.

Massage Consideration/s—The massage therapist needs to ask the client where the stretch marks are, how large an area of the body is involved, and how sensitive to pressure the areas are. Lighter pressure is indicated on stretch marks because of the risk of further damaging the tissues. Massage will not remove or reduce stretch marks because they are not a buildup of scar tissue.

Thrush (Oral Candidiasis) (ohr´·uhl kan`·duh·dai´·uh·sis)

L. Glowing White

Description—Caused by the fungus *Candida albicans*, thrush affects the oral mucosa. It is characterized by white plates of soft, curd-like material that may be wiped off, leaving a raw bleeding surface (Figure 3-60). Thrush usually affects sick or weak infants, individuals in poor health or who are immunocompromised, and occasionally individuals who have been treated with antibiotics.

Massage Consideration/s—The massage therapist needs to ask the client if the thrush is due to another disease or disorder and, if so, which one. Depending on the disease, massage may be contraindicated. If the thrush is not due to a contraindicated disease, massage may be performed.

Wart (Verruca) (vuh·roo´·kuh)

L. Wart

Description—A wart is a thickening of the epidermis resulting in a mass of cutaneous elevations caused by a contagious virus, papillomavirus (Figures 3-61 and 3-62).

Massage Consideration/s—Local massage is contraindicated because warts are contagious.

Xerosis (zuh·roh´·sis)

Gr. Dry; L. Skin

Description—Xerosis is abnormally dry skin. It may be caused by too frequent hot water bathing.

Massage Consideration/s—Massage can be performed. A number of different massage lubricants (oil versus lotion versus cream) may need to be tried to see which works best for the client's skin.

SKIN PIGMENTATIONS

In this section, we examine common skin pigmentations such as age spots, albinism, birthmarks, freckles, vitiligo, and chloasma. Some pigmentations are congenital, some are a response to hormones (i.e., the mask of pregnancy), and others

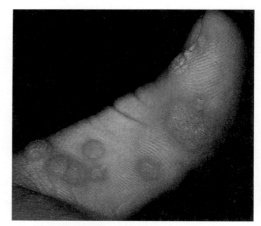

Figure 3-61. Warts on thumb.

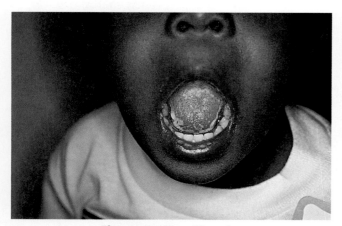

Figure 3-60. Thrush.

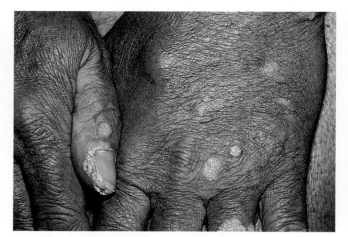

Figure 3-62. Warts on hands and fingers.

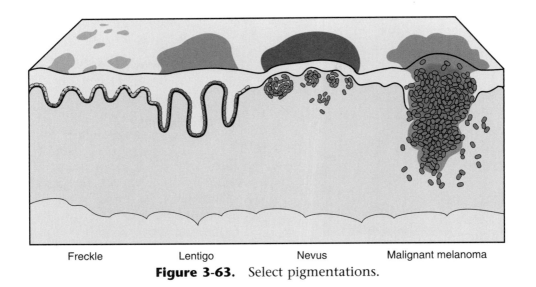

| Freckle | Lentigo | Nevus | Malignant melanoma |

Figure 3-63. Select pigmentations.

appear as a result of age or ultraviolet light such as sun exposure. Massage can be performed on individuals with skin pigmentations (Figure 3-63), unless the pigmentations present are due to a contraindicated disease.

Age Spots (Senile Lentigo, Liver Spots)
(see´·nail len´·tuh·goh)

L. Old; Freckle

🚦 **Description**—Age spots, a pigmented lesion, are tan or brown macules found on the skin of older people, especially those who have chronic and excessive exposure to the sun (Figure 3-64).

Albinism (al´·buh·ni`·zuhm)

L. White; Gr. Condition

🚦 **Description**—A congenital condition, albinism is characterized by total or partial lack of the pigment melanin in the skin, iris of the eyes, and hair. These individuals have white hair, typically pink eyes (because of visible blood vessels), and pale skin; they do not tan. Hence, albinos are prone to severe sunburn and skin cancer (Figure 3-65).

Birthmarks (Nevi, Moles) (ne´·vee)

L. Birthmark

🚦 **Description**—Birthmarks are any congenital pigmented blemish or spot on the skin, usually visible at birth or shortly thereafter (Figure 3-66). Birthmarks are usually benign but may become cancerous. Please refer to the section in this chapter on mole changes (Box 3-3). Any

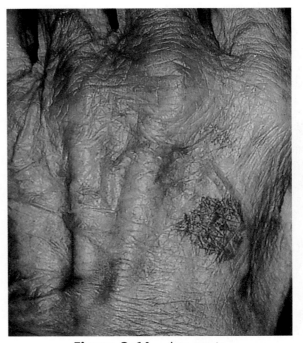

Figure 3-64. Age spots.

change in size, color, or texture, or itching or bleeding from a mole should be brought to the attention of the client, and the massage therapist needs to refer the client to the client's health care provider.

- Café au lait spots: These birthmarks are light brown (Figure 3-67).
- Port wine spots: These birthmarks are pink, red, or purplish-red. They are formed by a

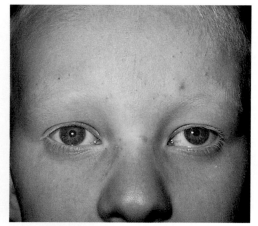

Figure 3-65.   Albino child.

collection of superficial capillaries. (See Figure 3-66, *A*.)

- Strawberry and cherry hemangiomas (capillary hemangioma): These birthmarks are small and bright red. They are a group of superficial blood vessels and 90% of them

disappear by the person's ninth birthday (Figure 3-68; also see Figure 3-66, *B* and *C*.)

Chloasma (Melasma, Mask of Pregnancy)
(khloh`·az´·muh) (muhl·az´·muh)

Gr. To Be Green

Description—Chloasma is formed by tan to brown spots, particularly on the nose, cheeks, and foreheads of pregnant women, menopausal women, or women taking oral contraceptives. The blotchy spots may also be found on the lips and neck. A similar pattern of pigmentation may be associated with chronic liver disease (Figure 3-69) and therefore may be seen in both genders.

Freckle (Ephelis) (e´·fuh·lis)

O. Norse. Freckle

Description—Freckles are benign, small, tan to brown macules occurring on sun-exposed skin, especially in children (Figure 3-70). Freckles tend to fade in adult life. The tendency to develop freckles is inherited and is seen most frequently in red-haired individuals.

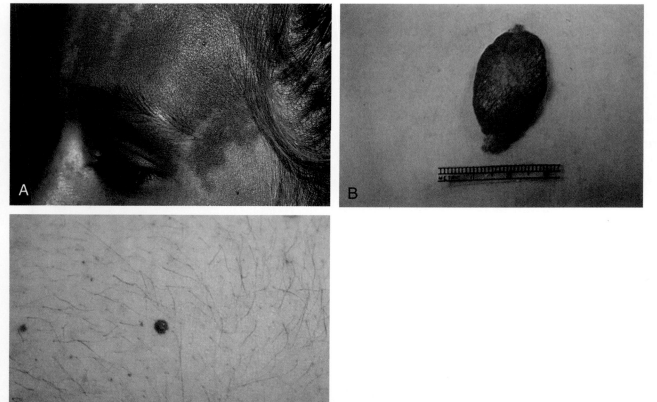

Figure 3-66.   Select birthmarks. **A,** Port wine stain. **B,** Strawberry hemangioma. **C,** Cherry hemangioma.

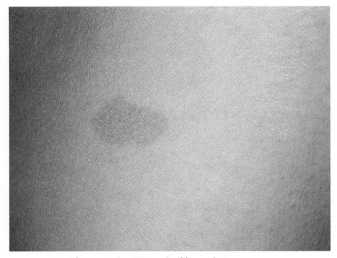

Figure 3-67. Café au lait spots.

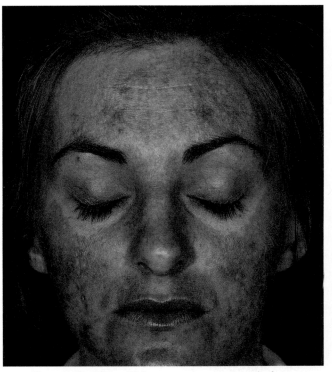

Figure 3-69. Chloasma on woman's face.

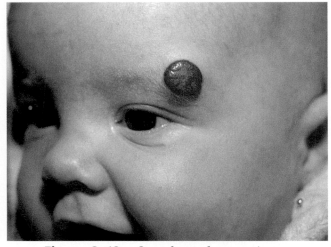

Figure 3-68. Strawberry hemangioma.

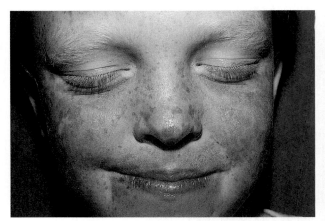

Figure 3-70. Freckled face.

Vitiligo (Leukoderma) (vi·tuh·lai´·goh)
(loo`·koh·der´·muh)

L. Blemish

Description—Vitiligo is an abnormal lack of skin pigmentation that usually occurs in patches (Figure 3-71). This condition is more noticeable on individuals with darker skin.

Resources

American Academy of Dermatology
930 North Meacham Road
Schaumburg, IL 60173
888.462.DERM (888-462-3376)

American Society for Dermatologic Surgery
800-441-2737
www.asds-net.org/

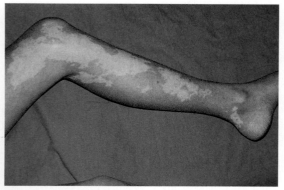

A

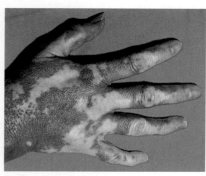

B

Figure 3-71. **A,** Vitiligo on leg. **B,** Vitiligo on hands.

National Arthritis and Musculoskeletal and Skin Diseases Information Clearinghouse
1 AMS Circle
Bethesda, MD 20892-3675
301-495-4484
www.nih.gov/niams

National Pediculosis (Lice) Association
PO Box 610189
Newton, MA 02161
781-449-NITS (781-449-6487)
www.headlice.org/

National Psoriasis Foundation
6600 SW 92nd Avenue, Suite 300
Portland, OR 97223
503-244-7404
www.psoriasis.org/

United Scleroderma Federation
89 Newbury Street, Suite 201
Danvers, MA 01923
800-722-4673

SUMMARY

The integumentary system is made up of the skin and its derivatives. The skin is divided into two distinct regions: the epidermis and the dermis. The epidermis is the most superficial layer and contains skin pigmentation cells, nails, and pores to allow passage for hair and secretions from specialized glands. The dermis is located beneath the epidermis and contains numerous blood vessels, adipose tissue, sensory nerve receptors, hair follicles, oil, and sweat glands.

One of the main functions of the skin is protection. Protection is achieved physically, biologically, and chemically. The skin acts as a physical barrier against scrapes and minor trauma. It is relatively waterproof and provides some protection from ultraviolet radiation. Intact skin provides some protection against pathogens such as bacteria and viruses. Other functions include absorption, vitamin synthesis, sensation, excretion, and temperature regulation.

Dermatological pathologies are numerous and include acne vulgaris, athlete's foot, blister, bruise, burns, cellulitis, chickenpox, contact dermatitis, corns, calluses, decubitus ulcers, eczema, folliculitis, furuncle, carbuncle, German measles, herpes simplex, hives, ichthyosis vulgaris, impetigo, jock itch, lice, measles, onychomycosis, open wounds, paronychia, psoriasis, ringworm, rosacea, scabies, scars, scleroderma, seborrheic dermatitis, seborrheic keratosis, shingles, skin tags, stretch marks, thrush, warts, and xerosis.

Dermatological pathologies may be suspected when symptoms include lumps, nodules, masses, persistent itching, signs of edema or dehydration, unhealed wounds, excessive bruising, hives or rashes of unknown origin, swollen lymph nodes, any suspicious looking moles or lesions, and areas of inflammation, cyanosis, or jaundice. Refer the client to a physician immediately when these symptoms are present. Other signs to look for during assessment include skin color, condition, and temperature.

List the letter of the answer to the term or phrase that best describes it.

A. Acne vulgaris
B. Athlete's foot
C. Cellulitis
D. Contact dermatitis
E. Decubitus ulcer
F. Eczema
G. Folliculitis
H. Furuncle
I. Herpes simplex
J. Hives
K. Impetigo
L. Lice
M. Onychomycosis
N. Psoriasis
O. Ringworm
P. Rosacea
Q. Scabies
R. Scleroderma
S. Sebaceous cyst
T. Seborrheic dermatitis
U. Shingles
V. Stretch marks
W. Wart

_____ 1. Characterized by dry, scaly material from the scalp or excessive scaly material from the skin; types include dandruff and cradle cap.

_____ 2. An acute or chronic inflammatory disorder of the skin characterized by redness, watery discharge, crusting, scaling, itching, and burning; there is no known cause, and it may be hereditary.

_____ 3. Inflammation of the hair follicles, often due to *Staphylococcus aureus*.

_____ 4. This highly contagious viral infection has the ability to remain dormant for extended periods without expressing any signs or symptoms of disease; flare-ups are characterized by cold sores on the skin and mucous membranes.

_____ 5. An acute infection of the subcutaneous tissues caused by staphylococci or streptococci characterized by localized swelling, redness, abscess formation, and warm, and tender skin.

_____ 6. A chronic inflammatory disorder affecting the blood vessels and hair follicles of the face, characterized by persistent redness and swelling; typically, only the middle third of the face is involved.

_____ 7. This condition is often due to allergic reactions of the skin when the skin comes into "contact" with various substances, creating an inflammatory response.

_____ 8. Characterized by red, flaky skin elevations covered by thick, dry, silvery scales; it is characterized by periods of remission and exacerbation.

_____ 9. This is a bacterial infection of the hair follicles and their associated sebaceous glands.

_____ 10. An autoimmune disorder affecting blood vessels and connective tissue with excessive collagen production of the connective tissue of the skin, lungs, and internal organs; the skin tightens and becomes fixed to underlying tissues.

_____ 11. A highly contagious parasitic insect that is typically found in hair and is diagnosed with the presence of egg sacs, called nits, on the hair shaft.

_____ 12. This is a boil or an abscess caused by staphylococci in the dermis or hair follicle and is characterized by pain, redness, and swelling.

_____ 13. A thickening of the epidermis resulting in a mass of cutaneous elevations caused by a contagious virus, papillomavirus.

_____ 14. This condition occurs as a reactivation of the herpes zoster virus and presents itself as painful groups of vesicles (blisters) in a striplike pattern along the affected nerves of a dermatome.

_____ 15. An infection involving the nails, usually caused by a combination of bacteria and fungi, particularly *Candida*.

_____ 16. A highly contagious infestation caused by parasitic mites that burrow and crawl under the skin's surface.

_____ 17. An inflammatory disorder consisting of localized edema, with development of wheals often caused by an allergic reaction to food, insect bites or stings, or medications.

_____ 18. Caused by staphylococci or streptococci, this inflammatory skin infection is characterized by raised, fluid-filled sores that itch or burn; it is most commonly seen in children, and occurs mainly around the mouth, nose, and hands.

_____ 19. A contagious superficial fungal infection of the foot characterized by discoloration of the skin and a ridge of red tissue.

_____ **20.** A common, benign swelling beneath the skin lined by keratinizing epithelium and filled with material composed of sebum and epithelial debris.

_____ **21.** A group of contagious fungal diseases characterized by itching, scaling, and sometimes painful lesions manifested as a raised red-ringed patch.

_____ **22.** Caused by local ischemia of tissues that have been subjected to prolonged pressure, which restricts normal blood supply to the skin, resulting in cell necrosis (death).

_____ **23.** Tearing, thinning, or overstretching of skin that actually reduces its thickness; these begin as red to pink streaks that eventually fade to silvery white.

4 Musculoskeletal Pathologies

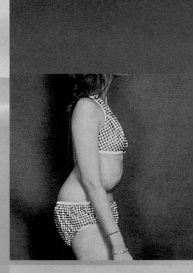

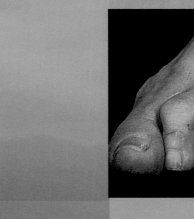

Aside from the skin and the circulatory system, the muscles and joints of the body are most directly affected by massage (Figure 4-1). Massage techniques not only loosen tight muscles, they can also

"smooth out," lengthen, and untwist the fascia surrounding the muscles, as well as increase blood and lymphatic flow locally within the tissues. Techniques such as stretches and joint mobilizations help nourish joints and increase range of motion. Although all of these effects are important in healthy clients, they are essential in clients with

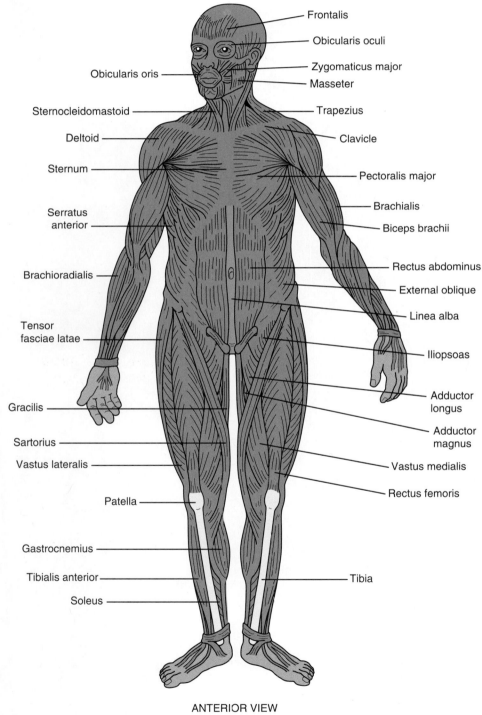

ANTERIOR VIEW

A

Figure 4-1. Muscles of the body. **A,** Anterior view.

various musculoskeletal disorders to maintain flexibility and mobility.

There are three types of muscle tissues: cardiac, smooth, and skeletal. See Table 4-1 for histological characteristics. Cardiac muscle tissue is found only in the heart and is responsible for its pumping action. It operates involuntarily; its contraction and relaxation are not consciously controlled. No nerves innervate the heart to make it contract. Instead, it has an intrinsic nervous system, a conduction system that initiates and maintains the heart's beat. The rate and force of contraction of the heartbeat are modified, however, by the sympathetic and parasympathetic divisions of the autonomic nervous system (see Chapter 5) and hormones such as epinephrine and norepi-

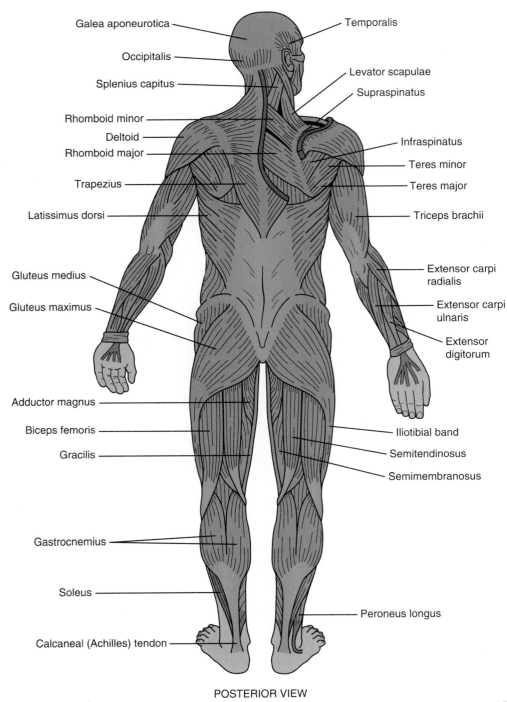

Figure 4-1, cont'd. B, Posterior view.

POSTERIOR VIEW

B

Table **4-1**   **MUSCLE HISTOLOGICAL TABLE**

HISTOLOGICAL CHARACTERISTICS	SMOOTH	CARDIAC	SKELETAL
Synonyms	Visceral	None	Voluntary
Striations	No	Yes	Yes
Number of nuclei	Mononucleate	Mononucleate (can be multinucleate)	Multinucleate
Location of nuclei	Centrally located	Centrally located	Peripherally located
Shape of nuclei	Oval-shaped	Oval-shaped	Small, elongated
Shape of fibers	Spindle-shaped	Y- or H-shaped	Cylindrical-shaped
Voluntary or involuntary	Involuntary	Involuntary	Voluntary (can be involuntary)
Fatigue rate: rapid, slow, or none	Slow	None	Rapid
Discussion	Forms the walls of hollow organs and tubes (e.g., stomach, bladder, blood vessel) controls the transport of materials, moving them along or restricting their flow	Located in the myocardium; possesses intercalated disks, which operate like an electrical synapse	Attaches to bones or related structures; is the "flesh" of the body; must be stimulated by a nerve impulse to contract

From Salvo S: Massage therapy: principles and practice, *ed 2, Philadelphia, 2003, WB Saunders.*

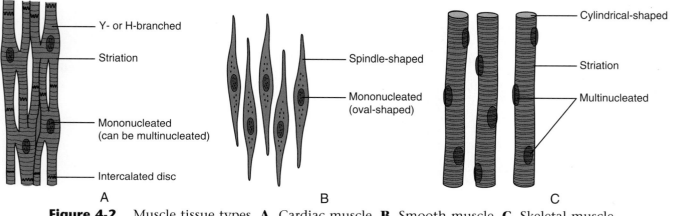

Figure 4-2.   Muscle tissue types. **A,** Cardiac muscle. **B,** Smooth muscle. **C,** Skeletal muscle.

nephrine. (See Chapter 6.) The heart is discussed in more detail in Chapter 7.

Smooth muscle tissue is found in the walls of hollow structures such as blood vessels, air passageways, and most abdominopelvic organs (Figure 4-2). It is also involuntary; its contractions are controlled by the autonomic nervous system.

Skeletal muscle tissue makes up skeletal muscles, most of which move the bones of the skeleton. Other skeletal muscles move the skin or other skele-

tal muscles. Skeletal muscle tissue is voluntary; it is consciously controlled by nerves from the somatic (voluntary) division of the nervous system (see Chapter 5). Some skeletal muscles are also controlled unconsciously. For example, the diaphragm, which is the main muscle of inspiration, continues to contract and relax even during sleep. Postural muscles are also controlled unconsciously.

A skeletal muscle consists of individual muscle cells called muscle fibers. Muscle fibers are bundled together into fascicles, which are wrapped in connective tissue. Connective tissue called fascia also wraps the entire muscle and comes off in sheets, turning into cords called tendons, which connect muscles to bones. These connections are called attachment sites, or origins and insertions of the muscle (Figure 4-3).

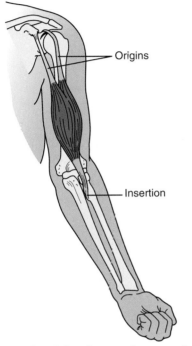

Figure 4-3. Muscle attachment sites.

Within muscle fibers are smaller filaments called myofibrils. The myofibrils contain sarcomeres, the contractile units of the muscle. Each sarcomere is made of contractile proteins or myofilaments called actin and myosin (Figure 4-4). Actin is thinner in diameter than myosin. Myosin attaches to actin and pulls on it, shortening the myofibrils, which shortens the muscle fibers and ultimately shortens the entire muscle (Figure 4-5). This process of muscular contraction is called the sliding filament theory. When the muscle contracts, it pulls on the tendons, which, in turn, pull on bones, and movement occurs.

Muscle tissue has four important functions. First, it produces body movements. Second, it stabilizes body positions such as standing or sitting. The third function of muscle tissue is to store and move substances within the body. Rings of smooth muscle called sphincters regulate the flow of substances through hollow structures such as the stomach and intestines. The urinary bladder holds urine until it is expelled with the help of sphincters. Cardiac muscle contracts to pump blood through blood vessels. Smooth muscle within the intestinal tube contracts to move food through the digestive tract. The flow of lymph and the return of blood to the heart are promoted by smooth muscle contractions. The last function of muscle tissue is the generation of heat. When muscle tissue contracts, it produces heat, which helps to maintain normal body temperature. When the body is cold, involuntary con-

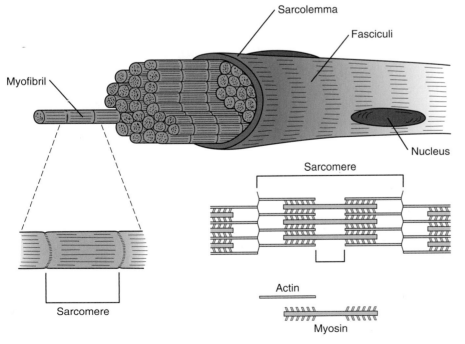

Figure 4-4. Fasciculi, myofibril, sarcomere, and myofilaments.

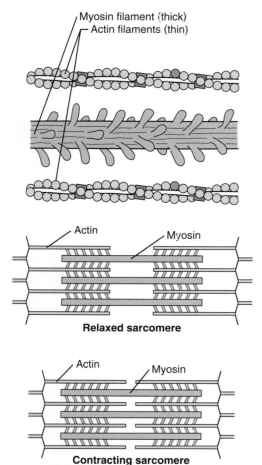

Figure 4-5. Sliding filaments.

tractions of skeletal muscles, called shivering, can increase heat production.

In the coordination of movement, muscles work in pairs and groups. Muscles involved in these groups are classified by function as agonists (prime movers), antagonists, synergists, and fixators (stabilizers). Within opposing pairs of muscles, the agonist or prime mover contracts to cause an action. The antagonist will relax and stretch to allow the agonist's action to occur. For example, in elbow flexion, an agonist is biceps brachii, and triceps brachii, as an antagonist, relaxes and stretches to allow flexion to occur. The roles of agonist and antagonist also switch places for different movements. In the case of elbow extension, triceps brachii becomes an agonist and biceps brachii becomes an antagonist. A synergist will contract to aid the movement caused by the agonist. Brachialis and brachioradialis are synergists to biceps brachii in elbow flexion. A chart of these movement relationships is located in Chapter 2. A fixator stabilizes attachment sites of the agonist so

that the agonist can contract more efficiently. For example, when the arm is in motion, fixators need to stabilize the scapula, which is an attachment site for muscles of arm movement. Muscles such as pectoralis minor, trapezius, serratus anterior, and rhomboids will stabilize the scapula, whereas deltoid contracts to abduct the arm.

The intricate structures of bone, cartilage, ligament, and joints make up the skeletal system (Figure 4-6). The skeleton acts as a supportive framework for the rest of the body systems. It protects delicate internal organs. For instance, the skull protects the brain and the ribcage protects the heart and lungs. The skeletal system acts as a storehouse for fats and vital minerals such as calcium, as well as being the site of blood cell production. The skeletal system also helps provide movement via muscle attachments.

Bones are living tissue. They are strong, flexible, and relatively light. Compact bone tissue consists of bone cells almost completely surrounded by dense material made of calcium and phosphate. There are few spaces in compact bone tissue. It forms the surface layer of all bones and the bulk of the shaft of long bones such as the humerus. It provides protection and support, and resists the stresses of weight and movement. Spongy bone tissue is made of lattices of thin columns of bone. There are many spaces in spongy bone, and it is filled with red bone marrow. Red bone marrow is where blood cells are made. Spongy bone makes up most of the inside of short, flat bones, and is inside the ends of long bones (Figure 4-7).

The human body has 206 bones. In a typical long bone, the diaphysis is the shaft. The epiphyses (epiphysis is singular) are the ends, and they have spongy bone tissue filled with red bone marrow. The epiphyses are also where the bone grows in length. The periosteum is the fibrous, dense, vascular connective tissue sheath around the bone. The medullary cavity is the hollow space within the center of the diaphysis. It contains yellow marrow, which is filled with fat. Articular surfaces, such as the epiphysis, are covered with hyaline cartilage. (Figure 4-8).

Bones can be classified according to shape. These categories are long, short, flat, irregular, and sesamoid (Figure 4-9). Long bones are longer than they are wide (e.g., humerus, femur, tibia, metacarpals, phalanges). Short bones are generally cube-shaped (e.g., carpals, tarsals). Flat bones are thin and flattened like pancakes (e.g., sternum, ribs, scapula). Irregular is a category for bones that do not fit in other categories (e.g., cranial and facial bones,

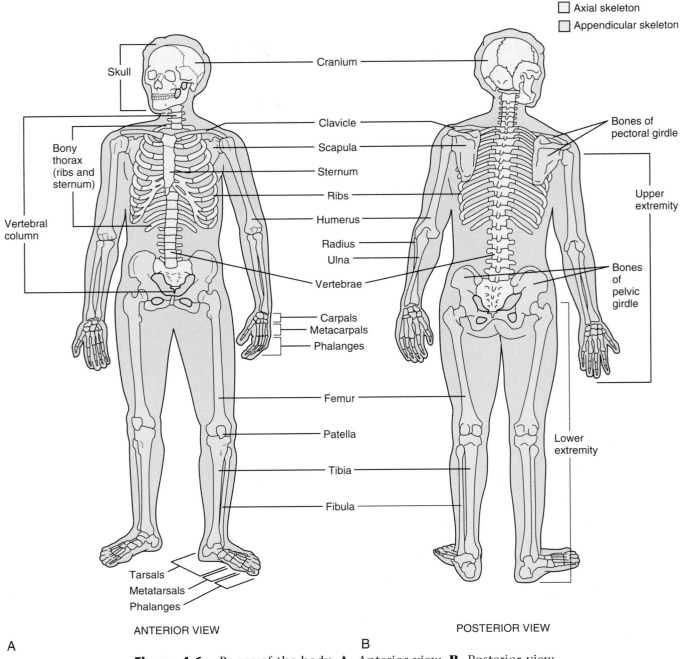

☐ Axial skeleton
☐ Appendicular skeleton

ANTERIOR VIEW

POSTERIOR VIEW

A
B

Figure 4-6.   Bones of the body. **A,** Anterior view. **B,** Posterior view.

vertebrae, hyoid bone). Sesamoid bones are small and round and are embedded in certain tendons (e.g., patella).

Where bones come together, a joint or articulation is formed. Another term for a joint is an arthrosis (arthroses are plural). A synarthrotic joint is an immovable joint. The joints between the skull bones, called sutures, are examples of synarthroses. An amphiarthrotic joint is a slightly movable joint. The pubic symphysis, where the anterior hip bones

join, is an example of an amphiarthrosis. A diarthrotic joint is a freely movable joint. All diarthroses are synovial joints. Synovial joints are different from synarthrotic and amphiarthrotic joints because they have a space between the articulating bones, called the synovial cavity (Figure 4-10). This allows for the free movement of the joint.

Synovial joints are responsible for movements of the body (Figure 4-11). Besides having a synovial cavity, synovial joints have articular (hyaline) carti-

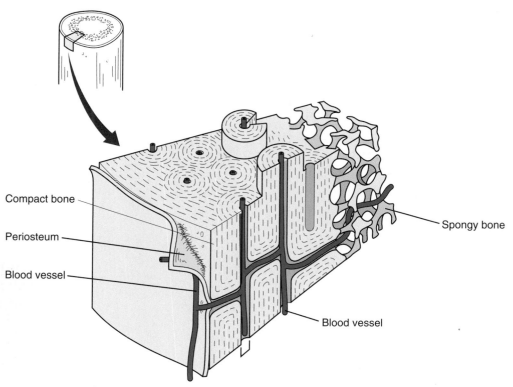

Figure 4-7. Microscopic cross-section of bone tissue.

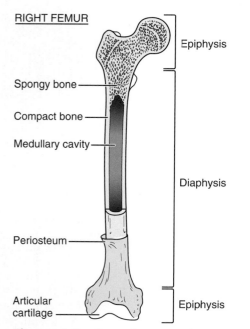

Figure 4-8. Long bone anatomy.

lage that covers the epiphyses of the articulating bones without joining them together. It is smooth and slippery, decreases friction, and helps absorb shock when the bones in the joint move.

A joint capsule forms a sleeve around the synovial joint. The outer layer is fibrous and forms ligaments, which connect the bones in the joint together. The inner layer of the capsule is called the synovial membrane. It secretes synovial fluid that lubricates and nourishes the joint. Many synovial joints also have accessory ligaments that further stabilize the joint. Menisci are pads of fibrous cartilage found between the ends of the articulating bones to help them fit together better.

Types of diarthrotic, or synovial joints are hinge, pivot, ellipsoidal, saddle, gliding, and ball-and-socket (Figure 4-12).

THERAPEUTIC ASSESSMENT OF THE MUSCULOSKELETAL SYSTEM

During the consultation, the massage therapist can conduct a general survey of the musculoskeletal system by observing and palpating the client. Chapter 2 provides specific instructions on how to conduct assessments. This section contains a list of pertinent questions to serve as a review of how to

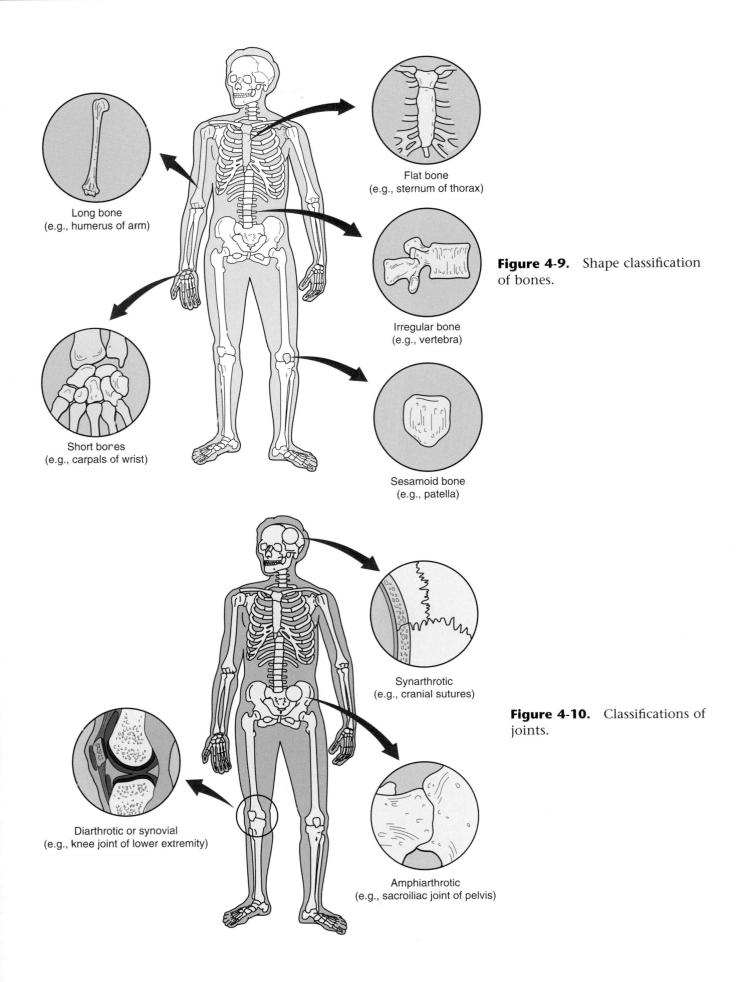

Figure 4-9. Shape classification of bones.

Long bone
(e.g., humerus of arm)

Flat bone
(e.g., sternum of thorax)

Irregular bone
(e.g., vertebra)

Short bores
(e.g., carpals of wrist)

Sesamoid bone
(e.g., patella)

Figure 4-10. Classifications of joints.

Synarthrotic
(e.g., cranial sutures)

Diarthrotic or synovial
(e.g., knee joint of lower extremity)

Amphiarthrotic
(e.g., sacroiliac joint of pelvis)

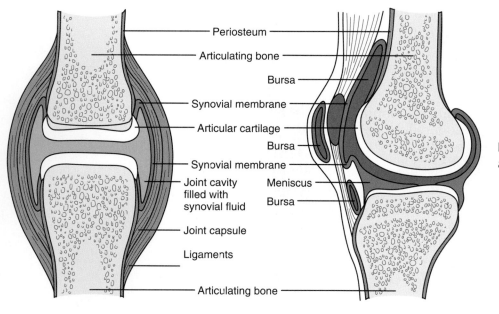

Periosteum
Articulating bone
Bursa
Synovial membrane
Articular cartilage
Bursa
Synovial membrane
Joint cavity filled with synovial fluid
Meniscus
Bursa
Joint capsule
Ligaments
Articulating bone

Figure 4-11. Synovial joint anatomy.

evaluate for abnormalities of both structure and function within the musculoskeletal system. Findings need to be documented.

The following observations can be used to assess structure:

- *When the client stands, does his or her bone structure appear bilaterally symmetrical in the frontal, midsagittal, and horizontal planes?* This will help the therapist ascertain imbalances.
- *Are there any spinal deviations?* See entries for Kyphosis, Lordosis, and Scoliosis.
- *When the client lies down, is one leg shorter/longer than the other?* If so, assess whether it is structural or functional. If the difference is due to muscles, treat them.

The following questions can be used to assess function:

Premassage interview:

- *Does the client have any localized muscle tension or muscle spasm? If so, is it due to trauma, overuse, a systemic disorder, or other?* Include techniques to affect muscle tension. If other pathologies are also present, take them into consideration.
- *Is the client taking any medication/s for musculoskeletal disorders?* Table 4-2 includes more information including possible side effects.

Premassage interview and massage treatment:

- *Does the client's contour formed by the major muscles appear bilaterally symmetrical?* If not,

determine whether it is due to lack of tone or pathology. Treat accordingly.

- *During palpation, are there areas of generalized tension and excessive tone? Does the musculature house localized tension or muscle spasm? During palpation, does the muscle twitch involuntarily?* This is called a local twitch response. An involuntary firing or twitching in a muscle can be a response to sensory stimulation on a trigger point.
- *During palpation, are there areas that lack tone or feel flaccid?* See entry for flaccid.
- *Does the skin glide easily or with difficulty when moved over the underlying structures?* The latter indicates adhesions of superficial fascia, which can be addressed with massage.
- *Does the client wince, jump, or verbalize when pressure is applied?* This often indicates pain or discomfort. Other signs to look for include changes in facial expression and breathing patterns, feet leaving the bolster, and fist tightening.

The following can be used to assess gait:

Premassage interview:

- *Does the client list or lean?* If so, the massage therapist needs to ask if it is due to pain, muscle weakness, structural abnormalities, brain disorders, or use of prosthesis (Figure 4-13). The low back, ankle, and foot are common problem areas.
- *How fast or slow does the client walk?* A slow gait may be pain-related, age-related, or an

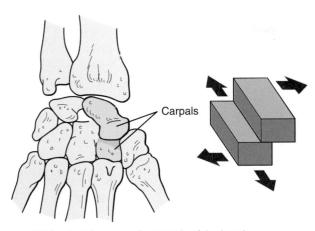

Gliding joint between the carpals of the hand

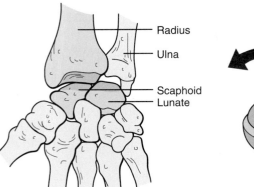

Ellipsoidal joint between radius and scaphoid and lunate bones (wrist)

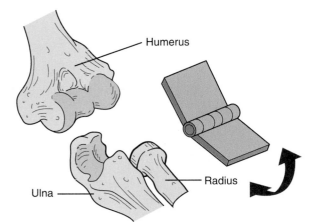

Hinge joint between humerus and ulna and radius at the elbow

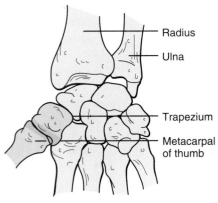

Saddle joint between trapezium (wrist) and metacarpal of thumb

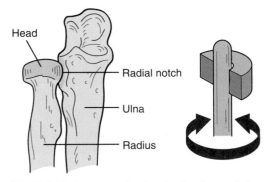

Pivot joint between proximal ends of radius and ulna

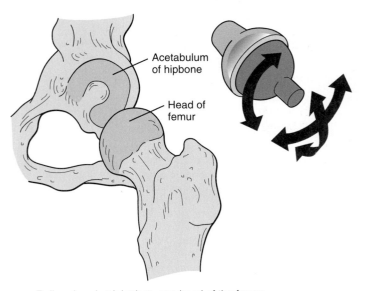

Ball and socket joint between head of the femur and acetabulum

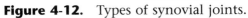

Figure 4-12. Types of synovial joints.

Table **4-2**   COMMONLY USED MUSCULOSKELETAL MEDICATIONS

MEDICATION CLASSIFICATION	MEDICATION NAME	POSSIBLE SIDE EFFECTS
Nonsteroidal antiinflammatory drugs (NSAIDs)*	Acetaminophen (Tylenol), acetylsalicylic acid (aspirin), Aleve, Celecoxib (Celebrex), Clinoril, diclofenac (Voltaren), ibuprofen (Motrin, Advil, Nuprin), Indocin, Naprosyn, naproxen (Anaprox), Nuprin, paclitaxel (Taxol), Relafen, vinblastine (Velban, Velsar), vincristine (Oncovin, Vincasar)	Abdominal cramps, allergic reaction, bruising, constipation, depression, diarrhea, disorientation, drowsiness, gastrointestinal irritation, headaches, hypertension, insomnia, lymphedema, nausea and vomiting, poor wound healing, shortness of breath, skin rashes, vertigo, weight loss
Narcotic analgesics (opiates)†	Buprenex, codeine, Darvocet, Darvon, Demerol, Dilaudid, Dolophine, Duragesic, Hydrocodone, Lorcet, Lortab, morphine, Nubain, OxyContin, Percocet, Percodan, pethidine, Roxanol, Stadol, Talwin, Tylox, Vicodin	Abdominal cramps, anxiousness, constipation, drowsiness, dry mouth, hypotension, irregular heartbeat, lethargy, low respiration rate, nausea and vomiting, skin rashes, vertigo, weight loss
Muscle relaxants (skeletal muscle relaxants)†	Cyclobenzaprine, dantrolene, diazepam (Valium), Equagesic, Flexeril, Lioresal, Norgesic Forte, Parafon Forte, Soma, Succinylcholine	Anxiousness, disorientation, drowsiness, dry mouth, facial flushing, fever, headaches, indigestion, insomnia, irregular heartbeat, lethargy, nausea and vomiting, skin rashes
Corticosteroids‡	Cortisone (Cortone), hydrocortisone (Cortef), prednisone (Delatsone, Orasone), prednisolone (Prelone, Pediapred, Orapred), triamcinoclone (Aristocort, Kenalog), methyl prednisolone (Medrol), dexamethasone (Decadron), betamethasone (Celestone)	Abdominal cramps, acne, bruising, gastrointestinal irritation, headaches, hypertension, lethargy, lymphedema, nausea and vomiting, poor immune response, vertigo

*When clients are taking NSAIDs, massage techniques such as deep effleurage (e.g., ironing), deep petrissage, ischemic compression, and deep, specific frictions (e.g., chucking, circular) should be carefully monitored or avoided. These specific techniques often produce a mild inflammatory response that usually resolves within 48 hours. Performing these techniques when a client is taking these medications may result in internal bleeding (bruising) and an excessive postmassage inflammatory response. Additionally, these medications can alter tissue integrity. In these cases, the therapist's ability to observe and palpate tissue is more reliable than the ability of the client to offer feedback on pressure.

†When clients are taking medications such as muscle relaxers and narcotic analgesics, caution is merited, as these medications depress sensory information entering the nervous system. During the massage, the therapist often relies on the client's ability to respond to internal and external stimuli to help gauge pressure. The client's response is also helpful when applying joint mobilizations or stretching. When the tissue does not respond by tightening, the sensory feedback loop is reduced or lost, and the client may be injured because of excessive pressure or aggressively applied joint movement or muscle stretch. These techniques must be applied carefully or eliminated from the routine in the event the client is taking the previously-mentioned medications.

‡When clients are taking corticosteroids, especially if the medication has been taken for more than 30 days, certain body tissues respond by losing their integrity. For example, muscles may atrophy, and connective tissues of the skin, ligaments, joints, bones, and tendons may weaken. Massage that stresses these structures, such as joint mobilizations, rib cage compressions, stretching, heavy percussion, skin rolling, wringing, and deep friction (cross-fiber, chucking, and circular), should be monitored or avoided. This is particularly true for women who have, or are at risk for, osteoporosis (i.e., postmenopausal women or older women). Furthermore, use of corticosteroids reduces the client's resistance to communicable diseases, so the massage therapist should not massage those clients when the massage therapist is ill.

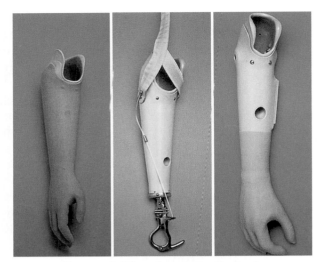

Figure 4-13. A prosthetic limb.

indication of a neurological disorder. The massage therapist needs to find out the cause of the slow gait from the client.

- *Does the client exhibit both balance and grace?* If not, suspect problems with the brain, muscles, or skeletal system. Conduct further assessments.
- *Does the client use a normal cross-pattern gait?* During a normal cross pattern gait, the arms hang freely at the sides and swing in opposition to the legs.
- *Does the client use short, shuffling steps?* This may be the result of weak quadriceps or a neurological disorder such as Parkinson's disease. The massage therapist needs to find out the cause of the short, shuffling steps from the client.
- *Are both arms swinging freely at the client's side?* Tight shoulder girdle or neck muscles prevent arm movement while walking.
- *Are one or both arms crossing the midline during stride?* If so, this indicates torquing or listing movements in the torso. See next bullet for more information.
- *Are both feet pointing forward?* If not, this indicates torquing or listing movements in the torso. This may also be due to pain in the low back, hip, knee, ankle, generalized leg pain, or tightness in the hip rotators. The massage therapist needs to ask the client where any pain and/or muscle tightness is felt.
- *Do the client's feet drag?* This is called foot-drop and can be an indicator of weakness in the ankle dorsiflexors. This may suggest a neurological disorder. The massage therapist

needs to find out the cause of the foot-drop from the client.

- *Does the client's gait pattern waddle?* This may be the result of complaints of pain in the lower back, hip, knees, ankle, or generalized leg pain, or improper use of prosthesis or orthotics. The massage therapist needs to ask the client where any pain and/or muscle tightness is felt.
- *Is the client limping or compensating?* This may be from a muscle cramp, bone spur, recent injury, neurological disorder, sacroiliac joint dysfunction, or a chronic condition such as sciatica. The massage therapist needs to ask the client the reason for limping or compensating.
- *While walking, does the client's facial expression indicate discomfort?* If so, ascertain the cause of discomfort.

The following can be used to assess joint range of motion:

During the massage treatment:

- *During active joint mobilizations, does the client guard movement?* The massage therapist needs to note any comments or reactions made by the client.
- *At the end of passive joint movements, is the endfeel hard or soft?* If a hard endfeel is felt at a joint that normally has a soft endfeel, this may indicate the presence of abnormal muscle contraction (i.e., contracture).
- *Are any crackling noises (crepitation) heard when the client's joints move?* This may indicate irregularities on articulating surfaces such as deterioration of cartilage or arthritis. Avoid joint mobilizations that cause pain, with or without crepitis.

GENERAL MANIFESTATIONS OF MUSCULOSKELETAL DISEASE

If a client has any of the following, the massage therapist needs to refer the client to a health care provider for diagnosis and treatment.

- Generalized severe or persistent pain
- Localized severe or persistent pain during palpation
- Pain accompanied by crepitation during joint mobilizations
- Severe distortion while walking, such as listing or leaning, shuffling or dragging feet, waddling or limping
- Evidence of local or general inflammation (heat, swelling, redness, pain, loss of

function) or ischemia (paleness or coolness)
- Body asymmetry while standing or lying down
- Lumps, nodules, masses, or lesions
- Loss of range of motion and/or loss of strength in the affected muscle

SPECIFIC MUSCULOSKELETAL PATHOLOGIES

In general, most musculoskeletal pathologies benefit from massage therapy.

Adhesive Capsulitis (Frozen Shoulder)
(ad·hee´·siv kap`·soo·lai´·tis)

L. Stuck To; Little Box; Gr. Inflammation

Description—The cause of adhesive capsulitis, or frozen shoulder, could be misalignment of the scapula with the humerus, as happens in kyphosis, or by trauma. It could also be caused by inflammation from lesions of the rotator cuff muscles and the related joint capsule. Other causes are arthritis or prolonged immobilization. Abduction, flexion, lateral rotation of the arm, and extension become difficult. There can be a gradual onset of a dull ache, with pain referring to C5-C6 (Figure 4-14). Adhesive capsulitis is most common in women more than 50 years old.

Massage Consideration/s—Appropriate goals of massage are to maintain and slowly increase the client's range of motion. This can be done by stretching/tractioning the capsule with the client's arm hanging over the side of the massage table. Shoulder girdle muscles, such as pectoralis major and minor, and the rotator cuff muscles need to be addressed with massage. Other muscles to focus on include biceps brachii, triceps brachii, and deltoid. If the client is also seeing a physical or occupational therapist, the massage therapist needs to work closely with him or her. The client can use ice at home to control inflammation and pain.

Amputation

L. To Cut Around

Description—An amputation is the surgical removal of a limb or outgrowth of the body. It may be done to treat recurrent infections, to remove necrosis (dead tissue) from gangrene or frostbite, to remove malignant tumors, and in cases of severe trauma. While the client is under anesthesia, the part is removed and a shaped flap is cut from muscular and cutaneous tissue to cover the exposed area.

Approximately 70% of all people with amputations experience *phantom limb sensation* (feeling pain and other sensations such as tingling or itching in all or part of an amputated limb). The onset of these sensations is generally within the first week but may occur several months or years after the amputation. One possible explanation of this phenomenon is that a neuroma (tumor found in nervous tissue) forms on the severed nerve ends of the amputated limb. Another theory states that abnormal sensory input along the afferent nerve in the amputated area enters the higher centers of the brain, resulting in unusual or uncomfortable sensations. Another postulation is that nerves in the central nervous system still send out signals along the length of the missing limb.

Massage Consideration/s—Once the client gives permission for massage of the amputation, the massage therapist needs information regarding the actual surgical procedure. For instance, if a mid-humeral amputation has a smooth stump with no protruding bone, knowing whether triceps brachii or biceps brachii was used to wrap the stump end (Figure 4-15) will help the therapist locate trigger points in the affected muscles. While massaging the stump, the massage therapist needs to ask the client if the area is sensitive or numb. Light percussion, towel friction, or mechanical vibration can desensitize any sensitive areas. Many practitioners of energy work, such as polarity and Reiki, treat the energy field of the missing limb as if it were still present.

Clients with leg amputations may walk using leg prosthetics, and at other times be on crutches or in a wheelchair. Some clients may not want to remove the prosthetic because of the time it takes to reattach it, whereas others are glad to be free of prosthesis for a while. The massage therapist needs to watch out for chafing or friction wounds where the prosthetic limb fits to the stump. Any inflamed areas, broken skin, or open wounds need to be avoided.

Ankylosing Spondylitis (ang`·ki·loh´·sing spawn`·duh·lai´·tis)

Gr. Stiff; Joint; Vertebrae; Inflammation

Description—Ankylosing spondylitis is an inflammatory disease leading to calcification and fusion of the joints between vertebrae or in the sacroiliac joint. It is more common in men between 20 and 40 years old. There is pain and stiffness in the hips and lower back that can progress upward along the spine. Inflammation can lead to loss of movement of the joints (ankylosis) and kyphosis (hunchback) (Figure 4-16). When the joints between the thoracic vertebrae and the ribs

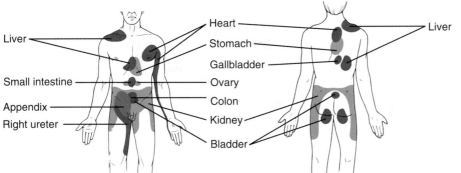

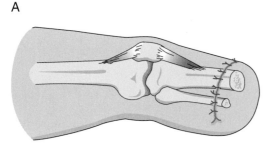

Figure 4-14. Referred pain patterns of miscellaneous organs.

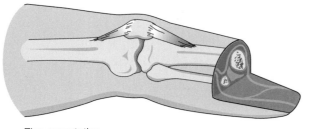

Flap amputation

A

Secured flap amputation

B

Figure 4-15. Amputation. **A,** Skin flap with attached muscle. **B,** Secured flap.

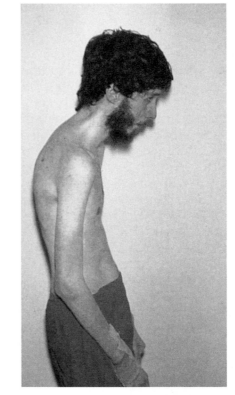

Figure 4-16. Typical posture of individual with ankylosing spondylitis.

are involved, the client may have difficulty in expanding the rib cage for inhalation.

Massage Consideration/s—The massage therapist needs to ask the client which positions are most comfortable so the client can be positioned properly. Clients who have kyphosis may need extra cushioning in the neck region while lying supine or in the side-lying position. The focus of massage treatments should be to retain joint mobility, strengthen weak muscles, and stretch tight ones. Kneading techniques, stretches, and joint mobilizations, all done within the client's tolerance, can help with these goals. Ankylosed joints should not be forced into movement. The back and limbs should be massaged gently. Heat packs will help ease pain. Breathing exercises may help mobilize the thorax. It

is important for the massage therapist to keep in open communication with the client regarding the pressure and effectiveness of techniques.

Anterior Compartment Syndrome

L. Front; To Share; Gr. Together Course

Description—Tibialis anterior, extensor hallicis longus, extensor digitorum longus, peroneus longus, as well as the peroneal nerve and blood vessels lie in the anterior compartment of the lower leg (Figure 4-17). Symptoms of anterior com-

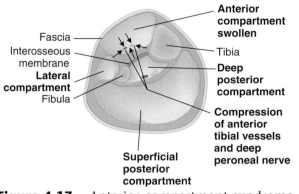

Figure 4-17. Anterior compartment syndrome.

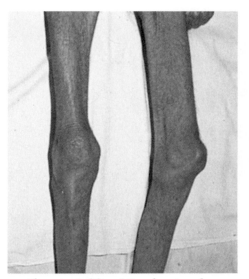

Figure 4-18. Muscle atrophy.

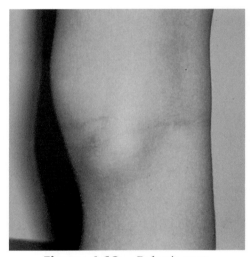

Figure 4-19. Baker's cyst.

partment syndrome include pain and tenderness of these muscles, numbness, tingling, and edema. These symptoms develop slowly and progress steadily. The cause is overuse and repetitive stress of the anterior compartment muscles. Shin splints, if they are not addressed, can be a precursor to anterior compartment syndrome (see Shin Splints).

Massage Consideration/s—The massage therapist needs to ask the client how severe the symptoms are. If the client reports intense, stabbing pain, medical attention is needed before the massage. If the client reports more of a dull, aching pain, the limb should be elevated to assist the movement of venous blood flow and lymph out of the area. Gliding strokes and kneading of the upper and lower leg are helpful. Heat and friction may help to loosen up the fascia and relax tight muscles. If the area is hypersensitive, only moderate to light gliding strokes should be used. Ice application should end the treatment, and the client can use ice at home to control inflammation and pain.

Arthritis (See entries of osteoarthritis, juvenile rheumatoid arthritis, rheumatoid arthritis, gouty arthritis, and Lyme Disease)

Atrophy

Gr. Without; To Grow

Description—Atrophy is a decrease in the size of muscle fibers; a wasting away of muscles as a result of poor nutrition, lack of use, motor unit dysfunction, or lack of motor nerve impulses (Figure 4-18).

Massage Consideration/s—Massage strokes should be slow, superficial, and soothing, with intermittent use of manual vibration and cross-fiber hacking percussion. The massage therapist needs to

communicate with the client about the pressure and effectiveness of techniques.

Baker's Cyst

William Baker; British Surgeon; 1839-1896

Description—A Baker's cyst is a cyst behind the knee caused by escape of synovial fluid that becomes enclosed in a membranous sac. It may appear only when the knee is extended (Figure 4-19).

Massage Consideration/s—Local massage is contraindicated because over the area may be painful, or the pressure of massage may injure the site.

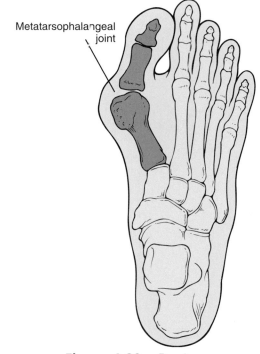

Metatarsophalangeal joint

Figure 4-20. Bunion.

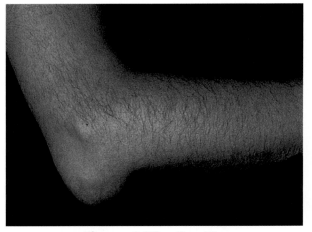

Figure 4-21. Bursitis.

Bunion (Hallux Valgus) (ha´·luhks val´·guhs)

Gr. Turnip

Description—Bunions are an abnormal enlargement of the joint of the great toe. Bunions are characterized by pain, swelling, thickening of skin, and medial displacement of the big toe. However, bunions can also be found on the lateral side of the foot. They are caused by chronic irritation and pressure from poorly fitting shoes (Figure 4-20).

Massage Consideration/s—The massage therapist needs to ask the client how sensitive the area is. If it is not sensitive, light gliding strokes can be done over the area. If the area is painful and/or inflamed, local massage is contraindicated because of the pain and because massage will worsen the inflammation.

Bursitis

L. Little Sac; Gr. Inflammation

Description—Acute or chronic inflammation of the bursae is called bursitis. It can be caused by arthritis, infection, injury, tremendous strain, or trauma. There is severe pain with movement of the affected joint. In acute bursitis, the damage is recent and is accompanied by pain and inflammation. Chronic bursitis is also accompanied by pain, and there may be calcium deposits that need to be removed surgically (Figure 4-21). The

most common types of bursitis are subacromial bursitis (Figure 4-22), subcoracoid bursitis, subscapular bursitis, olecranon bursitis (Figure 4-23), ischial bursitis (Figure 4-24), trochanteric bursitis (Figure 4-25), prepatellar bursitis (Figure 4-26), and calcaneal bursitis (Figure 4-27).

Massage Consideration/s—In the acute stage, local massage is contraindicated until swelling has subsided. Cold packs can be applied to reduce swelling. In chronic bursitis, the massage therapist needs to assess the client for joint mobility and amount of pain with movement. If the client is pain-free, joint mobilizations and stretches can be done to maintain mobility of the joint. Friction can also be done, with ice packs applied afterward. The client can use ice at home to control inflammation and pain.

Chondromalacia Patellae (Patellofemoral Syndrome) (kawn`·droh`·muh·lay´·shee·uh puh·te´·lay)

Gr. Cartilage; Softness

Description—Chondromalacia patellae is a softening of the articular cartilage, most frequently on the posterior patella. This may occur after knee injury, and is characterized by pain and crepitus, particularly in knee flexion, along with swelling and joint degeneration changes.

Massage Consideration/s—If the knee is inflamed and painful, local massage is contraindicated. Otherwise, massage is fine, especially on the quadriceps femoris group as the patella is embedded in the tendons. Effective techniques include kneading, deep friction, myofascial release techniques, and ischemic compression on trigger points. The massage therapist needs to communicate with the client about the pressure and effectiveness of techniques.

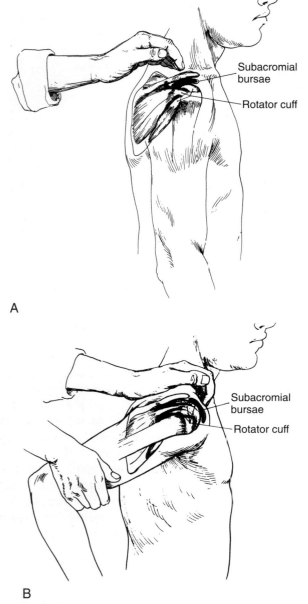

A

B

Figure 4-22. Subacromial bursae. **A,** Location of subacromial bursae. **B,** Palpation of subacromial bursae.

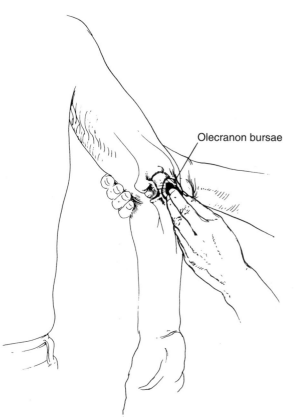

Figure 4-23. Palpation of olecranon bursae.

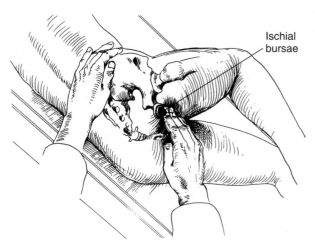

Figure 4-24. Palpation of ischial bursae.

Clubfoot

Nonapplicable

Description—A clubfoot is a congenital deformity of the foot, which is twisted out of shape or position resulting from variances in the metatarsals (Figure 4-28). Ninety-five percent of clubfoot deformities are medial deviations accompanied by plantar flexion; the rest are lateral deviations accompanied by dorsiflexion (either outward from or inward toward the midline of the body).

Massage Consideration/s—Light pressure, using gliding strokes and possibly kneading, over the affected area is indicated.

Contracture

L. A Pulling Together

Description—Contracture is an abnormal, usually permanent, condition of a joint in which the muscle is a flexed and fixated posi-

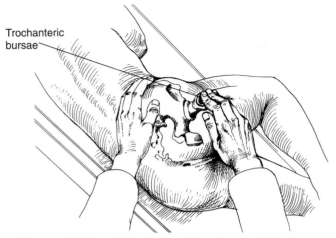

Figure 4-25. Palpation of trochanteric bursae.

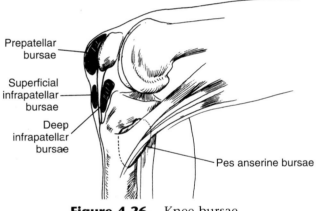

Figure 4-26. Knee bursae.

tion (Figure 4-29). It may be the result of spasm, paralysis, or formation of fibrotic tissue surrounding a joint. A contracture can also be brought on by medication.

Massage Consideration/s—It is important for the massage therapist to ask about the quality of pain the client is experiencing. The massage therapist also needs to communicate with the client about the pressure and effectiveness of techniques. Broad strokes to increase blood flow in the affected area can be used. Friction can be used to reduce adhesions. The muscles should be kneaded thoroughly to stretch the fascia. Myofascial release techniques are helpful. Slow and gentle stretches may help elongate the muscles. The client can use ice at home to control inflammation and pain.

Dupuytren's Contracture (doo´·pyuh·trenz` kuhn·trak´·chuhr)

Baron Guillaume Dupuytren; French Surgeon; 1777-1835

Description—Fibrosis of the palmar fascia, resulting in a shortening and thickening of the palm that produces a flexion deformity of a finger, is Dupuytren's contracture (Figure 4-30). This type of contracture may be used to refer to flexion deformity of a toe caused by involvement of the plantar fascia.

Massage Consideration/s—Deep moist heat may help soften the fascia. Broad strokes help increase circulation to the forearm muscles. The palms can be kneaded, and gentle tractioning and joint mobilizations can be applied to the fingers

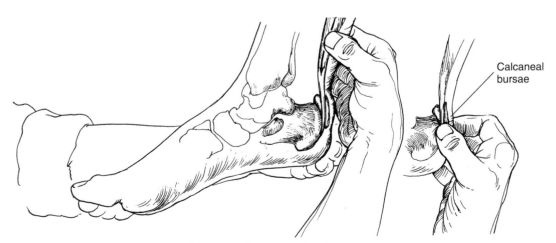

Figure 4-27. Palpation of calcaneal bursae.

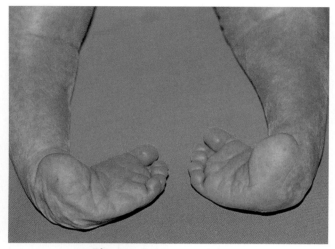

Figure 4-28.   Clubfoot.

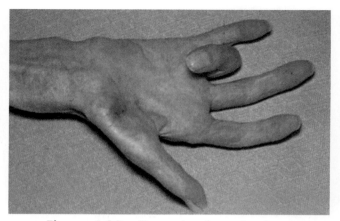

Figure 4-30.   Dupuytren's contracture.

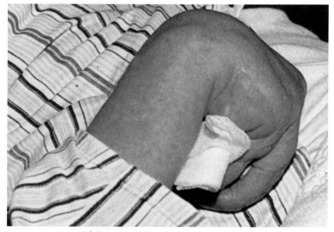

Figure 4-29.   Contracture.

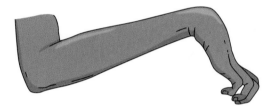

Figure 4-31.   Volkmann's (ischemic) contracture.

and wrist, all within the client's tolerance. If the foot is involved, apply the same massage consideration to the lower leg musculature, toes, feet, and ankle.

Volkmann's Contracture (Ischemic Contracture) (vohlk´·muhnz` kuhn·trak´·chuhr)

Richard Von Volkmann; German Surgeon; 1830-1889

Description—Volkmann's contracture refers to contracture of the fingers and sometimes the wrist after severe injury (Figure 4-31). This may occur in instances of overexposure to cold, excessive pressure as in a tight bandage, or improper use of a tourniquet, which interferes with the muscle's blood supply.

Massage Consideration/s—Same as for Dupuytren's contracture.

Cubital Tunnel Syndrome

L. Elbow; Gr. Channel; Together Course

Description—Cubital tunnel syndrome is a stretching or compression of the ulnar nerve resulting from overuse of the elbow, prolonged elbow flexion, or adhesions. Symptoms include pain, and/or paresthesia (numbness, tingling or "pins and needles" sensation) in the medial side of the hand and fingers. This syndrome is common in people who chronically lean on their elbows, perform manual labor, or play sports that involve throwing.

Massage Consideration/s—If the area is inflamed, local massage is contraindicated because massage will only worsen the inflammation. If inflammation is not present, massage techniques such as gliding strokes and kneading can be used on the forearm muscles and muscles in the palm of the hand, within the client's tolerance. Gentle stretching of the anterior and posterior forearm muscles to maintain flexibility is also helpful.

de Quervain's Tendonitis (de Quervain's Disease) (duh·kwer´·vaynz ten`·duh·nai´·tis)

Fritz de Quervain; Swiss surgeon; 1868-1940

Description—de Quervain's tendonitis is a type of tendonitis resulting from narrowing of the tendon sheath surrounding abductor pollicis longus and extensor pollicis brevis.

Massage Consideration/s—If the area is inflamed, local massage is contraindicated because massage will only worsen the inflammation. Otherwise, massage can loosen the affected muscles. Good techniques to use include gliding strokes, kneading, and gentle stretching. The massage therapist needs to communicate with the client about the pressure and effectiveness of techniques.

Dislocation

L. Apart; To Place

Description—A dislocation (luxation) occurs when bones are forced out of their normal position in the joint cavity (Figure 4-32). Associated ligaments, tendons, articular capsules, and blood vessels are torn in the process. An incomplete or partial dislocation is known as a subluxation.

Massage Consideration/s—Local massage, especially joint mobilizations, is contraindicated for recent dislocations because massage will only worsen the inflammation. However, once the inflammation is gone and the healing is complete, deep specific friction and cross-fiber friction can help increase mobility of the joint. Dislocations often leave the affected joint with permanent laxity, so avoid traction and joint mobilizations of the area.

Fibromyalgia (Myofascial Fibrocystitis, Fibrositis, Muscular Rheumatism)

L. Fiber; Gr. Muscle; Pain

Description—Fibromyalgia is a chronic inflammatory disease that affects muscle and related connective tissues. Pain, joint stiffness, and the presence of tender points or trigger points are involved in this condition (Figure 4-33). During diagnosis, the health care provider evaluates 18 tender points on the body; if 11 of these 18 points are painful, the diagnosis of fibromyalgia is often made. This condition frequently develops after emotional trauma (client may not have dealt with an emotional situation and it manifests as physical pain), local or general infections, or even changes in climate. The symptoms vary from individual to individual and may range from pain, insomnia, headaches, depression, gastrointestinal tract and urinary system disturbances, to lethargy. Fibromyalgia may go into remission, only to flare up at a later date, or it may not flare up at all.

Massage Consideration/s—Massage is currently the best treatment for this condition. Massage should be tailored to how the client is feeling at the time of the treatment because symptoms vary from day to day. The massage therapist needs to ask the client to assess the symptoms each time he or she comes in for a massage therapy treatment. Some clients want deep pressure and others can withstand only light pressure.

Flaccid (fla´·sid)

L. Flabby

Description—Flaccid muscles are lacking normal tone. They are loose and flattened rather than rounded. Flaccidity is often considered the first stage of muscular atrophy. Muscles will become flaccid if they are not used and exercised regularly.

Massage Consideration/s—Friction and kneading techniques may help increase muscle tone, along with intermittent use of manual vibration and cross-fiber hacking percussion. Flushing gliding strokes will increase blood flow and assist in the removal of metabolic wastes.

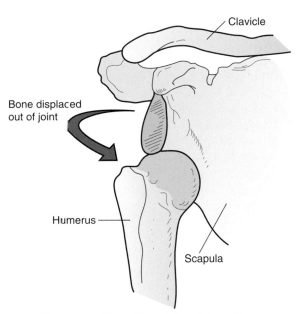

Clavicle

Bone displaced out of joint

Humerus

Scapula

Figure 4-32. Shoulder dislocation.

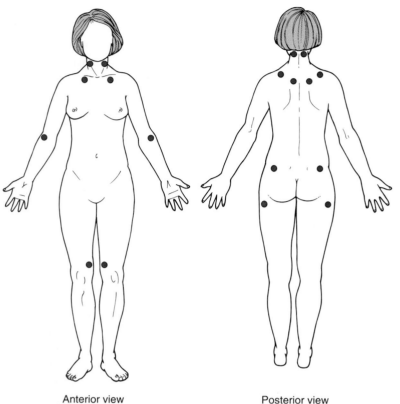

Anterior view   Posterior view

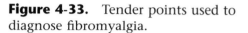

Figure 4-33. Tender points used to diagnose fibromyalgia.

Fractures

L. To Break

Description—A fracture is a break, chip, crack, or rupture in a bone. Osseous tissue is highly vascularized, but healing sometimes takes months because calcium and phosphorus are deposited slowly in new bone. The three most common types of fractures are *simple fractures*, *open fractures*, and *stress fractures*. Simple fractures, also known as closed fractures, occurs when the bone is broken, but does not protrude through the skin. Open fractures, also known as compound fractures, occurs when the broken end of the bone breaks through the skin and soft tissue. Stress fractures are accumulated microfractures (small cracks in a bone). Stress fractures are often a result of repeated activity such as running on a hard surface or high-impact aerobic dance. A common place for stress fractures is the metatarsal bones (Figure 4-34).

Massage Consideration/s—While a bone is immobilized, the fractured area is a local contraindication, but massage proximal and distal to the fracture can help maintain circulation and muscle tone and can reduce edema. The massage therapist should elevate the affected limb to help with drainage. Massaging muscles close to the immobilized part can decrease spasms and reduce pain. A full-body massage can help reduce the client's stress. The massage ther-

apist needs to communicate with the client about the pressure and effectiveness of techniques. Once healing is complete and bone union has occurred, as determined by the client's health care provider, massage, stretching, and joint mobilizations can help the client regain joint mobility and increase tone in muscles that have atrophied. Massage should begin slowly and gently, about a week after the cast has been removed. The massage therapist should gradually increase massage pressure to the client's tolerance.

Ganglion Cyst

Gr. Knot

Description—A ganglion cyst is a benign tumor occurring on a flat tendon (aponeurosis) or on a cordlike tendon, as in the wrist or dorsum of the foot; it consists of a thin fibrous capsule enclosing a clear fluid (Figure 4-35).

Massage Consideration/s—Local massage is contraindicated because pressure from the massage over the area can be painful, and/or it may damage the tissue.

Gouty Arthritis (Gout)

L. Drop

Description—Gout is characterized by an abnormal accumulation of uric acid in the body. Uric acid is produced when nucleic acids

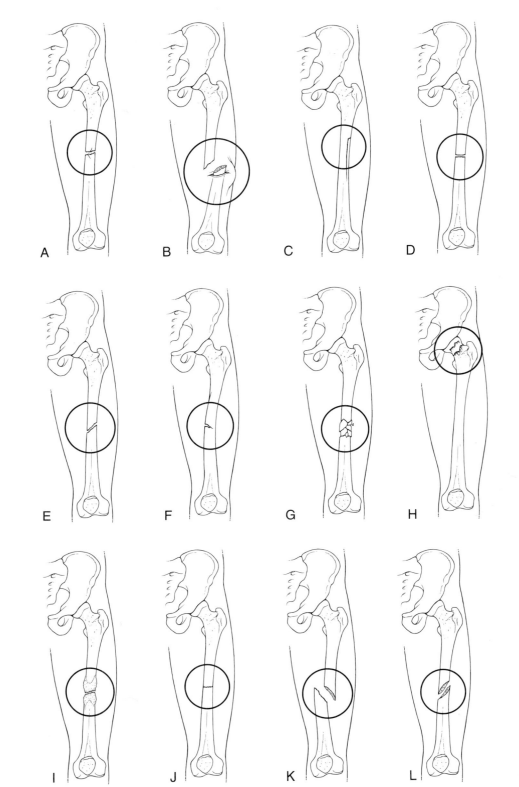

Figure 4-34. Fracture types. **A,** Closed, or simple. The overlying skin is intact. **B,** Open, or compound. The skin overlying the bone ends is not intact. **C,** Longitudinal. The fracture extends along the length of the bone. **D,** Transverse. The fracture is at right angles to the axis of the bone. **E,** Oblique. The fracture extends in an oblique direction. **F,** Greenstick. The fracture is on one side of the bone; the other side is bent. **G,** Comminuted. The bone is splintered or crushed. **H,** Impacted. The fractured ends of the bone are driven into each other. **I,** Pathological. The fracture results from weakening of the bone by disease. **J,** Nondisplaced. The bone ends remain in alignment. **K,** Displaced. The bone ends are out of alignment. **L,** Spiral. The fracture results from a twisting mechanism, causing the break to wind around the bone in a spiral.

Continued

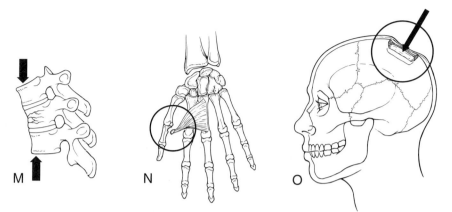

M

N

O

Figure 4-34,   cont'd. M, Compression. Excessive pressure causes the bone to collapse. **N,** Avulsion. Tearing away of a muscle or a ligament is accompanied by tearing away of a bone fragment. **O,** Depression. Bone fragments of the skull are driven inward.

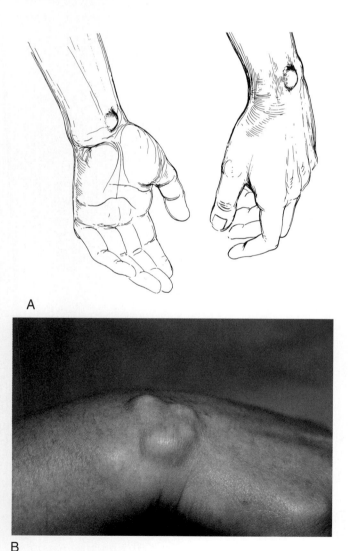

A

B

Figure 4-35.   Ganglion cyst on wrist.

are metabolized; the uric acid is then converted to monosodium urate crystals. In most cases, uric acid is eliminated in the urine. Some individuals, usually males, either produce excessive amounts or are unable to excrete uric acid, resulting in abnormally high levels of uric acid in the bloodstream. The sodium urate crystals eventually settle in soft tissue around the joints, typically the feet and toes, but the hands may be involved as well. Typically, the first joint affected is the metatarsophalangeal joint of the great toe. Initial bouts may last just a few days; later bouts may last several weeks (Figures 4-36 and 4-37).

Massage Consideration/s—Local massage is contraindicated because of the pain and inflammation. Massage will only make the pain and inflammation worse.

Hammertoe

Nonapplicable

Description—A hammertoe is a condition in which the proximal phalanx of a toe (most commonly the second toe) is extended and the second and distal phalanges are flexed, causing a clawlike appearance (Figure 4-38).

Massage Consideration/s—Gentle massage, using gliding strokes, over the affected area is indicated to help loosen the tissue. The massage therapist needs to communicate with the client about the pressure.

Headaches (Cephalalgia, Cephalgia)

(se·fuh·lal´·jee·uh) (suh·fal´·jee·uh)

Nonapplicable

Description—Headaches are a pain in the head from any cause. Types of headaches are muscular contraction or tension headaches, cluster headaches, and migraine headaches (Figure 4-39). Migraine headaches and cluster headaches are addressed in Chapter 7.

Massage Consideration/s—The massage therapist needs to ask the client the cause of the headaches, as well as their frequency and duration.

If headaches are caused by a condition that is a massage contraindication, massage is contraindicated for these headaches as well. For severe, frequent, and/or long-term headaches, the massage therapist needs to refer the client to his or her health care provider for evaluation. For headaches caused by muscular contraction or tension, the goals of massage are to relax the neck, shoulder, and back muscles involved and to relieve the pressure on the nerves and blood vessels. Muscles to address are trapezius, levator scapulae, splenius capitis and cervicis, suboccipitals, scalenes, and sternocleidomastoid. Moist heat may help to loosen the myofascial component before massage. The massage therapist can then use techniques such as deep gliding strokes, kneading, deep friction, and gentle stretches. The massage therapist needs to communicate with the client about pressure.

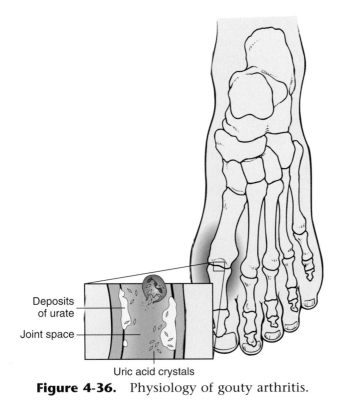
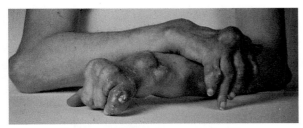
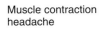

Deposits of urate

Joint space

Uric acid crystals

Figure 4-36. Physiology of gouty arthritis.

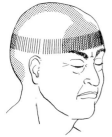

Figure 4-37. Gouty arthritis.

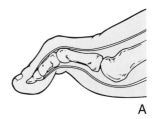

A

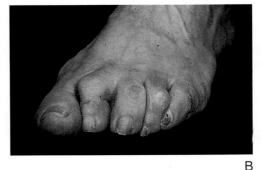

B

Figure 4-38. **A,** Skeletal structure of a hammertoe. **B,** Photograph of a hammertoe.

Muscle contraction headache

Cluster headache

Migraine headache

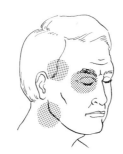
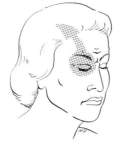

Figure 4-39. Types of headaches and associated pain patterns.

Herniated Disk (Ruptured Disk, Slipped Disk)

L. Rupture; Gr. Flat Plate

Description—Protrusion of the nucleus pulposus from the annulus fibrosus of an intervertebral disk is called a herniated disk (Figure 4-40). The protruding disk may impinge on nerve roots, causing numbness and pain. This may be a result of improper lifting or direct trauma.

Massage Consideration/s—Because there are many causes that contribute to a herniated disk, it is important for the massage therapist to get clearance from the client's health care provider and proceed with massage only if it is safe to do so. Massage does little for a herniated disk, and massage in the area of the disk is contraindicated. It can relieve pain from the muscles splinting around the area (which functions to limit movement). Muscles to treat are the iliopsoas, erector spinae, transversospinalis, and quadratus lumborum. Heat can be used for its analgesic affect, as long as the massage therapist follows its use with application of ice for 20 minutes. Traction or mobilization of the involved area should be avoided. The client can use ice at home to control inflammation and pain.

Juvenile Rheumatoid Arthritis (Still's Disease)

L. Young; Gr. Discharge; Shape; Gr. Joint; Inflammation

Description—Juvenile rheumatoid arthritis is a type of rheumatoid arthritis usually affecting the larger joints of children less than 16 years old (Figure 4-41). Because growth in children is dependent on the epiphyseal plates, bone growth and development may be impaired if these structures are affected (Figure 4-42).

Massage Consideration/s—See entry for rheumatoid arthritis in this chapter.

Kyphosis (Humpback, Hunchback, Hyperkyphosis) (kai·foh´·sis)

Gr. Humpback; Condition

Description—Kyphosis is an exaggeration of the normal posterior thoracic curve (Figure 4-43). Typically, the chest appears caved in, the arms tend to hang in the front of the body, and the head moves forward. Kyphosis may be caused by rickets (resulting from vitamin D deficiency), degeneration of the intervertebral disks as can happen in older adults, osteoporosis, or chronic spasticity of the pectoralis major and minor, and serratus anterior muscles, or weak rhomboid major and minor muscles. Mild to moderate back pain often accompanies this spinal condition. Rounded shoulders and a dowager's hump are occasionally classified as a mild form of kyphosis.

Massage Consideration/s—Position the client for comfort. Some relief can be gained by massage of the involved muscles (pectoralis major/minor, serratus anterior, rhomboids major/minor) using

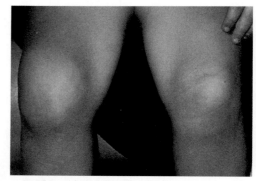

Figure 4-41.   Juvenile rheumatoid arthritis (knee).

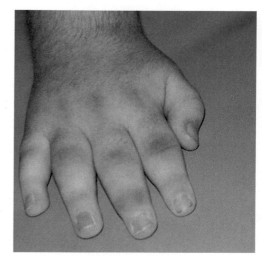

Figure 4-42.   Juvenile rheumatoid arthritis (hand).

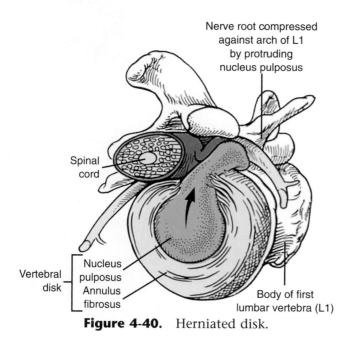

Figure 4-40.   Herniated disk.

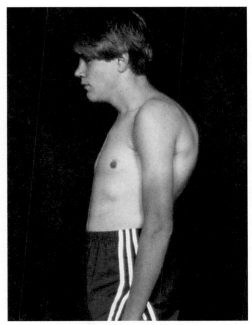

Figure 4-43. Kyphosis.

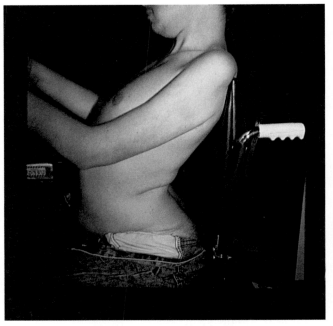

Figure 4-44. Lordosis.

techniques such as deep gliding strokes, kneading, and deep friction. The massage therapist should take care not to overstretch the spine. If the cause is osteoporosis, a lighter massage is indicated.

Lordosis (Swayback, Hyperlordosis)
(lohr·doh´·sis)

Gr. Bent Forward; Condition

Description—Lordosis is an exaggeration of the anterior curvature of the lumbar concavity (Figure 4-44). A tightening of the back and hip muscles (such as the iliopsoas), followed by a weakening of the abdominal muscles, is typical. Increased weight gain or pregnancy may cause or exacerbate this spinal condition. Because of the anterior tilt of the pelvis, hamstring problems are common.

Massage Consideration/s—Position the client for comfort. The massage therapist needs to treat the muscles of both anterior and posterior pelvic tilt. These include the abdominal muscles, quadratus lumborum, psoas major, and erector spinae. Techniques such as deep gliding strokes, kneading, deep friction, and myofascial release techniques can be helpful. The massage therapist can remind the client to strengthen the abdominal muscles and not to gain excess weight.

Lyme Disease (Lyme Arthritis)

Named after the community of Lyme, Connecticut

Description—Lyme disease is a recurrent form of arthritis caused by the bacterium *Borrelia burgdorferi*, which is transmitted by a tick

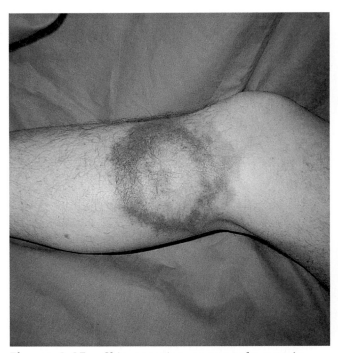

Figure 4-45. Skin eruption commonly seen in Lyme disease.

bite. The condition was originally described in the community of Lyme, Connecticut, but has been reported throughout North America and in other countries. Large joints, such as the knee and hip, are most commonly involved, with local inflammation and swelling. Headaches, fever, and a scaly red skin eruption (erythema) (Figure 4-45) often precede the joint manifestations (Figure 4-46).

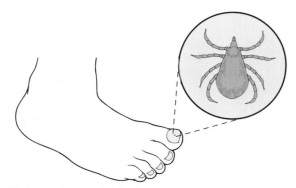

Figure 4-46. Tick that causes Lyme disease.

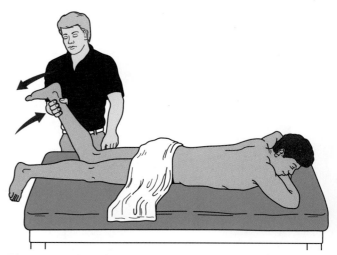

Figure 4-47. Reciprocal inhibition. The therapist is resisting knee extension.

Massage Consideration/s—Because the disease is chronic (lasting months or years), the massage needs to be tailored to the client's individual symptoms. The massage therapist should inquire about client symptoms before each massage treatment. Massage is contraindicated if the client is experiencing widespread inflammation. Generally, a gentle, full-body massage is indicated. Passive stretching and joint mobilizations, within the client's tolerance, will retain joint mobility.

Muscle Spasm (Muscle Cramp)

L. Mouse; Gr. Convulsion

Description—An increase in muscle tension with or without shortening, resulting from excessive motor nerve activity, may result in a rigid zone (i.e., knot) in the muscle called a spasm. Muscle spasms cannot be alleviated by voluntary relaxation. Cramping is often associated with mineral deficiency or muscle fatigue and is usually short lived.

Massage Consideration/s—The massage therapist needs to ask the client the cause of the muscle spasm to help determine all of the muscles involved. Massage can increase local circulation to a muscle spasm/cramp and mechanically lengthen and spread muscle fibers apart. If the muscle spasm is acute, reciprocal inhibition techniques can be used. The massage therapist needs to communicate with the client about the pressure and effectiveness of techniques (Figure 4-47).

Muscular Dystrophy

L. Mouse; Gr. Bad; Nourishment

Description—A collection of genetic diseases, muscular dystrophy is characterized by the progressive atrophy of skeletal muscles without any indication of neural degeneration or damage (Figure 4-48). All forms of muscular dystrophy involve a loss of muscular strength, disability, and deformity.

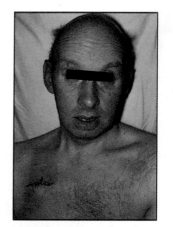

Figure 4-48. Muscular dystrophy.

Massage Consideration/s—Massage may slow muscular atrophy. The massage therapist can use massage techniques such as gliding strokes, kneading, and superficial warming friction to increase blood flow. Vibration and percussion will activate muscle spindles in weak muscles (if they are functional). Active and passive stretching and joint mobilizations may be helpful. This disorder also affects involuntary muscles, including those of the large intestine. Abdominal massage may help with resulting constipation.

Osgood-Schlatter Disease (Osteochondrosis)

(ahz´·guud-shla´·ter duh·zez´)
(ahs`·tee·oh·kuhn·droh´·sis)

Robert B. Osgood; US Physician; 1873-1956
Carl Schlatter; Swiss Surgeon; 1864-1934

Description—Osgood-Schlatter disease results from overuse of the quadriceps muscle (knee extension). The anterior knee region becomes irritated and inflamed; the tibial tuberosity may even become partially separated (Figure 4-49). This condition is seen primarily in muscular, athletic adolescents and is marked by swelling and tenderness over the tibial tuberosity that increases with any activity that extends the knee.

Massage Consideration/s—Local massage is contraindicated during the acute phase because massage would only worsen the pain and inflammation. Once the inflammation has abated, friction around the knee can reduce adhesions. Deep gliding strokes, kneading, and friction can be used to reduce tension in the quadriceps.

Osteoarthritis (OA, Degenerative Joint Disease, DJD) (aws´·tee·oh·ahr·thrai´·tuhs)

Gr. Bone; Joint; Inflammation

Description—Osteoarthritis is a chronic, progressive erosion of the articular cartilage resulting from chronic inflammation. Often called "wear and tear" arthritis, the most common affected areas are weight–bearing joints, which may eventually become immovable. OA, which is more frequently seen than rheumatoid arthritis, is most common in the older population (Figures 4-50 through 4-52).

Massage Consideration/s—Deep pressure massage, stretching, and joint mobilizations are contraindicated because these movements may injure the client. The massage therapist needs to ask the client about depth of pressure at the site of the arthritis. Techniques that can be helpful are gliding strokes, light kneading, light vibration, and superficial warming friction, within the client's tolerance, which can warm and loosen surrounding tissues.

Osteomyelitis (ahs`·tee·oh·mai·lai´·tis)

L. Bone; Marrow; Inflammation

Description—Inflammation of the bone is called osteomyelitis. It is caused by infection (usually staphylococci) that can remain localized or spread throughout the bone involving the marrow and periosteum. The infection can be introduced by trauma, surgery, a nearby infection, or through the bloodstream (Figure 4-53).

Massage Consideration/s—In clients with infectious wounds, local massage is contraindicated because massage can spread the infection, cause pain, and further damage the tissues. In clients who have well-healed wounds, massage may help increase strength of the muscles surrounding the

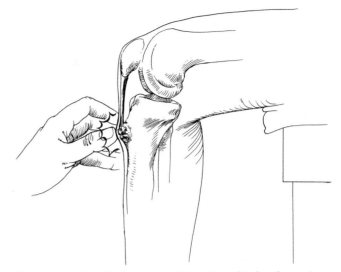

Figure 4-49. Palpation of tender tibial tuberosity seen in Osgood-Schlatter disease.

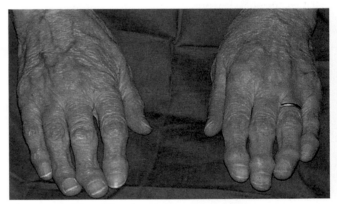

Figure 4-50. Hands with osteoarthritic involvement.

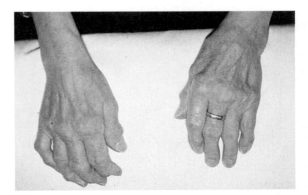

Figure 4-51. Hands with advanced osteoarthritis.

affected area and improve joint range of motion. Good techniques to use include gliding strokes, kneading, joint mobilizations, and gentle stretches. The massage therapist needs to communicate with the client about the pressure and effectiveness of techniques.

Osteoporosis

Gr. Bone; Passage; Condition

Description—Osteoporosis is characterized by decreased bone mass and increased susceptibility to fractures; 80% of people with osteo-

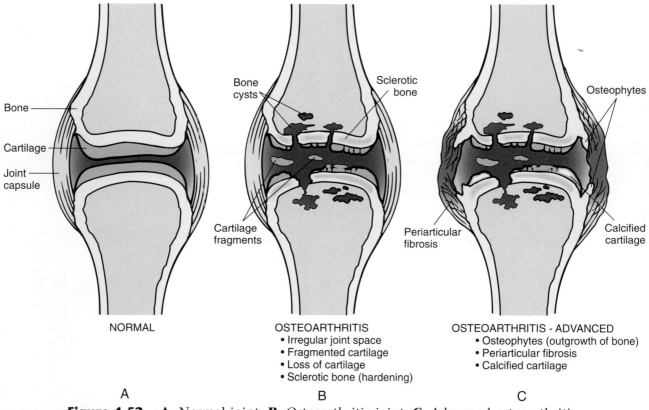

Figure 4-52. **A,** Normal joint. **B,** Osteoarthritic joint. **C,** Advanced osteoarthritis.

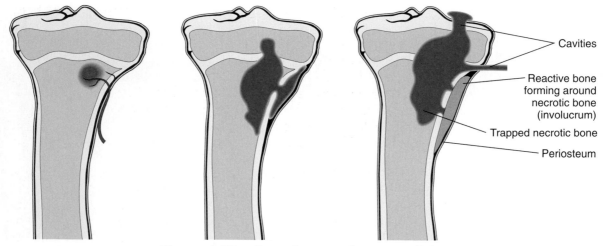

Figure 4-53. Bone damage of osteomyelitis.

porosis are women. As women age, they produce much smaller amounts of estrogen. The decreased estrogen levels result in less calcium being deposited in bones; this causes a decrease in bone mass. Parathyroid production from the parathyroid glands may also decrease. Bone mass may become so depleted that the skeleton can no longer withstand mechanical stress. Osteoporosis is responsible for hip and other fractures, shrinkage of the backbone, height loss, age-related kyphosis, and considerable pain (Figure 4-54).

Massage Consideration/s—Gentle massage, while avoiding undue pressure over bones, is indicated. The massage therapist needs to communicate with the client about pressure tolerance. Joint mobilizations should be limited or avoided.

Paget's Disease (Osteitis Deformans)
(ays`·tee·ai´·tis duh·fohr´·muhnz)

Sir James Paget; British Surgeon; 1814-1899

Description—Paget's disease is a bone disease marked by repeated episodes of bone destruction followed by excessive or unorganized attempts at bone repair. These cycles result in weakened deformed bones of increased mass. Individuals living with this disease tend to be middle-aged and older people. Individuals with this disease experience pain, leg deformity (bowlegged), deafness, and kyphosis (Figures 4-55 and 4-56).

Massage Consideration/s—A gentle, relaxing massage is indicated. The massage therapist needs to communicate with the client about pressure tolerance. Gentle gliding strokes would be the most effective techniques.

Plantar Fasciitis (Calcaneal Spur)
(plan´·tuhr fa`·shee·ai´·tis)

L. Sole of Foot; Fascia; Gr. Inflammation

Description—Plantar fasciitis is inflammation of the plantar fascia at the calcaneus, medial aspect of the foot, and insertions of tibialis posterior. Symptoms are "pain in the heel" and/or pain on dorsiflexion. Clients will often state that they cannot walk comfortably because of pain when their heels strike the floor. The pain frequently goes away, only to return the next morning. If the condition is prolonged, the client

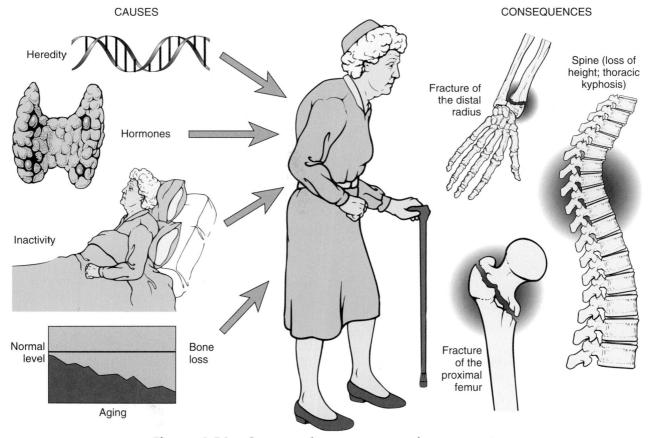

CAUSES

Heredity

Hormones

Inactivity

Normal level

Bone loss

Aging

CONSEQUENCES

Fracture of the distal radius

Spine (loss of height; thoracic kyphosis)

Fracture of the proximal femur

Figure 4-54. Causes and consequences of osteoporosis.

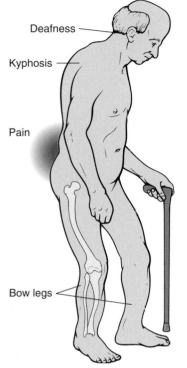

Figure 4-55.   Individual with Paget's disease.

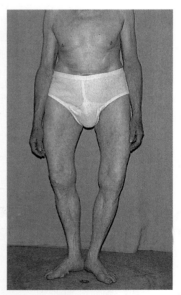

Figure 4-56.   Leg deformity of Paget's disease.

may not be able to withstand pressure applied to the heel (Figure 4-57).

   Massage Consideration/s—Cross-fiber friction on the calcaneus, within the client's tolerance, may reduce adhesions, and muscles of the leg should be massaged thoroughly. The client can use ice at home to control inflammation and pain. The massage therapist can suggest an activity to the

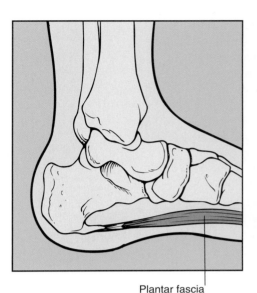

Figure 4-57.   Attachment of plantar fascia on calcaneus.

client that does not involve putting pressure on the heel, such as biking or swimming.

Repetitive Strain Injury (RSI, Repetitive Motion Injury)

Nonapplicable

   Description—Repetitive strain injuries (RSIs) are self-inflicted injuries related to inefficient biomechanics, which include general posture, sporting movements, and work habits. A repetitive or constant motion, combined with compressive forces or joint hyperextension, causes damage to soft tissues. This injury type encompasses a broad spectrum of injuries. The most common types of repetitive motion injuries are carpal tunnel syndrome (see Nervous Pathologies, Chapter 5), thoracic outlet syndrome (see Nervous Pathologies, Chapter 5), tennis elbow (see Tendinitis in this chapter), and rotator cuff problems (see Strain, Tendinitis, and Bursitis in this chapter). The symptoms and damage are progressive, unless the inefficient biomechanics or repetitive strain is altered. General symptoms are related to the inflammation response: pain, redness, heat, swelling, and limited range of motion. The progression of injury typically goes from muscle soreness to increased tonus to the formation of multiple trigger points, and in some cases to nerve entrapment. Chronic RSIs may result in neuropathy, subluxation, deterioration, or trauma to the joints, including bursitis, arthritis, and even stress fractures of involved bones.

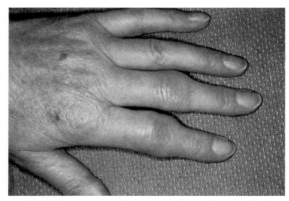

Figure 4-58. Early rheumatoid arthritis of the hands.

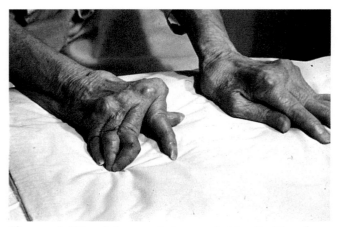

Figure 4-59. Advanced rheumatoid arthritis of the hands.

Massage Consideration/s—Massage considerations are tailored to the type of RSI. The massage therapist needs to ask the client the cause of the RSI. In general, local massage is contraindicated until inflammation is gone because massage will only make the inflammation worse. Afterward, deep pressure massage, broad flat strokes, and friction, within the client's tolerance, on the affected muscles are helpful.

Rheumatoid Arthritis (RA)

Gr. Discharge; Shape; Joint; Inflammation

Description—Rheumatoid arthritis is a systemic arthritis characterized by inflammation that destroys the synovial membranes of joints, especially the hands and feet (Figure 4-58). The membranes are replaced by fibrous tissues that add to the joint stiffness already present. This process greatly reduces the person's range of motion. Usually there is bilateral involvement with a high incidence of crippling deformity (Figure 4-59). The cause of RA is unknown, but it is believed to be an autoimmune disease. Persons who have RA experience flare-ups and remissions (Figures 4-60 and 4-61).

Massage Consideration/s—Massage is contraindicated when a client has a flare-up because massage will only worsen the inflammation. When the client's RA is in remission, massage can be administered safely. Massage can help reduce stress, and gentle stretches and joint mobilizations can help increase joint mobility. The massage therapist needs to communicate with the client about pressure and tolerance of joint mobilizations. If the client is on painkillers and/or antiinflammatory medications that may result in inadequate feedback, a shorter, lighter massage is indicated. See Table 4-2 for more information.

Scoliosis (skoh·lee·oh´·sis)

Gr. Crookedness

Description—Scoliosis is the lateral deviation or curvature in the normally straight vertical line of the vertebral column, usually in the thoracic region (Figure 4-62). Causes of scoliosis include congenital malformations of the spine; poliomyelitis; paralysis; chronic spasticity of the iliopsoas, quadratus lumborum, and the paraspinal muscles; and postural deviations such as poor posture, distorted rib cage, and leg length discrepancy (Figure 4-63). Unequal position of the hips or shoulders may be one indication of this condition. Early detection and intervention may prevent progression of the curvature. The vast majority of people who have scoliosis are female (80%).

Massage Consideration/s—If scoliosis is caused by a condition that is a massage contraindication, massage is contraindicated for this as well. Otherwise, position client for comfort. Treatment should include work on iliopsoas, quadratus lumborum, and the paraspinal muscles. Deep muscle stripping, myofascial release techniques, and gentle stretches are indicated. The spine should not be overstretched. The massage therapist needs to communicate with the client about the pressure and effectiveness of techniques.

Separation

L. To Separate

Description—A separation is almost the same as a dislocation, but the joint structure is simply pulled and stretched, causing a subluxation; the bone is not displaced out of the joint capsule. (See prior entry for dislocation.)

Massage Consideration/s—The massage therapist needs to ask the client how the separation

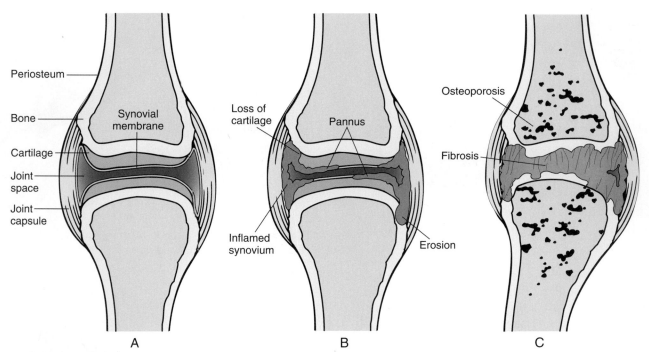

Figure 4-60. **A,** Normal joint. **B,** Rheumatoid arthritic joint. **C,** Advanced rheumatoid arthritis.

occurred, which joint is involved, and what positions on the massage table are comfortable. Afterward, position the client for comfort and use gentle massage around the area, avoiding undue pressure over the separated bones. Massage can facilitate the healing process by increasing local blood flow. Joint mobilizations of the affected joint are contraindicated until the client is completely healed.

Shin Splints

AS. Shin; MD. A Wedge

Description—Shin splints are a strain of either the anterior or posterior tibial muscles marked by pain along the tibia. It is often the result of running or jumping on hard surfaces. During these activities, the tibia and fibula are jarred on top of the talus bone, causing one or both of the tibia and fibula to migrate laterally. This action tears the interosseous membrane between these two lower leg bones as well as the muscles attaching to all three structures (tibia, fibula, and interosseous membrane). Pain is usually referred to the anterior tibialis, located along the lateral edge of the tibia.

Massage Consideration/s—The massage therapist needs to ask the client how recently the pain has been felt and what the quality of the pain is to determine whether the condition is acute. Sharp, stabbing pain indicates acute shin splints; dull, throbbing pain indicates chronic shin splints.

When the condition is acute, RICE (rest, ice, compression, elevation) is helpful, and local massage should be postponed. If the condition is not acute, massage of the tibialis anterior is helpful. Although the tibialis posterior is too deep a muscle to access easily, deep kneading of the calf may bring some pain relief. RICE (rest, ice, compression, elevation) can also be helpful for chronic shin splints, along with wearing proper athletic shoes and performing athletic activity on a yielding surface.

Spasticity

Gr. A Convulsion

Description—Spasticity is characterized by increased muscle tone and stiffness. A spastic muscle resists stretching and typically involves the arm flexors and leg extensors, and effects can range from mild to severe. In severe cases, movement patterns become uncoordinated or impossible and usually involve a neurological dysfunction.

Massage Consideration/s—Clearance from the client's health care provider is recommended if symptoms are severe. The massage therapist needs to use caution during the massage, as sensations may be impaired and the client may not be able to give accurate feedback. Joint mobilizations should be avoided, as they may induce the stretch reflex, causing muscle contraction. Cross-fiber friction can be used around joints to prevent adhesions and

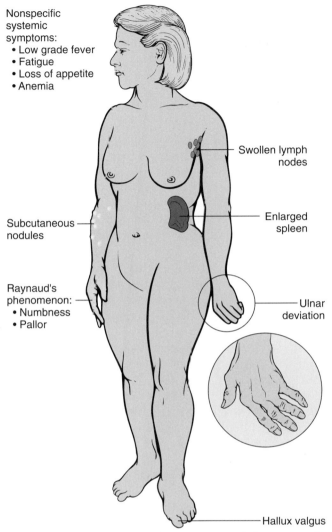

Nonspecific systemic symptoms:
• Low grade fever
• Fatigue
• Loss of appetite
• Anemia

Swollen lymph nodes

Enlarged spleen

Subcutaneous nodules

Raynaud's phenomenon:
• Numbness
• Pallor

Ulnar deviation

Hallux valgus

Figure 4-61. Signs and symptoms of rheumatoid arthritis.

Scoliosis

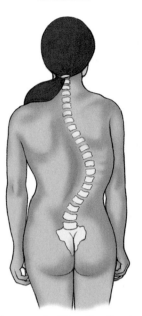

Figure 4-62. Scoliosis.

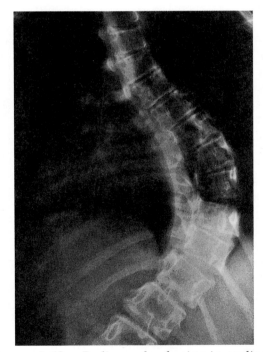

Figure 4-63. Radiograph of spine in scoliosis.

contractures. The massage therapist should concentrate on the spastic muscles as well, using a gentle to moderate pressure. Ongoing massage treatments can be helpful. The massage therapist needs to communicate with the client about the pressure and effectiveness of techniques.

Spondylolisthesis (spahn`·duh·luh·lis´·thuh·sis)

Gr. Vertebra; A Slipping

Description—Spondylolisthesis is an anteriorly displaced vertebra, usually the fifth lumbar vertebra over the first sacral vertebra. This condition can range from mild to severe. Severe cases deform the spine (Figure 4-64).

Massage Consideration/s—The massage therapist needs to ask the client about the severity of the condition. Gliding strokes, using gentle to moder-

ate pressure, can help loosen tight erector spinae muscles and the latissimus dorsi. Tight muscles in the area can be stretched, but should not be forced. The massage therapist needs to communicate with the client about the pressure and effectiveness of techniques.

Spondylosis (spahn·duh·loh´·sis)

Gr. Vertebra; Dissolution

Description—Spondylosis is a general term for degenerative of the spine often resulting from osteoarthritis. It is frequently called arthritis of the spine.

Massage Consideration/s—The massage therapist needs to ask the client about the severity of the condition, and what positions on the massage table are comfortable. Gentle to moderate massage of the back using gliding strokes, avoiding undue pressure over the spine, can be helpful. The massage thera-

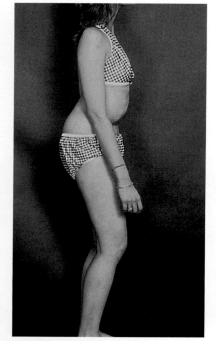

Figure 4-64. Severe spondylolisthesis.

pist needs to communicate with the client about the pressure and effectiveness of techniques.

Sprain

O. Fr. To Wrench

Description—Joint trauma that stretches or tears the ligamentous attachments without bone displacement is called a sprain. Sprains cause pain and possible temporary disability. Depending on the severity of the injury, it is not uncommon for a ligamentous sprain to take 6 months to a year to completely rehabilitate because ligaments have a limited blood supply (Figure 4-65). Acute ligament sprains can be classified into three grades or degrees of severity: first, second, and third degree.

First degree is the stretching of the ligament without tearing. The area has minimal pain and swelling, and there is a risk of re-injury. The joint structures can maintain efficient motion and hold against resistance.

In a second-degree sprain, the ligament partially tears. The joint structures cannot hold against moderate resistance. Edema is typically found and the muscles surrounding the strain or sprain are splinted to restrict painful movement.

In a third-degree sprain, the ligament tears completely, and a "snap" is often heard at the time of injury. A piece of the bone may be torn away as well (avulsion fracture). A depression in the area of the torn muscle can be felt and is usually painful to touch. Function is greatly altered in third-degree tears.

Massage Consideration/s—Massage should not be performed until the client receives medical clearance. The injured area should not be stretched.

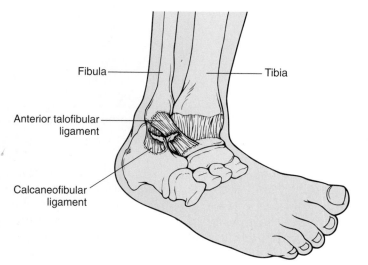

Fibula

Tibia

Anterior talofibular ligament

Calcaneofibular ligament

Figure 4-65. Ankle sprain.

The massage therapist needs to ask the client how the sprain occurred to determine which joint and muscles are involved, and how recent the injury is. Initially, RICE (rest, ice, compression, elevation) can help bring down the swelling. When the inflammation has subsided or 72 hours after the initial injury, whichever comes first, light effleurage and light friction around the area are helpful massage techniques. Cross-fiber friction is an excellent rehabilitation technique. The client can use ice at home to control inflammation and pain.

Strain (Pull)

AS. Offspring

Description—A strain is an injury of a muscle or tendon resulting from a violent contraction, forced stretching, or synergistic failure. Most muscle strains occur on the antagonist, or the muscle that must resist the muscle creating the action. When the antagonist is hypotonus or in spasm, it cannot stretch easily and may become injured. Acute muscle strains can be classified into three grades or degrees of severity: first, second, and third degree (Figure 4-66).

First-degree strains involve stretching of fibers with no palpable defects. There is typically mild pain at the time of injury, and there may be mild swelling and localized tenderness. The joint structures can maintain efficient motion and hold against resistance.

When the muscle or tendon is torn partially, it is classified as a second-degree strain. A palpable defect is noted and the joint structures cannot hold against moderate resistance. Edema is typically

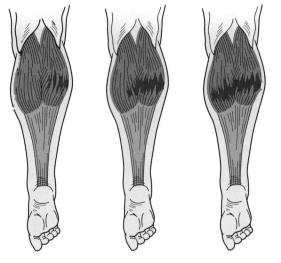

GRADE I   GRADE II   GRADE III

Figure 4-66. Calf pull with degrees of severity.

found, and the muscles surrounding the strain splint to restrict painful movement.

In third-degree tears, the muscle and/or tendon are completely avulsed, and a "snap" is often heard at the time of injury. Third-degree tears may represent a complete rupture of the involved structures. An avulsion fracture occurs when a tendon is pulled away from a bone, taking a bone fragment with it. A depression in the area of the torn muscle can be palpated and is usually painful to touch. Function is greatly altered in third-degree tears.

Massage Consideration/s—Massage should not be performed until the client receives medical clearance. The massage therapist needs to ask the client how the strain occurred, what area of the body is involved, and how recent the injury is. Initially, RICE (rest, ice, compression, elevation) can help reduce the swelling. When the inflammation has subsided or 72 hours after the initial injury, whichever comes first, gliding strokes on muscles around the affected area can reduce muscle spasms. Massage should not be done distal to the injury site, as massage increases local blood flow and may, in fact, make the swelling worse. The massage therapist can move joints passively to maintain range of motion, and must be careful not to stretch the injured area. After the acute stage, cross-fiber friction can prevent adhesion formation. Gentle stretches to realign fibers can also be done. Initially, treatments of shorter duration are indicated and can become longer as injury heals. The client can use ice at home to control inflammation and pain.

Temporomandibular Joint Dysfunction (TMJD)
(tem`·puh·roh·man·di´·byuh·luhr joint´ dis·funk´·shuhn)

L. A period of time; Lower Jawbone; A Joining; Gr. Bad; L. A Performance

Description—TMJD is a common ailment afflicting the jaw joint, its musculature, or both. Its chief symptoms are pain (in the jaws, toothache, headache, and earache), clicking of the joint, and limited range of motion. Causes of TMJD include trauma to the joint, chewing hard objects, especially if only on one side of the mouth, biting fingernails, teeth clenching or grinding (bruxism) whether awake or asleep, poor alignment of the upper and lower teeth, and emotional stress. It is estimated that 60% of the population either clench or grind their teeth, but only 25% of this group is aware of it.

Massage Consideration/s—For TMJD, advanced techniques that require the donning of rubber gloves to intraorally treat some of the jaw musculature can be helpful. The massage therapist can use ischemic compression to address the muscles of the jaw such as masseter, temporalis, medial and lateral pterygoids, and neck and shoulder muscles such as trapezius, rhomboids, levator scapula, scalenes, splenius muscles, and suboccipitals. Because the majority of all TMJD cases are associated with clenching or bruxism, which is often stress related, general massage techniques can also be helpful for stress management.

Tendinitis

Gr. Tendon; Inflammation

Description—Inflammation of the tendon, accompanied by pain and swelling, is called tendinitis. This may be a result of chronic overuse, direct trauma, or even a sudden pull of the muscle. When inflammation also involves the tendon sheath, it is referred to as tendosynovitis.

Massage Consideration/s—The massage therapist needs to ask the client where the tendonitis is occurring and how recent the onset is. If tendinitis is the result of injury, local massage is contraindicated for 72 hours because of the inflammation. Massage will only make it worse. Afterward, massage should include stripping the muscle, cross-fiber friction on the involved tendons, and a 20-minute follow-up period with ice. The client can use ice at home to control inflammation and pain.

Tetanus (Lockjaw)

Gr. Stretched

Description—Tetanus is an acute, often fatal infection of the central nervous system caused by the bacillus *Clostridium tetani*. It is characterized by irritability, headache, fever, and painful spasms of the muscles resulting in lockjaw; eventually, every muscle of the body is in tonic spasm. This bacillus is one of the most lethal poisons known and enters the body through contaminated wounds. *C. tetani* is commonly found in topsoil where barn animals live because *C. tetani* is a normal inhabitant of the intestinal tracts of animals such as cows and horses. Barnyards and fields fertilized with manure are heavily contaminated.

Massage Consideration/s—Massage is contraindicated. This is a life-threatening condition that requires medical attention.

Torticollis (Wryneck) (tohr·tuh·koh´·luhs)

L. Twisted; Neck

Description—Torticollis involves spasms of the sternocleidomastoid (SCM) muscles. The scalenes, trapezius, and the splenius muscles

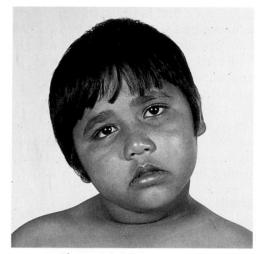

Figure 4-67. Torticollis.

may also be involved. This condition may cause vertigo because of the many sensory and positional receptors located in the SCM. Because this muscular condition is often unilateral, a tilt or rotation of the head is often noted (Figure 4-67).

Massage Consideration/s—Local massage can be helpful. Firm gliding strokes, within the client's tolerance, along the SCM, trapezius, scalenes and the splenius muscles may help loosen them. Moist heat can reduce spasms and loosen connective tissues. The massage therapist needs to communicate with the client about the pressure and effectiveness of techniques.

Whiplash

Nonapplicable

Description—Whiplash is a sprain/strain of cervical spine and spinal cord at the junction of the fourth and fifth cervical vertebrae, occurring as the result of rapid acceleration (causing extension) or deceleration (causing flexion) of the head and neck. Because of their greater mobility, the four upper vertebrae act as the lash, and the lower three act as the handle of the whip. Symptoms may include headaches, dizziness, pain, dysphagia (difficulty swallowing), and inflammation. Upper and lower vertebral segments may be involved.

Massage Consideration/s—Other prevailing disorders, such as a luxation of a vertebra, need to be ruled out by the client's health care provider, and clearance needs to be given before massage can be performed. The massage therapist needs to ask the client how the whiplash occurred, and how recent the injury is. Local massage is contraindicated for

72 hours after initial injury because massage will only worsen the pain and inflammation. If it is an anterior/posterior whiplash, the muscles involved could include longus colli, scalenes, splenius muscles, SCM, levator scapula, and upper trapezius. If it is a lateral whiplash, scalenes and SCM could be the primary muscles involved. Broad, gliding strokes and gentle stretches, within the client's tolerance, can be helpful. The massage therapist needs to communicate with the client about the pressure and effectiveness of techniques. The session can be followed with ice for 20 minutes, and the client can use ice at home to control inflammation.

SUMMARY

The functions of the muscular system are to provide external and internal motility, to produce heat, and to maintain posture. There are three different types of muscle tissue: smooth, cardiac, and skeletal. Skeletal muscles are composed of bundles of muscle fibers, which are bound together individually and collectively with layers of fascia. The muscle is attached to bones by two or more tendons. As the muscle contracts, the tendons are drawn closer together. This changes the joint position and produces movement of the skeletal system. To achieve this movement, the muscles must work in pairs or groups that either act to produce movement (agonists), oppose or resist movement (antagonists), assist movement (synergists), or stabilize muscle attachments so that movement can occur (fixators).

The skeleton itself functions as a supportive and protective framework for the body and is composed of bone. Where the bones come together, a joint is formed. The joints give flexibility to the skeleton and are moved by muscular contraction. Types of joints are synarthrotic, amphiarthrotic, and diarthrotic. Types of diarthrotic or synovial joints are hinge, pivot, ellipsoidal, saddle, gliding, and ball-and-socket.

Common pathologies of the musculoskeletal system include adhesive capsulitis, amputation, ankylosing spondylitis, anterior compartment syndrome, arthritis, atrophy, Baker's cyst, bunion, bursitis, chondromalacia patellae, clubfoot, contracture, cubital tunnel syndrome, de Quervain's tendonitis, dislocation, fibromyalgia, flaccid, fractures, ganglion, gout, hammertoe, headaches, herniated disk. juvenile rheumatoid arthritis, kyphosis, lordo- sis, Lyme disease, muscle spasm, muscular dystrophy, Osgood-Schlatter disease, osteoarthritis, osteomyelitis, osteoporosis, Paget's disease, plantar fasciitis, repetitive strain injury, rheumatoid arthritis, scoliosis, separation, shin splints, spasticity, spondylolisthesis, spondylosis, sprain, strain, temporomandibular joint dysfunction, tendinitis, tetanus, torticollis, and whiplash.

Musculoskeletal pathologies may be suspected when symptoms include generalized severe pain, persistent pain, pain accompanied by crepitation during joint mobilizations, severe postural distortion while walking (e.g., listing, leaning, shuffling or dragging feet, waddling, limping), evidence of localized or generalized inflammation, ischemia, body asymmetry while standing or lying down, lumps, nodules, masses, or lesions, loss of range of motion, and loss of strength in the affected muscle. The massage therapist needs to refer the client to a physician immediately when these symptoms are present. Other signs to look for during intake and assessment include structural asymmetries, increased or decreased muscular tonus, trigger points, adhesions, abnormal gait patterns, muscle guarding, hard endfeel during joint movement, and medications for musculoskeletal pathologies.

Resources

Ankylosing Spondylitis Association
800-777-8189
Arthritis Foundation
3400 Peachtree Road NE
Atlanta, GA 30329
404-320-3333
800-283-7800
www.arthritis.org
Lyme Disease Foundation
One Financial Plaza, 18th Floor
Hartford, CT 06103
860-525-2000
800-886-LYME (24 hours a day)
www.lymenet.org
Muscular Dystrophy Association
3300 East Sunrise Drive
Tucson, AZ 85718
800-572-1717
Myositis Association of America
755 Cantrell Avenue, Suite C
Harrisonburg, VA 22801
540-433-7686
www.myositis.org
maa@myositis.org

National Arthritis and Musculoskeletal and Skin Diseases Information Clearinghouse
1 AMS Circle
Bethesda, MD 20892-3675
301-495-4484
www.nih.gov/niams

National Fibromyalgia Research Association
P.O. Box 500
Salem, OR 97302

National Headache Foundation
428 West St. James Place
Chicago, IL 60616
800-843-2256
800-523-8858 (in Illinois)
www.headaches.org

National Osteoporosis Foundation
1150 17th Street, NW, Suite 500
Washington, DC 20036-4603
202-223-2226
www.nof.org
www.orbdnrc@nof.org

National Scoliosis Foundation
3 Cabot Place
Stoughton, MA 02072
617-341-6333
scoliosis@aol.com

SELF-TEST

List the letter of the answer to the term or phrase that best describes it.

A. Ankylosing spondylitis
B. Baker's cyst
C. Bunion
D. Bursitis
E. de Quervain's tendonitis
F. Fibromyalgia
G. Ganglion cyst
H. Gout
I. Headache
J. Herniated disk
K. Kyphosis
L. Lordosis
M. Muscular dystrophy
N. Osteoarthritis
O. Osteoporosis
P. Plantar fasciitis
Q. Rheumatoid arthritis
R. Scoliosis
S. Shin splints
T. Spondylolisthesis
U. Spondylosis
V. Sprain
W. Temporomandibular joint dysfunction
X. Tendinitis
Y. Torticollis
Z. Whiplash

_____ 1. A condition affecting either the jaw joint, its musculature, or both.

_____ 2. A chronic inflammatory disease that affects muscle and related connective tissues. Pain, joint stiffness, and the presence of tender points or trigger points are involved in this condition.

_____ 3. Inflammation of a tendon accompanied by pain and swelling.

_____ 4. A benign tumor occurring on a flat tendon or on a cordlike tendon; it consists of a thin fibrous capsule enclosing a clear fluid.

_____ 5. A chronic, progressive erosion of the articular cartilage resulting from chronic inflammation; often called "wear and tear" arthritis.

_____ 6. An abnormal accumulation of uric acid in the body.

_____ 7. An inflammatory disease leading to calcification and fusion of the joints between the vertebrae or in the sacroiliac joints.

_____ 8. A systemic arthritis characterized by inflammation that destroys the synovial membranes of joints, especially the hands and feet.

_____ 9. An exaggeration of the normal posterior thoracic curve.

_____ 10. A collection of genetic diseases characterized by the progressive atrophy of skeletal muscles without any indication of neural degeneration or damage.

_____ 11. A condition that involves spasms of the sternocleidomastoid muscles.

_____ 12. Abnormal enlargement and medial displacement of the joint of the great toe.

_____ 13. Inflammation of the plantar fascia at the calcaneus, medial aspect of the foot, and insertions of tibialis posterior.

_____ 14. A strain of either the anterior or posterior tibial muscles marked by pain along the shin bone.

_____ 15. Protrusion of the nucleus pulposus from the annulus fibrosus of an intervertebral disk.

_____ 16. Acute or chronic inflammation of the bursae.

_____ 17. An anteriorly displaced vertebra, usually the fifth lumbar vertebra over the first sacral vertebra.

_____ 18. Joint trauma that stretches or tears the ligamentous attachments without bone displacement.

_____ 19. A type of tendonitis due to narrowing of the tendon sheath surrounding abductor pollicis longus and extensor pollicis brevis.

_____ 20. A sprain/strain of cervical spine and spinal cord at the junction of the fourth and fifth cervical vertebrae, occurring as the result of rapid acceleration (causing extension) or deceleration (causing flexion) of the head and neck.

_____ 21. A cyst behind the knee caused by escape of synovial fluid that becomes enclosed in a membranous sac.

_____ 22. A general term for degeneration of the spine often caused by osteoarthritis; frequently called arthritis of the spine.

_____ 23. Condition characterized by decreased bone mass and increased susceptibility to fractures.

_____ 24. Pain in the head due to any cause.

_____ 25. An exaggeration of the anterior curvature of the lumbar concavity.

_____ 26. A lateral deviation in the normally straight vertical line of the spinal column, usually in the thoracic region.

5 Nervous Pathologies

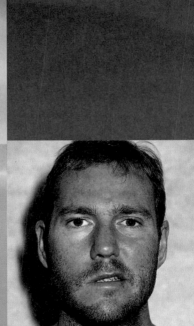

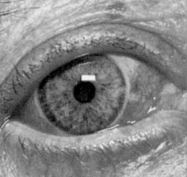

NERVOUS SYSTEM OVERVIEW

The nervous system is an important system for massage therapy. Massage can directly affect the nervous system and help promote client relaxation and muscle release. Gliding strokes can be soothing to the nervous system; percussion can stimulate the nervous system initially and, with continued use, eventually soothe the nervous system; stretches and joint mobilizations help "reset" specialized nerve receptors within muscles and joints so that muscles can release tension and elongate. Additionally, massage can give an overall sense of well-being and help in the connection between mind and body.

Along with the endocrine system, the nervous system helps maintain homeostasis. The nervous system responds to changes in the body rapidly, using nerve impulses to cause changes in the body. The endocrine system responds more slowly, using hormones as chemical messengers to cause physiological changes in body cells.

In addition to helping maintain homeostasis, the nervous system is responsible for mental processes such as perceptions, cognition, and memory; for behaviors; and for emotional responses such as joy, excitement, anger, and anxiety.

The nervous system has a highly organized structure. It is made up of billions of neurons (nerve cells) and supporting cells called neuroglia. Neurons generate nerve impulses or action potentials. There are three main parts to a neuron. (Figure 5-1) Dendrites receive a nerve impulse from another neuron or detect a stimulus and create an action potential. The cell body of the neuron has a nucleus, mitochondria, and other organelles. Axons carry the nerve impulse away from the neuron toward another neuron, muscle cell, or gland. The junction of the neuron and other neuron, muscle, or gland is called a synapse. The neuron does not actually touch the other neuron, muscle, or gland. Instead, there is a space between them called the synaptic cleft (Figure 5-2). The neuron releases chemicals called neurotransmitters into the synaptic cleft to carry the nerve impulses across. Acetylcholine is the most common neurotransmitter. After the neurotransmitter travels across the synaptic cleft, it binds with receptor sites on the adjacent neuron, muscle, or gland. This binding can cause the impulse to either continue or not continue in the adjacent neuron, muscle, or gland.

The nervous system has enormously complex activities. Everything it does, however, can be grouped into three basic functions:

- *Sensory function.* Sensory receptors are either dendrites of neurons or separate, specialized cells. They detect changes, or stimuli, inside the body such as lowered blood sugar levels, or outside the body, such as an increase in temperature. Sensory receptors respond to stimuli by generating nerve impulses along sensory or afferent neurons that travel into the spinal cord and brain.
- *Integrative function.* The spinal cord and brain integrate or process sensory information. They analyze it, store some of it, and decide on an appropriate response. Interneurons are found between sensory and motor neurons (discussed next), and they participate in integrative functions. Most of the neurons of the body are interneurons.
- *Motor function.* The motor function of the nervous system is to respond to integrative decisions. Motor or efferent neurons carry nerve impulses from the brain and spinal cord to smooth muscle, cardiac muscle, skeletal muscle, and glands. These are called effectors.

The spinal cord and brain together make up the central nervous system (CNS). The brain is housed in the skull, and the spinal cord is housed inside the vertebral column. In addition to this bony protection, the brain and spinal cord are protected by meninges and cerebrospinal fluid. Meninges are connective tissue coverings deep to the skull and vertebral column (Figure 5-3). The innermost layer is attached to the surface of the brain and spinal cord. It is a delicate, transparent layer called the pia mater. The middle layer is an arrangement of collagen and elastic fibers that looks like a spider's web. It is called the arachnoid mater. The most superficial layer is dense connective tissue and is called the dura mater.

Cerebrospinal fluid is derived from the blood. It is a clear substance that supplies the tissues of the brain and spinal cord with oxygen and nutrients, and carries away wastes. It also acts as a shock absorber. After it circulates through cavities in the brain and spinal cord, it is reabsorbed into the bloodstream.

In addition to being an integrating center, the spinal cord acts as an information highway. It conveys sensory information from peripheral nerves up to the brain, and it conveys motor information from the brain out to peripheral nerves.

The brain consists of four main parts (Figure 5-4):

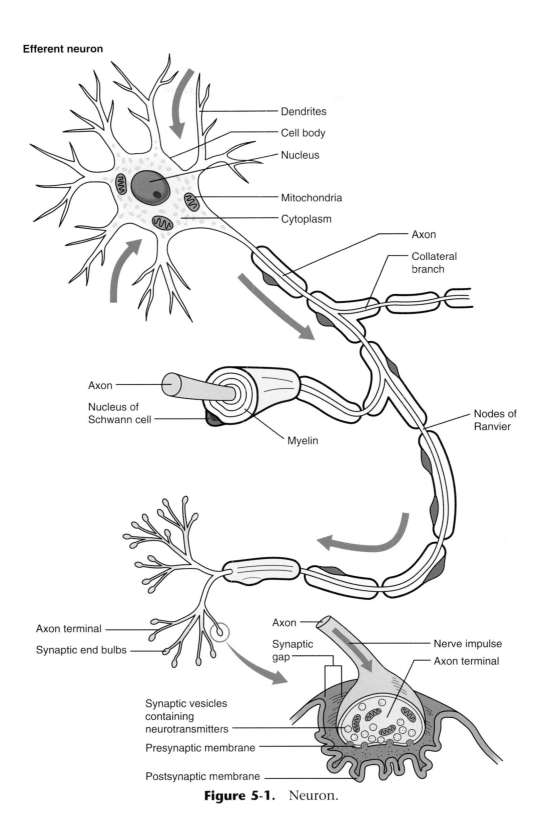

Figure 5-1. Neuron.

Efferent neuron

Dendrites
Cell body
Nucleus
Mitochondria
Cytoplasm
Axon
Collateral branch
Nodes of Ranvier

Axon
Nucleus of Schwann cell
Myelin

Axon terminal
Synaptic end bulbs
Axon
Synaptic gap
Nerve impulse
Axon terminal
Synaptic vesicles containing neurotransmitters
Presynaptic membrane
Postsynaptic membrane

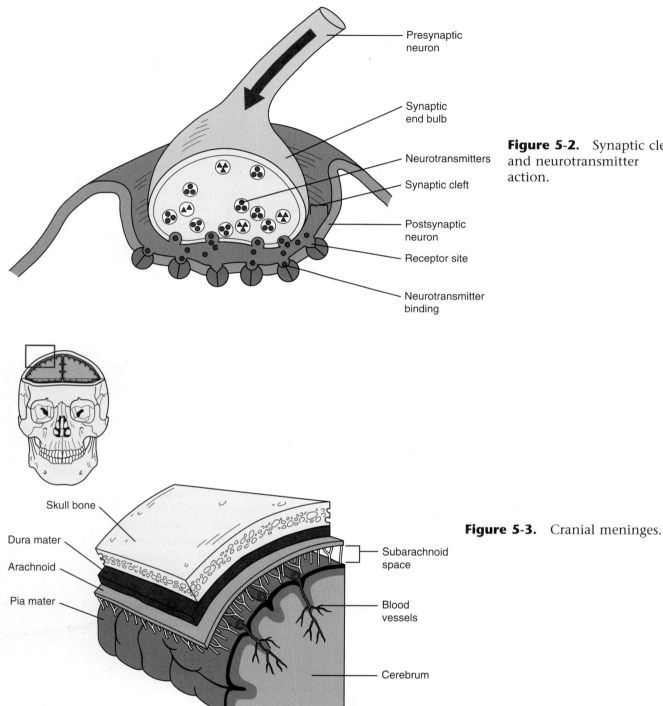

Figure 5-2. Synaptic cleft and neurotransmitter action.

Presynaptic neuron

Synaptic end bulb

Neurotransmitters

Synaptic cleft

Postsynaptic neuron

Receptor site

Neurotransmitter binding

Figure 5-3. Cranial meninges.

Skull bone

Dura mater

Arachnoid

Pia mater

Subarachnoid space

Blood vessels

Cerebrum

- *Brainstem.* The brainstem is continuous with the spinal cord and has three main divisions. The medulla oblongata conducts sensory and motor impulses between other parts of the brain and spinal cord. It also contains vital centers that regulate heartbeat, breathing, blood vessel diameter, swallowing, vomiting, coughing, sneezing, and hiccupping. The pons relays nerve impulses from one side of the cerebellum (discussed later) to another. It also has areas that help control breathing. The midbrain conducts nerve impulses from the cerebrum (discussed later) to the pons, and conducts sensory impulses from the spinal cord to the thalamus (discussed later). It also has centers

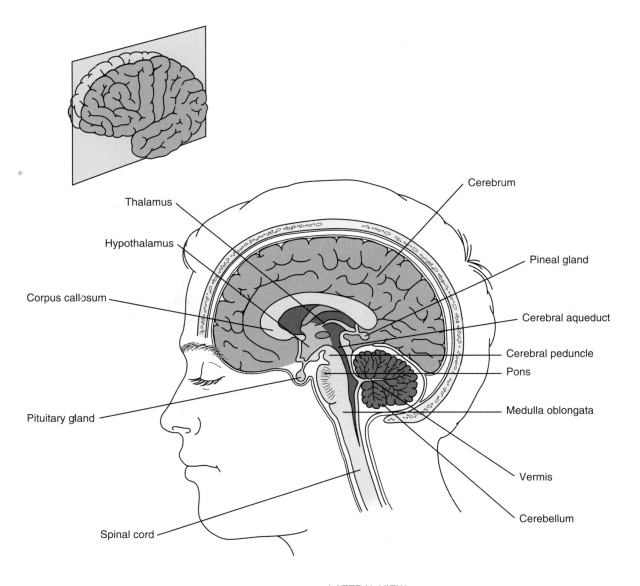

LATERAL VIEW

Figure 5-4. Miscellaneous structures located in a sagittal section of the brain.

to control movements of the eyes, head, and neck in response to visual and auditory stimuli. The substantia nigra in the midbrain helps control movements as well. An area called the reticular activating system is found throughout the entire brainstem. It functions in waking the person up from sleep and maintaining consciousness.

- *Cerebellum.* The cerebellum consists of two connected lobes found on the posterior and inferior part of the brain. It helps coordinate complex movements, and regulates posture and balance.
- *Diencephalon.* The diencephalon is found in the center of the brain. The two main parts

are the thalamus and hypothalamus. The thalamus relays sensory information to appropriate parts of the cerebrum (discussed later). The hypothalamus regulates and integrates the autonomic nervous system (discussed later) and the pituitary gland (see Chapter 6). The hypothalamus also controls behavioral patterns and the person's 24-hour cycle called the circadian rhythm. It controls body temperature and sleep patterns, and, along with the reticular activating system, maintains consciousness.

- *Cerebrum.* The largest part of the brain, the cerebrum is the area where sensations such as vision, smell, taste, and body movements

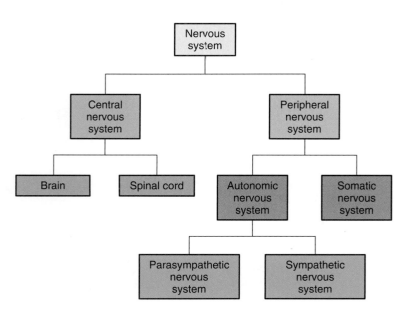

Figure 5-5. Nervous system divisions.

are consciously perceived, where skeletal muscle motor movements are initiated, and where emotional and intellectual processes occur. It is the area where decisions are made. Sensory areas interpret sensory input, and motor areas control muscular movement. Language centers that interpret written and spoken words, and initiate speech are located in the cerebrum. The limbic system within the cerebrum governs emotional aspects of behavior needed for survival, such as sexual feelings, rage, and docility.

All nervous tissue outside the CNS is considered part of the peripheral nervous system (PNS) (Figure 5-5). Peripheral nerves arising from the brain are called cranial nerves; there are 12 pairs of them. Peripheral nerves arising from the spinal cord are called spinal nerves; there are 31 of them. Most of the peripheral nerves have sensory and motor neurons within them.

The PNS can be further subdivided into the somatic nervous system and the autonomic nervous system. The somatic nervous system has sensory neurons that carry information from bones, muscles, joints, and the skin, as well as from sensory receptors for the special senses of vision, hearing, taste, and smell into the CNS. Motor neurons in the somatic nervous system carry impulses from the CNS out to skeletal muscles. Because these motor responses can be consciously controlled, they are considered voluntary.

The autonomic nervous system has sensory neurons that carry information from the visceral

organs such as the heart and intestines (Figure 5-6). The autonomic nervous system motor neurons carry nerve impulses from the CNS to smooth muscle, cardiac muscle, and glands, all found within the viscera. The motor portion of the autonomic nervous system can be divided further into the parasympathetic division and the sympathetic division. The nickname of the parasympathetic division is *rest-and-digest*; it dominates at rest and supports body functions that conserve and restore body energy, such as digestion. The sympathetic division overrides the parasympathetic division during physical exertion or emotional stress; thus it has the nickname *fight-or-flight*. Sympathetic responses require body energy. Effects include pupil dilation; an increase in heart rate, force of heart contraction, and blood pressure; dilation of airways; and constriction of blood vessels in the digestive tract so that more blood can be moved to dilated blood vessels in the active skeletal muscles and the heart.

Because the nervous system involves cognition, emotional and mental disorders are included in this chapter. Some of these conditions are related to a person's responses to life's challenges, some are age-related, some are linked to chemical imbalances, and others are associated with genetics.

THERAPEUTIC ASSESSMENT OF THE NERVOUS SYSTEM

The following list of pertinent questions can serve as a review of how to evaluate the nervous system. Findings need to be documented.

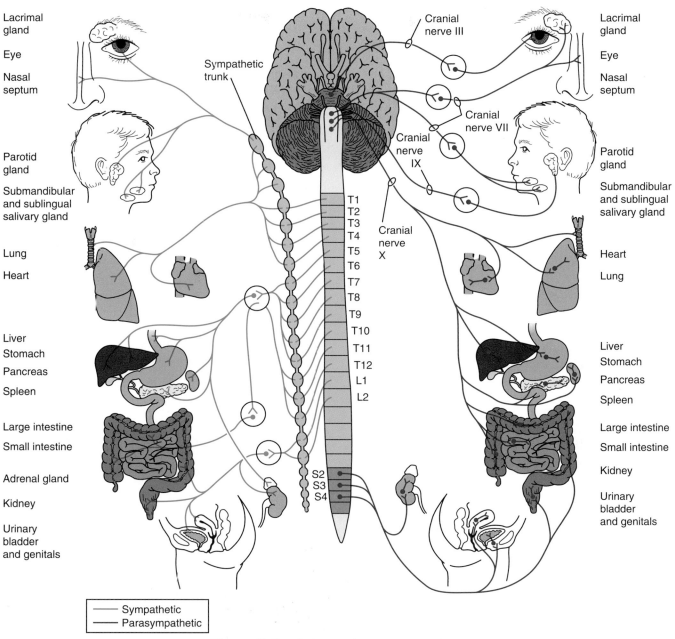

Sympathetic division   Parasympathetic division

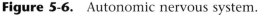

— Sympathetic
— Parasympathetic

Figure 5-6. Autonomic nervous system.

Questions to ask the client in the premassage interview:

- *During consultation, does the client mention any paralysis?* See entry for paralysis.
- *Does the client discuss changes in sensory abilities such as speech or hearing? Do mental abilities seem impaired?* This may denote a neurological problem or the aftermath of an injury. Query the client.

- *Is the client experiencing frequent or persistent headaches?* This may be due to stress or tension or an underlying diseased state. Ascertain the cause of the headaches.
- *Does the client experience feelings of fatigue, depression, insomnia, or anxiety?* Any of these are possible symptoms of mental/emotional conditions.

- *Is the client experiencing any pain? Where is it? Is it generalized or confined to a localized area? Does pressure on the painful area produce or refer sensations elsewhere? If so, where does it refer? Describe the sensations felt.* These areas often need to be addressed during treatment.
- *On a scale from 1 to 5, how intense is the client's pain?* Chapter 2 has a pain scale.
- *Can the client describe how the pain feels? Is it sharp or dull? Does it burn, itch, or ache? Does the area go numb? Does the pain feel like tingling, shooting, or like electricity?* These symptoms may indicate nerve entrapment, nerve compression, or perhaps a severe neurological disorder.
- *What makes the client's pain better? Does anything make it worse?* This can include anything from a specific movement, to rest, to activity/exercise. If the client exercises and pain is exacerbated, exercise should be modified or stopped immediately. Alternatively, if the client has been inactive, this will often give rise to pain. Moderate activity is recommended.
- *When did the client's pain begin? Is the pain continuous, or does it come and go?* If the pain is due to injury or other trauma, the client needs to consult his or her health care provider before the massage. Continuous pain requires a medical diagnosis and clearance from the client's health care provider before massage therapy can be performed.
- *Does the client consume caffeine daily? How much or how often?* These and other neurostimulants increase pain perception. Reduced usage of these substances is recommended.
- *Is the client taking any medication/s for mood or mental/emotional disorders?* Table 5-1 has more information including possible side effects.

Observations to make during the premassage interview and during the massage treatment:

- *Does the client move with grace and balance?* If not, suspect problems with the brain, nerves, muscles, or skeletal system. Conduct further assessments.
- *Are there any involuntary movements?* This often indicates neurological or medication problems.
- *Does the client exhibit changes in sensory abilities such as speech, vision, or hearing? Do mental abilities seem impaired?* This may denote a neurological problem or the aftermath of an injury. See Box 5-2 for more information on visually impaired clients.
- *Are the client's breathing patterns slow and deep? Shallow and rapid?* The latter may indicate stress or anxiety.
- *During the client consultation, is the client focused and attentive?* If the client is focused and attentive, that can indicate health and vigor. Stress, illness, pain, and anxiety can all be projected through body language and be shown as distraction.

GENERAL MANIFESTATIONS OF NERVOUS SYSTEM DISEASE

If a client has any of the following, the massage therapist needs to refer the client to the client's health care provider for diagnosis and treatment:

- Dizziness
- Tremors
- Loss in mental abilities
- Any sensory impairment or paralysis
- Loss of coordination
- Loss of range of motion and/or loss of strength in the affected muscle
- Sensations of numbness, coldness, tingling, or itching that may or may not be accompanied by loss of motor control
- Persistent headaches or one that becomes progressively worse
- Acute, persistent, or progressive pain
- Unexplained radiating pain down the arm or leg

NERVOUS PATHOLOGIES

Alzheimer's Disease (alz´·hai`·merz duh·zeez´)

Alois Alzheimer, German Neurologist; 1864-1915

Description—Alzheimer's disease is characterized by confusion, memory failure, disorientation, restlessness, delusions, speech disturbances, and an inability to carry out purposeful movements (Figure 5-7). Persons with Alzheimer's disease may refuse food, lose bowel or bladder control, and become delirious or violent. The disease usually begins in later middle life with slight defects in memory and behavior and then gradually progresses.

Massage Consideration/s—A full body massage helps relax and soothe the client. The length of the massage should be determined by the client's

Table **5-1** **MEDICATIONS USED TO MANAGE MOOD DISORDERS**

MEDICATION CLASSIFICATION	MEDICATION NAME	POSSIBLE SIDE EFFECTS THAT MAY AFFECT TREATMENT
Atypical Antipsychotics*	Aripiprazole (Abilify), clozapine (Clozaril), olanzapine (Zyprexa), risperidone (Risperdal), sertindole (Serlect) (sertindole is not yet available in the United States), quetiapine (Seroquel), ziprasidone (Geodon)	Drowsiness, dry mouth, edema, fever, irregular heartbeat, joint pain, migraine headaches, seizures, shortness of breath
Benzodiazepines*	Alprazolam (Xanax), diazepam (Valium), lorazepam (Ativan), ketazolam (Loftran) (ketazolam is not available in the United States), chlordiazepoxide (Librium), clonazepam (Klonopin), estazolam (ProSom), flurazepam (Dalmane), midazolam (Versed), oxazepam (Serax), temazepam (Restoril), triazolam (Halcion)	Constipation and diarrhea, disorientation, drowsiness, dry mouth, headaches, hypotension, lethargy, nausea and vomiting, skin rashes, vertigo
Buspirone HCl (BuSpar)*	Nonapplicable	Diarrhea, dizziness, drowsiness, dry mouth, edema, fever, numbness, shortness of breath, skin rashes

When clients are taking medications for mood disorders, caution is merited, as these medications depress sensory information entering the nervous system. During the massage, the therapist often relies on the client's ability to respond to internal and external stimuli to help gauge pressure. The client's response is also helpful when applying joint mobilizations or stretching. When the tissue does not respond by tightening, the sensory feedback loop is reduced or lost and the client may be injured because of excessive pressure or aggressively applied joint movement or muscle stretch. These techniques must be applied carefully or eliminated from the routine in the event the client is taking these medications.

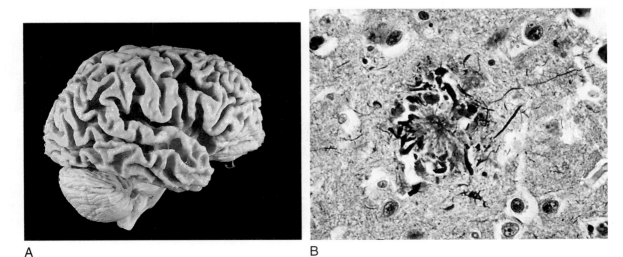

A   B

Figure 5-7. Alzheimer's disease. **A,** Narrowing of the gyri seen in Alzheimer's disease. **B,** Plaque found in the central nervous systems of persons with Alzheimer's disease.

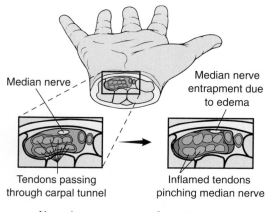

Figure 5-8. Physiology of carpal tunnel syndrome.

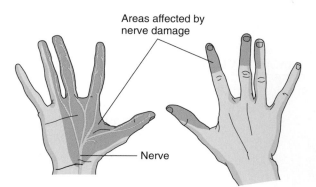

Figure 5-9. Distribution of median nerve.

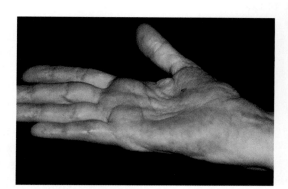

Figure 5-10. Atrophy of the hand in carpal tunnel syndrome.

tolerance, but should not exceed 90 minutes. As Alzheimer's disease progresses, the aim of the massage should be to prevent joint stiffening and muscle contractures and to maintain mobility. Passive joint mobilizations and stretching is indicated, as well as friction around the joints to prevent adhesions. The massage therapist should be aware of and avoid bedsores (see Chapter 3) and bring them to the attention of the client's caregiver.

Carpal Tunnel Syndrome (CTS)

Gr. Wrist; Channel; Together; Course

Description—CTS is a painful repetitive strain injury of the hand and wrist. The carpal tunnel is formed where the transverse carpal ligament connects across carpal bones (anterior wrist). The tendons of the wrist flexors and the median nerve pass through this tunnel into the hand (Figure 5-8). CTS occurs when the size of the carpal tunnel decreases, or the size of the contents of the tendons increase. Both of these scenarios cause compression on the median nerve, resulting in pain, numbness, tingling, and weakened muscles (Figure 5-9). Tendinous sheaths may become swollen and irritated through an improper arm-to-wrist angle and overuse. As these tendons become irritated, extra synovial fluid is secreted. The accumulated fluid decreases the size of the carpal tunnel, which also compresses the median nerve. Chronic inflammation causes the tendon sheath to thicken, increasing the size of the contents of the carpal tunnel and compounding the problem. This condition may cause muscle atrophy of the hand (Figure 5-10). Other problems may mimic CTS such as brachial plexus nerve compression (thoracic outlet syndrome) and neck/shoulder injuries.

Massage Consideration/s—For clients with this syndrome, local massage over the wrist is contraindicated if there is acute inflammation because massage will make the inflammation worse. In chronic conditions, edema can be reduced by elevating the limb and using centripetal gliding strokes or lymphatic drainage techniques. Penetrating moist heat can help soften and allow stretching of fibrous adhesions. Cross-fiber friction loosens scar tissue. Passive movement of the elbow, wrist, and finger joints maintains joint range of motion. It is also essential to massage the neck, shoulders, upper chest, and arms. The massage therapist should help the client identify and avoid risk factors such as improper arm-to-wrist angle and excessive wrist flexion or extension.

Because CTS is an occupational hazard for massage therapists, preventive measures must be applied such as keeping wrists neutral while working, and massaging forearms, hands, and neck regularly (Figure 5-11). (See Box 5-1 for stretching and joint mobilizations for the massage therapist.) To prevent repetitive strain injuries such as CTS, massage therapists need to strengthen

Box **5-1**

Stretching and Joint Mobilizations for the Massage Therapist

The following exercises are designed to assist the therapist in preparing her shoulders, elbows, and hands for the physical exertion involved in massage therapy.

- **Warm-up.** Begin by rubbing your palms and fingers together, creating friction and warmth; then vigorously rub the backs of your hands and arms. Shake your hands and fingers at the wrists and then drop your hands to your sides and roll your shoulders forward for 10 repetitions. Reverse this direction and rotate your shoulders backward. Do this movement sequence 10 times. This quick warm-up is effective for preparing the hands right before a massage or before other hand-developing exercises. Remember to breathe as you move.

- **Hand swishing.** Press your palms and fingers together at chest level with fingertips pointing up to your chin. Quickly rotate your fingers forward until they are pointing downward toward the toes and then reverse back to the starting position. This motion should be playful, quick, and vigorous. NOTE: The elbows and shoulders remain fixed while the wrists rotate together.

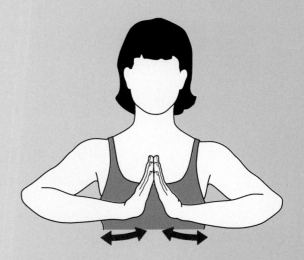

- **Wrist circles.** Begin with your arms at your sides. Flex the elbows while lifting your hands in front of you to chest level. With your fingers extended, circle both wrists in one direction for 10 revolutions and then reverse the direction for 10 revolutions. Repeat the wrist circles in both directions, but this time, close your hands into a fist. Do 10 revolutions in both directions.

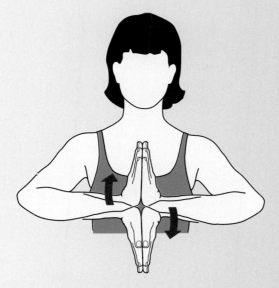

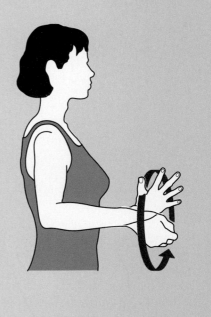

- **Digit stretch.** Press your fingertips together as you keep your wrists apart about 6 to 8 inches. Release this pressure while maintaining contact. Repeat the fingertip press-and-release sequence 10 times.

Box **5-1**

Stretching and Joint Mobilizations for the Massage Therapist—cont'd

- **Grab and stretch.** Start with your open palms at your sides. Pull your hands up to chest height, closing the palms into fists. Without stopping, continue the upward thrust of your hands over your head, stretching your fingertips out and inhaling simultaneously. Reverse the direction, bringing your arms back down. Close your hands as you pass your chest and reopen them as they reach your sides, exhaling forcefully. Keep your pace slow and your movements graceful. Repeat the sequence five times. Stop immediately if you become lightheaded.

- **Ball squeeze.** Place a tennis ball or a racquet ball in the palm of your hand and wrap your fingers around it. Squeeze the ball as hard as you can for 10 seconds. Repeat 10 times. Switch hands and repeat the sequence.

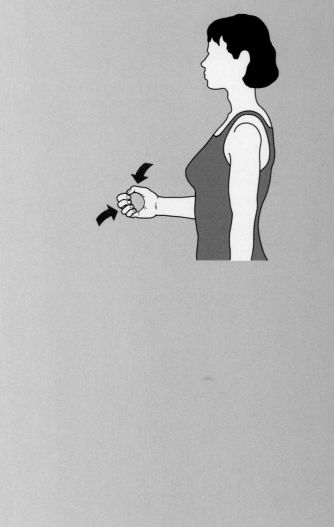

Adapted from Salvo S: Massage therapy: principles and practice, *ed 2, Philadelphia, 2003, WB Saunders.*

forearm and hand muscles using isometric and isotonic contractions (Figure 5-12). Also, using a variety of strokes during the massage, resting hands by spacing clients, stretching between sessions, and adjusting the height of the massage table can help prevent CTS. Lowering table height will decrease the risk of wrist hyperextension and thus decrease the risk of carpal tunnel injury/irritation (Figure 5-13).

Cataract

Gr. To Flow Down

Description—Cataracts are a partial or complete lack of transparency in the lens or lens capsule of the eye that can impair vision or cause blindness. A gray-white opaqueness can be seen within the lens and behind the pupil (Figure 5-14). Most cataracts occur after a person is 50 years of age. The tendency to develop cataracts is inher-

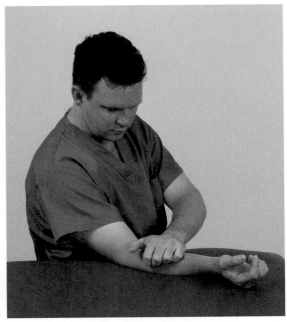

Figure 5-11. Therapist massaging forearms.

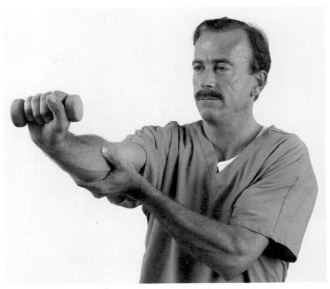

Figure 5-12. Therapist doing strengthening exercises to prevent carpal tunnel syndrome.

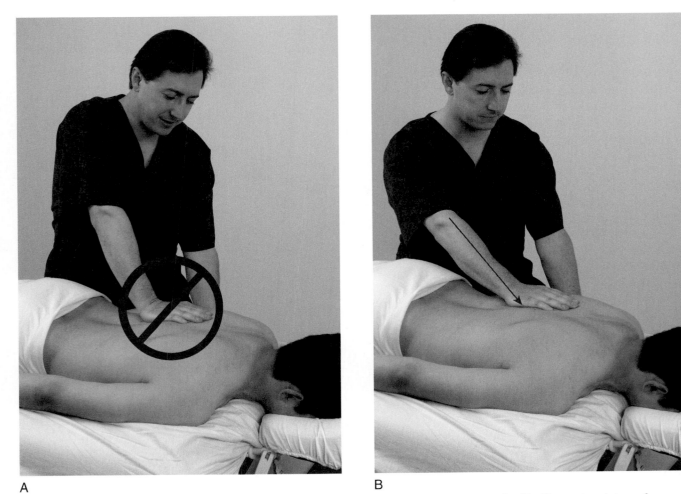

A

B

Figure 5-13. Correct and incorrect wrist angles. **A,** Incorrect wrist angle. **B,** Correct wrist angle.

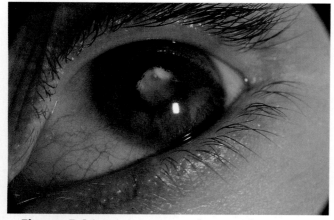

Figure 5-14. Appearance of eye with cataract.

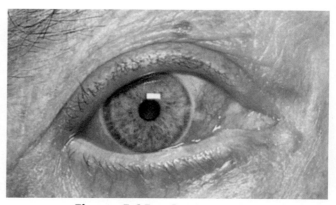

Figure 5-15. Conjunctivitis.

ited. However, trauma, such as a puncture wound to the eyes or blow to the head, contact with chemicals, excess exposure to sunlight, and diabetes mellitus may later result in cataract formation.

Massage Consideration/s—Massage can be performed on clients with cataracts. If the client is visually impaired, the massage therapist needs to explain everything that happens during the massage verbally, and establish verbal feedback. Box 5-2 has more information on visually impaired clients.

Conjunctivitis (Pinkeye) (kuhn·junk´·tuh·vai`·tis)

L. To Join Together; Gr. Inflammation

Description—Inflammation of the conjunctiva of the eye, or conjunctivitis, is caused by a bacterial or viral infection, allergy, or environmental factors such as debris. Red eyes, a thick discharge, sticky eyelids in the morning, and inflammation, are characteristic (Figure 5-15).

Massage Consideration/s—Massage is contraindicated because this is often a contagious disease.

Detached Retina

O. Fr. To Unfasten; L. Net

Description—Retinal detachment involves separation of the retina from the pigmented epithelium in the back of the eye (Figure 5-16). Most cases are associated with the aging process. Retinal reattachment requires surgery.

Massage Consideration/s—Massage can be performed on clients with surgically reattached retinas. Massage considerations are the same as for cataracts.

Encephalitis (en`·se`·fuh·lai´·tis)

Gr. Brain; Inflammation

Description—Inflammation of the brain, or encephalitis, is usually caused by a virus, but can also result from exposure to bacteria or

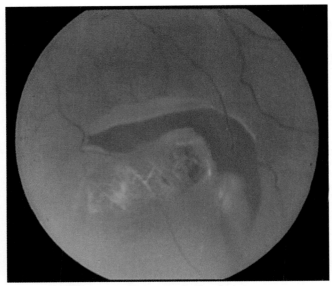
Figure 5-16.   Detached retina.

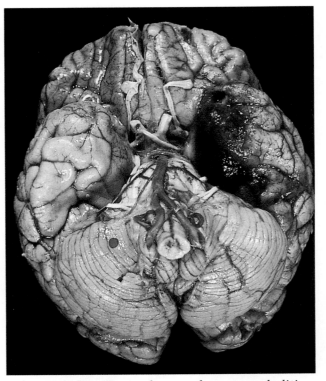
Figure 5-17.   Brain damage from encephalitis.

fungi. The mode of transmission is a mosquito bite or bite from a rabid animal. Less frequent causes of encephalitis are ingested lead or other type of poisoning, or as a secondary complication of another condition (Figure 5-17). This condition is characterized by headaches, fever, vertigo, nausea, and vomiting. In severe cases, encephalitis causes seizures, paralysis, and coma.

Massage Consideration/s—Massage is contraindicated because this is a life-threatening disorder. The person will be under medical treatment and will be debilitated.

Glaucoma (glah·koh´·muh)

L. Cataract

Description—Glaucoma is a group of eye diseases characterized by an elevated pressure within the eye/s resulting from an obstruction of the outflow of aqueous humor (Figure 5-18). This increased pressure causes pathological changes in the optic disc and defects in the field of vision.

Massage Consideration/s—Massage can be performed on clients with glaucoma. Massage considerations are the same as those for cataracts. The massage therapist needs to avoid pressure over the eyes when doing facial massage so as not to put undue pressure on sensitive eyes. The massage therapist needs to ask if the client is comfortable lying prone with the face in the face cradle. If the client is not comfortable, the face cradle should not be used, and the posterior body should be massaged in the side-lying position.

Guillain-Barré Syndrome (GBS, Acute Idiopathic Polyneuritis) (gee·lan´ bah·ray´ sin´·drohm)

Georges Guillain, French Neurologist; 1876-1961
J.A. Barré, French Neurologist, 1880-1967

Description—Guillain-Barré syndrome is a rapidly progressive peripheral nerve paralysis. Although the cause is unknown, many cases follow a viral infection. From 1976 to 1977, an increase in the number of cases of GBS occurred after the swine flu vaccination program. The accompanying neuritis usually begins in the feet, spreading upwardly to the trunk, down the arms, and up toward the head. Some people may have minimal symptoms; others have severe symptoms and may require critical care. Muscles may atrophy due to paralysis. The disease resolves itself, but recovery may take months or years.

Massage Consideration/s—The massage therapist needs to obtain clearance for massage from the client's health care provider. During recovery, the goals of massage are to prevent muscle contractures and increase muscle tone of flaccid muscles. Passive joint mobilizations, stretching, and friction around joints help to reduce adhesions and can help improve client mobility.

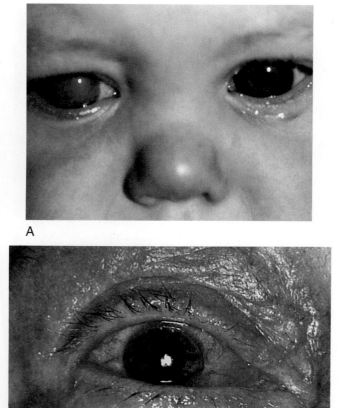

A

B

Figure 5-18. **A,** Congenital glaucoma. **B,** Acute glaucoma.

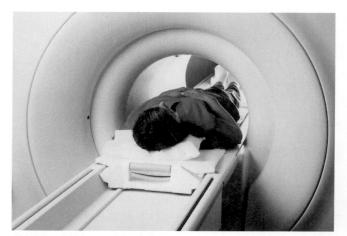

Figure 5-19. Clinical setting for magnetic resonance imaging.

A more vigorous massage can be done as the client more fully recovers. The massage therapist needs to communicate with the client about the pressure of the massage and effectiveness of techniques.

Head Injury

Description—Head injuries may result from any blunt or penetrating trauma to the skull. Blood vessels, nerves, and the meninges can be torn. Types of head injuries are contusions, concussions, and epidural and subdural hematomas.

Contusion

L. To Bruise

Description—A contusion, or bruising of brain tissue, results from direct trauma to the head and often results in loss of consciousness. It is usually associated with a skull fracture. Contusions are often evident on computed tomography (CT)

or magnetic resonance imaging (MRI) (Figure 5-19).

Massage Consideration/s—Because a contusion results from head trauma and is a serious condition, massage is contraindicated. Once the client has completely healed, obtain clearance from the client's health care provider before beginning the first massage.

Concussion

L. Shaken Violently

Description—A concussion is a brief loss of brain function with or without loss of consciousness and may occur after a violent jarring or shaking of the head, usually caused by a blow or explosion. In mild concussions, there may be a temporary impairment of higher mental functions and retrograde amnesia. In severe concussions, there is often prolonged unconsciousness with brainstem involvement, such as temporary loss of respiratory reflex, vasomotor activity, and pupil dilation. CT scans and MRIs are usually normal. However 3% of patients with concussions will have intracranial hemorrhage.

Massage Consideration/s—Because a concussion is a serious condition, massage is contraindicated. Once the client has completely healed, obtain clearance from the client's health care provider before beginning the first massage.

Epidural Hematoma

Gr. Upon; L. Hard; Blood; Tumor

Description—When blood from a hemorrhage accumulates in the epidural space, it results in an epidural hematoma. The epidural space is between the bones of the skull and dura mater. The most common cause is head trauma resulting in a fractured skull. The accumulation of blood in the epidural space compresses the brain, causing brain dysfunction and possibly death.

Massage Consideration/s—Because an epidural hematoma is a serious condition, massage is contraindicated. Once the client has completely healed, obtain clearance from the client's health care provider before beginning the first massage.

Subdural Hematoma

L. Below; Hard; Blood; Tumor

Description—Blood accumulating in the subdural space is called a subdural hematoma. The subdural space is between the dura mater and the arachnoid mater. Subdural hematomas can result from a laceration of the brain and a tear in the arachnoid mater. In severe cases, both blood and cerebrospinal fluid enter the space and compress the brain, causing brain dysfunction and possibly death. In less severe cases, blood gradually enters the subdural space and may take weeks to detect and locate.

Massage Consideration/s—Because a subdural hematoma is a serious condition, massage is contraindicated. Once the client has completely healed, obtain clearance from the client's health care provider before beginning the first massage.

Huntington's Chorea (Huntington's Disease, Chronic Chorea)

George Huntington, United States Surgeon, 1850-1916; Gr. Dance

Description—A rare, hereditary condition, Huntington's chorea is characterized by chronic, progressive chorea and mental deterioration (Figure 5-20). Chorea is a condition characterized by a wide variety of involuntary, purposeless, rapid, and jerky motions such as flexing and extending the fingers, raising and lowering the shoulders, or grimacing. In some forms, the person is also irritable, emotionally unstable, weak, restless, and fretful. An individual afflicted with the condition usually shows the first signs in his or her 40s and typically dies within 15 years.

Massage Consideration/s—As Huntington's chorea is a debilitating disorder, massage should be performed only under medical supervision. The massage therapist needs to ask the client what positions on the table are comfortable, and special propping may be needed to ensure the client is

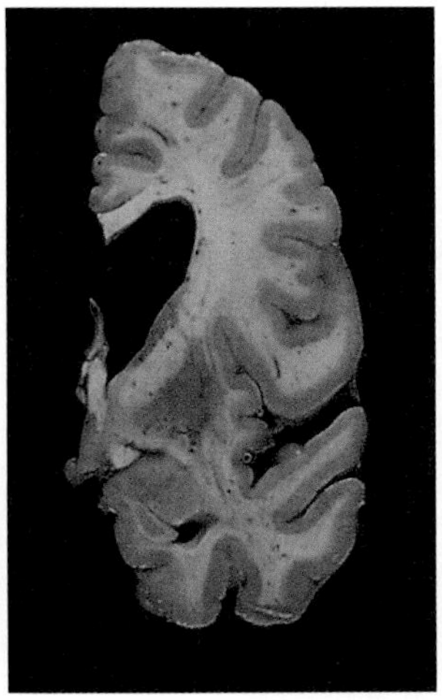

Figure 5-20. Lateral ventricle dilation seen in brain of patient with Huntington's chorea.

comfortable and safe on the massage table. If the client uses a wheelchair and is not able to get on the table, the massage may need to be performed while the client is in the wheelchair. Gentle, gliding strokes to help the client relax may be the most effective. The massage therapist needs to communicate with the client about the pressure of massage and effectiveness of techniques. Pressure sores may form in clients who use wheelchairs. The massage therapist should be aware of and avoid bedsores (see Chapter 3) and bring the bedsores to the attention of the client's caregiver.

Lou Gehrig's Disease (Amyotrophic Lateral Sclerosis, ALS) (ay`·mai`·uh·troh´·fik la´·tuh·ruhl skluh·roh´·sis)

Lou Gehrig, American Baseball Player (who died of the disease) 1903-1941
Gr. Without; Muscle; Tone; L. Side; Gr. Hardening

Description—A degeneration of motor neurons, Lou Gehrig's disease is characterized by weakness and muscle atrophy of the hands, forearms, and legs, spreading to involve most of the body. It often begins in life's middle years, progresses rapidly, and causes death within 2 to 5 years. In most cases, the cause of ALS is unknown. However, in 5% to 10% of cases, the disease is genetic.

Massage Consideration/s—As ALS is a debilitating disorder, massage should be performed only under medical supervision. The massage therapist needs to ask the client what positions on the table are comfortable, and special propping may be needed to ensure the client is comfortable and safe on the massage table. If the client uses a wheelchair

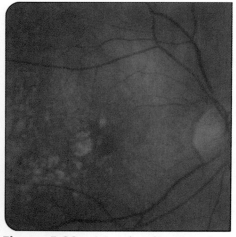

Figure 5-21. Macular degeneration.

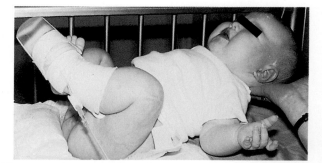

Figure 5-22. Neck stiffness commonly seen in meningitis.

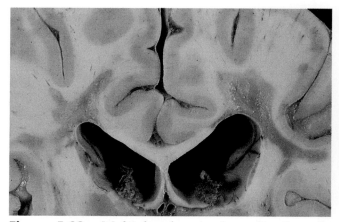

Figure 5-23. Multiple sclerosis: demyelination of the white matter in the brain.

and is not able to get on the table, the massage may need to be performed while the client is in the wheelchair. Gentle, gliding strokes to help the client relax may be the most effective. The massage therapist needs to communicate with the client about the pressure of massage and effectiveness of techniques. The massage therapist should be aware of and avoid bedsores (see Chapter 3) and bring the bedsores to the attention of the client's caregiver.

Macular Degeneration

L. Spot; To Become Unlike Others

Description—Associated with the aging process, macular degeneration is a progressive deterioration of the retinal maculae (Figure 5-21). This condition may also be a secondary complication from other diseases.

Massage Consideration/s—Massage can be performed on clients with macular degeneration. Considerations are the same as those for cataracts.

Meningitis

Gr. Membrane; Inflammation

Description—Meningitis is an infection or inflammation of the meninges, often characterized by a sudden severe headache, vertigo, stiffness of the neck (Figure 5-22), and severe irritability. As the condition progresses, individuals experience nausea, vomiting, and mental disorientation. An elevated body temperature, pulse rate, and respiration rate are often noted. Meningitis can be life threatening.

Massage Consideration/s—As this is often a contagious disease, massage is contraindicated. The person will be undergoing medical treatment and will be debilitated.

Multiple Sclerosis (MS)

L. Many; Folded; Hardening

Description—Multiple sclerosis is an autoimmune disorder in which there is a progressive destruction of myelin sheaths in the CNS (similar to an electrical wire stripped of its insulation). The myelin sheaths deteriorate to scleroses, which are scars or plaques (Figure 5-23). The symptoms of pain and loss of function in various parts of the body depend on the areas within the CNS that are most laden with plaque (Figure 5-24). There are several types of MS. Some types do not worsen with time; however, the most common type usually begins slowly in young adulthood with symptoms of weakness in muscles, abnormal sensations, or double vision. It worsens throughout life with periods of flare-up and remission. Remission occurs because the damaged axons heal and normal function resumes. The interim between flare-ups grows shorter as the disease advances. Women tend to be affected more often than men.

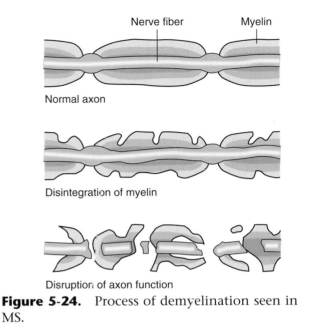

Figure 5-24. Process of demyelination seen in MS.

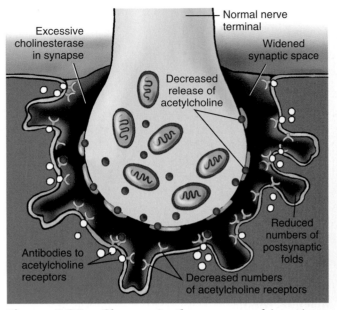

Figure 5-25. Changes in the myoneural junction seen in myasthenia gravis.

Massage Consideration/s—Massage is contraindicated during flare-ups because massage would only make the client feel worse. While in remission, massage may be performed. The client should be assessed thoroughly at every visit because symptoms may change from day to day. The goal of massage treatments is to lessen exacerbations, relax the client, decrease tone in rigid muscles, and prevent stiffness and contractures. Treatments should be slow and gentle and of shorter duration if the client tires easily. Heat and cold therapies are contraindicated because temperature extremes can make symptoms worse, and the client may not be able to give accurate feedback about the temperature. The massage therapist needs to communicate with the client about the pressure of massage and effectiveness of techniques.

Myasthenia Gravis (mai`·uhs·thee´·nyuh gra´·vis)

Gr. Muscle; Weakness; L. Pregnant

Description—Myasthenia gravis is an autoimmune disorder, resulting in a loss of acetylcholine receptors at the junction between the neuron and muscle cell. It is characterized by muscle weakness and fatigue (Figure 5-25). The onset of myasthenia gravis is gradual, with an initial drooping of the upper eyelids, throat, and facial muscles (Figure 5-26). The weakness may extend to the respiratory muscles. Muscular exertion may exacerbate this condition and is not advised.

Massage Consideration/s—The massage therapist needs to obtain clearance for massage from the

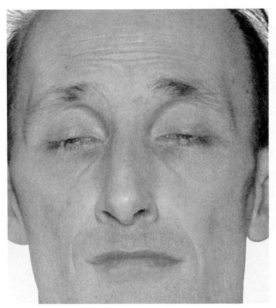

Figure 5-26. Myasthenia gravis.

client's health care provider if symptoms are severe. Gliding strokes and gentle kneading may slow the muscle atrophy. Also, passive joint mobilizations and stretching may be helpful in maintaining flexibility. The massage therapist needs to communicate with the client about the pressure of massage and effectiveness of techniques.

Nerve Compression (Nerve Impingement)

L. Sinew; L. To Press Together

Description—Nerve compression is caused by pressure against the nerve as a result of contact with hard tissues such as bone or cartilage. Common nerve compressions are found when vertebral disks "bulge" or "herniate" from between the bodies of adjacent vertebrae and migrate into the nerve root branching from the spinal cord. (See Chapter 4 for herniated disk.) The symptoms of nerve compressions include sharp radiating pain and sensations of burning, numbness, or tingling. Compression may occasionally result in weakness or the loss of strength or dexterity.

Massage Consideration/s—The massage therapist needs to obtain clearance for massage from the client's health care provider. Although deep pressure should not be applied to vertebral disks and bony surfaces, massage may be performed on the muscles in the area of the compression or muscles that are innervated by the nerve being compressed. Gentle gliding and kneading strokes may help relax these muscles. The massage therapist needs to communicate with the client about the pressure of massage and effectiveness of techniques.

Nerve Entrapment

L. Sinew; O. Fr. To Catch In A Trap

Description—Nerve entrapments result from pressure against the nerves from adjacent soft tissues such as muscle, tendon, fascia, and ligaments. The entrapment can be caused by muscle tightness and shortening resulting from injury or overuse. These tight soft tissues can affect the nerve in two ways. They may press an underlying nerve against hard tissues such as bone, disrupting normal nerve function (e.g., thoracic outlet syndrome caused by either the scalene or pectoralis minor muscles pressing the brachial plexus against the ribcage). The other type of entrapment occurs when a nerve actually passes through the belly of a muscle and is constricted by the tightening muscle, much like a rubber band stretched between two fingers (e.g., triceps brachii entrapment of the radial nerve or piriformis entrapment of the sciatic nerve). Both types of entrapment may have symptoms of sharp radiating pain (especially in the extremities) and sensations of burning, numbness, pins and needles, or weakness in the affected muscles.

Massage Consideration/s—The main goal of the massage treatment is reduction of tension in the involved muscles. It is helpful for the massage therapist to have a library that includes trigger point manuals and charts to help identify the muscles involved based on pain referral patterns. Many clients will already have a medical diagnosis that may specifically name the nerve or muscles implicated (e.g., piriformis syndrome). The massage therapist can work deeply, but briefly, to release the tissues responsible for the entrapment; overworking the affected area may further traumatize it. Helpful techniques include kneading, ischemic compression on trigger points, deep friction, and stretches.

Neuropathy (nuh·rah´·puh·thee)

L. Sinew; Gr. Disease

Description—Neuropathy is an inflammation or degeneration of the PNS. Symptoms vary from numbness to tingling to burning to the inability to detect vibration or the position of certain joints. The cause is often unknown. Some known causes are chronic inflammation, noninflammatory lesions, complications of diseases such as diabetes, or harmful substances such as lead. Neuropathies may be specifically named for nerves (e.g., ulnar neuropathy, femoral neuropathy), for the number of nerves involved (e.g., mononeuropathy, poly neuropathy), or for the specific structures involved (myelopathy).

Massage Consideration/s—Any client who has undiagnosed numbness or tingling needs to be referred to the health care provider. Massage is contraindicated until the cause of the neuropathy has been diagnosed. If the health care provider gives the massage therapist clearance for massage, either avoid massage or apply only light pressure over the area affected by the neuropathy because the client is unable to give accurate feedback about pressure.

Palsy

L. Paralysis

Description—Palsy is an abnormal condition characterized by paralysis. The three most common forms are Bell's palsy, cerebral palsy, and Erb's palsy.

Bell's Palsy

Sir Charles Bell; Scottish Physician, 1774-1842

Description—Bell's palsy is unilateral facial paralysis of sudden onset caused by inflammation of the facial nerve. Paralysis causes distortion of the face and may be so severe that the person may not be able to either open or close an eye or control salivation on the affected side

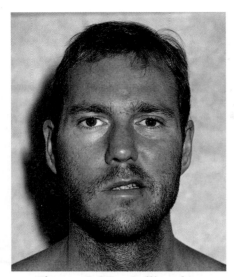

Figure 5-27. Bell's palsy.

(Figure 5-27). The symptoms may be transient (lasting only a few months) or permanent. Many cases involving Bell's palsy were preceded by an upper respiratory tract infection.

Massage Consideration/s—Light gliding strokes on the face, directed upward, can be helpful. Light kneading, percussion, and vibration may help stimulate paralyzed muscles. The client could also massage his or her own face two to three times a day to maintain muscle tone.

Cerebral Palsy (CP)

L. Brain; Paralysis

Description—Cerebral palsy is a group of motor disorders resulting in muscular incoordination and loss of muscle control. It is caused by damage to the brain's motor areas during fetal life, birth, or infancy. Causes include rubella infection, toxemia, or malnutrition during pregnancy, or damage during birth in which oxygen to the baby is reduced. Cerebral palsy is not progressive, but the damage is irreversible. Intelligence may or may not be affected, but speech may be impaired. The muscles may be spastic and hyperexcitable. Even small movements, touch, muscle stretch, pain, or emotional stress can increase spasticity (Figure 5-28).

Massage Consideration/s—The massage therapist needs to obtain clearance for massage from the client's health care provider if symptoms are severe. If the client is unable to speak, the massage therapist and client need to devise a code in which they are able to communicate about both comfort while the client is on the table and the pressure of massage. The code could be as simple as raising a finger or blinking the eyes once to indi-

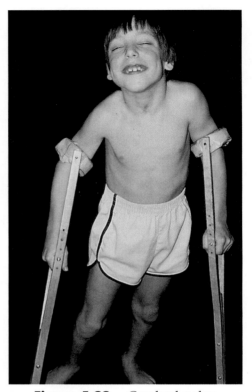

Figure 5-28. Cerebral palsy.

cate "yes" to a question, or raising two fingers or closing eyes to indicate "no" to questions. Special propping may be needed to ensure the client is comfortable and safe on the massage table; inquire about positions that are most comfortable. If the client uses a wheelchair and is not able to get on the table, the massage may need to be performed while the client is in the wheelchair. Relaxing massage treatments with light strokes and gentle kneading helps reduce spasms and involuntary movements. Passive stretching and joint mobilizations help to prevent muscle contractures. Force should not be used to stretch muscles in spasm. Pressure sores may form in clients who use wheelchairs. The massage therapist should be aware of and avoid bedsores (see Chapter 3) and bring the bedsores to the attention of the client's caregiver.

Erb's Palsy

Wilhelm H. Erb, German Neurologist; 1840-1921

Description—Often caused by birth trauma, Erb's palsy is due to injury of the upper brachial plexus, causing paralysis in the arm. One or more cervical nerve roots may also be involved (Figure 5-29).

Massage Consideration/s—Massage can be performed on clients with Erb's palsy. The massage therapist needs to ask the client what positions are comfortable on the massage table, and may need to prop the client under the affected arm. Gliding strokes and gentle kneading can assist with increasing muscle function and reducing swelling and contracture. Because these clients cannot give feedback about their affected limb/s, a lighter pressure is indicated on these areas.

Paralysis

Gr. To Disable

Description—Paralysis is the loss of muscle function, as in motor paralysis, or loss of sensation, as in sensory paralysis. Paralysis is often caused by spinal cord injuries resulting from trauma during a vehicular accident, sporting incidents, gunshot wounds, or from disease or poisoning. Types of paralysis are paraplegia, hemiplegia, and quadriplegia (Figure 5-30).

Paraplegia

Gr. Beside; Striking At The Side
Description—Paralysis of the lower extremities and trunk is called paraplegia (see Figure 5-30, *A*).

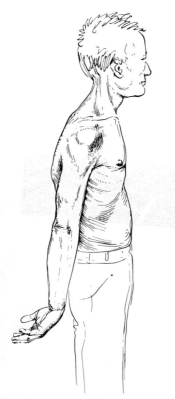

Figure 5-29. Erb's palsy.

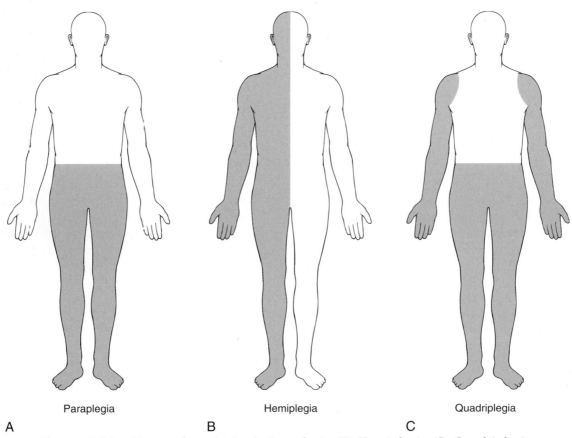

Paraplegia

Hemiplegia

Quadriplegia

A   B   C

Figure 5-30. Types of paralysis. **A,** Paraplegia. **B,** Hemiplegia. **C,** Quadriplegia.

Massage Consideration/s—See entry for Quadriplegia.

Hemiplegia

Gr. Half; Striking At The Side
Description—When the paralysis is restricted to one side of the body, it is called hemiplegia or unilateral paralysis (see Figure 5-30, *B*).
Massage Consideration/s—See entry for Quadriplegia.

Quadriplegia

L. Fourth; Gr. Striking At The Side
Description—Paralysis of the arms and legs is called quadriplegia (see Figure 5-30, *C*).
Massage Consideration/s—Massage can be performed on clients with paralysis. However, the massage therapist needs to keep the following precautions in mind. The longer the client has been inactive, the weaker the bones and muscles will usually be. When massaging legs or arms that have little or no sensation, the therapist must use light pressure, just enough to increase circulation, but not enough to cause any bruising or discomfort; pressure cannot be discerned by a client with sensory paralysis. Sometimes only motor nerves have been damaged, leaving the client immobile but able to feel some sensations such as pressure and vibration. Other clients who have had sensory nerve or total spinal cord separation may be paralyzed and sensory impaired, but may be able to feel vibrations in other parts of their body. The massage therapist needs to ask the client directly for valuable feedback regarding pressure, body warmth, and comfort on the table. All joint mobilizations and stretches, especially on the neck, spinal column, and hip joints, need to be avoided. Electrical vibrators should not be used. The massage therapist will need to assist the client on and off the table, because most clients with these conditions use wheelchairs. Be prepared to massage the client in the wheelchair. Clients with paralysis may also be prone to pressure sores. The massage therapist should be aware of and avoid bedsores (see Chapter 3) and bring the bedsores to the attention of the client's caregiver.

Parkinson's Disease

James Parkinson, English Physician; 1755-1824
Description—Parkinson's disease is a progressive, degenerative, neurological disorder marked by the destruction of dopamine-producing neurons in the brain resulting in depletion of the neurotransmitter dopamine. The neurotransmitter acetylcholine remains disproportionately high. It is thought that the imbalance of too little dopamine and too much acetylcholine causes most of the symptoms of Parkinson's disease (Figure 5-31). Muscles may alternately contract and relax, causing tremors, whereas other muscles contract continuously, causing rigidity of the involved part. Other symptoms include stooped posture, shuffling gait, and an expressionless face. Injections of dopamine are useless because the blood-brain barrier does not permit passage of this neurotransmitter. Levodopa, a dopamine precursor that does cross the blood-brain barrier, is often used to treat this disease.
Massage Consideration/s—The massage therapist needs to obtain clearance for massage from the client's health care provider if symptoms are severe. The goal of massage treatments is to reduce rigidity. Gentle, slow massage of shorter duration is indicated. Gliding strokes and gentle kneading can be helpful. Passive movements of joints after the massage are also indicated, but force should not be used. Symptoms may be reduced, although only temporarily. The massage therapist needs to communicate with the client about the pressure of massage and effectiveness of techniques.

Poliomyelitis (poh`·lee·oh·mai`·lai´·tis)

Gr. Gray; Marrow; Inflammation
Description—Poliomyelitis, or polio, is an infectious disease caused by the poliovirus. It is transmitted through fecal contamination or nasal secretions. Symptoms range from relatively asymptomatic to severe paralysis. Factors that influence the susceptibility to the viruses are gender, stress, and age. In spinal poliomyelitis, the virus

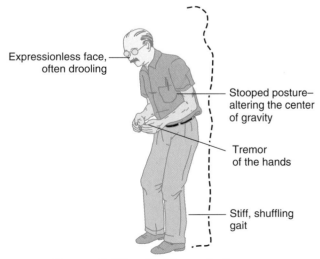

Expressionless face, often drooling

Stooped posture– altering the center of gravity

Tremor of the hands

Stiff, shuffling gait

Figure 5-31. Parkinson's disease.

attacks the anterior horn of the spinal cord, causing inflammation and eventual destruction of the spinal neurons, resulting in paralysis of certain voluntary muscles.

Massage Consideration/s—Massage therapists are most likely to encounter adults in the chronic noninfective stage. A lighter massage is indicated because the skin may be dry and fragile. Paralysis of one group of muscles causes antagonist muscles to increase in tone. The increased tone results in excessive stretch and adhesions of the affected muscle group. Kneading can help reduce contractures; passive joint mobilizations help retain joint mobility. Cross-fiber friction over joints and atrophied muscle helps loosen adhesions. It is important for the massage therapist to remember that the loss of motor function is irreversible. The massage therapist needs to communicate with the client about the pressure of massage and effectiveness of techniques.

There may be pressure sores in clients who wear braces or use crutches (Figure 5-32). The massage therapist should be aware of and avoid bedsores (see Chapter 3) and bring the bedsores to the attention of the client's caregiver.

Postpolio Syndrome (Postpoliomyelitis Syndrome, Postpoliomyelitis Sequela)

L. After; Gr. Gray; Together; Course

Description—Postpolio syndrome is a collection of symptoms seen in individuals who seem to have recovered from poliomyelitis. These symptoms may not show up for several years. Symptoms include weakness, fatigue, pain, involuntary movements, and muscle atrophy that is either generalized or limited to the areas previously affected by the poliomyelitis.

Massage Consideration/s—Massage considerations are the same as for poliomyelitis.

Rabies

L. To Rage

Description—Rabies is an acute infection that is frequently fatal. This condition is caused by the rhabdovirus often transmitted by animals (dogs, cats, bats, and raccoons) to people by infected blood, tissue, or, most commonly, saliva. The incubation period for individuals infected with the rabiesvirus is between 10 days and 1 year. Early symptoms include headaches, fever, and loss of sensation. The individual develops encephalitis, painful muscle spasms induced by the slightest sensations, seizures, paralysis, and coma. Death usually follows these symptoms. Because swallowing water causes throat spasms, rabies is also called hydrophobia, or "fear of water."

Massage Consideration/s—Because rabies is a life-threatening disorder, massage is contraindicated.

Radiculopathy (ruh·di`·kyuh·lah´·puh·thee)

L. Root; Gr. Disease

Description—Radiculopathy is a group of diseases involving spinal nerve roots. They are often named for the nerve root or roots affected (e.g., cervical radiculopathy). Other pathologies, such as spondylotic caudal radiculopathy, or compression of the cauda equina resulting from a narrowing of the spinal canal, may promote this disease. This narrowing may be a complication of spondylosis (see Chapter 4) and result in neural disorders of the lower extremity.

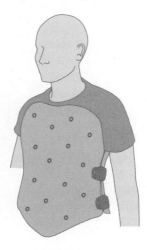

Molded thoracolumbo-sacral orthosis

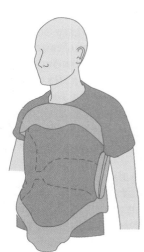

Hyperextension brace

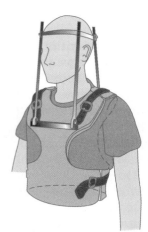

Halo vest

Figure 5-32. Types of braces.

Massage Consideration/s—The massage therapist needs to obtain clearance for massage from the client's health care provider. Because the client may not be able to give accurate feedback about pressure, only gentle gliding over the affected area is indicated.

Reflex Sympathetic Dystrophy (RSD)

L. Bend Back; Gr. To Feel With; Bad; Nourishment

Description—Reflex sympathetic dystrophy is a complex disorder or group of disorders affecting the limbs that may develop as a result of trauma (accident, repetitive motion, or surgery). It is characterized by pain, sensory and motor dysfunction, localized abnormal blood flow, and the inability of the body to control pain messages to the brain.

Massage Consideration/s—The massage therapist needs to obtain clearance for massage from the client's health care provider. Because symptoms vary from treatment to treatment, the massage therapist needs to ask the client what symptoms he or she is experiencing before every massage treatment. If the client is experiencing acute symptoms, local and possibly general massage is contraindicated because the pressure of massage may make the pain worse. Also, the client may not be able to give accurate feedback about pressure. With less severe symptoms, a gentle massage is indicated. Deeper pressure may make the symptoms worse. Passive joint mobilizations can help increase joint mobility.

Sciatica

Gr. Hip

Description—Inflammation of the sciatic nerve, or sciatica, is a type of neuritis often experienced as a dull pain and tenderness in the buttock region with sharper radiating pain or numbness down the leg. The pain is felt along the path of the sciatic nerve. As inflammation increases, motor function may be affected, with the knee becoming "rubbery" or unstable. Branches of the sciatic nerve may also be affected. Sciatica may be a result of nerve compression (caused by bone or cartilage) or nerve entrapment (caused by muscle/soft tissues; most likely the piriformis and other hip outward rotators). Sciatica may be unilateral or bilateral, and can be brought on by injury, overuse, or excessive emotional stress.

Massage Consideration/s—The massage therapist should assess the client's motor and sensory function before each massage treatment and keep a record of it. Massage needs to be modified according to the cause. For example, if the sciatica is due to a herniated disk, massage in the area of the disk is contraindicated. However, treatment of quadratus lumborum and psoas major using gliding strokes and deep friction, within the client's tolerance, may be helpful. If the sciatica is due to a tight piriformis muscle, deep specific work in the area using deep friction, kneading, and ischemic compression trigger points can be helpful. The aim is to relax muscles, reduce atrophy, prevent spasms, and reduce edema. The massage therapist needs to communicate with the client about the pressure of massage and effectiveness of techniques.

Seizure Disorders (Epilepsy) (e´·puh·lep´·see)

O. Fr. To Take Possession Of

Description—Seizure disorders are the presence of abnormal and irregular discharges of cerebral electrical activity; billions of neurons in the brain fire at once. It is viewed as a "lightning storm in the brain." During these episodes, the individual may experience sensory disturbances, seizures, abnormal behavior, and loss of consciousness. The causes of most seizure disorders are unknown, but they have been linked to cerebral trauma, brain tumors, cerebrovascular disturbances, and chemical imbalances. Epilepsy is a term that once described all seizure disorders.

Massage Consideration/s—Massage can be performed on clients who have a history of seizure disorders. The massage therapist needs to ask if the client is aware of specific triggers for a seizure. The massage therapist then needs to make sure none of the triggers occur during the client's treatment. For example, certain odors can trigger a seizure; therefore, aromatherapy is contraindicated. If a seizure occurs during a massage, the therapist should try to place the client on his or her side and provide light immobilization to prevent the client from falling off the table. The massage therapist needs to be aware that he or she may be injured by the client's movements; the therapist should, therefore, use best judgment for self-protection. The therapist should call 911 only if the seizure lasts more than 5 minutes.

Shingles (Herpes Zoster, Postherpetic Neuralgia) (pohst`·her·pe´·tik nu·ral´·gee·uh)

Gr. Creeping Skin Disease; a Girdle

See entry in Chapter 3.

Spina Bifida

L. Thorny; To Cleave

Description—Spina bifida is a congenital defect characterized by a lack of bone development in the lamina (posterior vertebral arch). It usually occurs in the lumbar spine. This condition may be mild (i.e., only a small deformed lamina with a gap), or it may be associated with the complete absence of laminae surrounding a large area. It may be identified externally by a skin depression, dark tufts of hair, dilation of superficial blood vessels called telangiectasis, or soft, subcutaneous lipomas at the site (Figure 5-33). In the more severe cases, the meninges and spinal cord protrude, producing a saclike appearance in the region. The severe forms cause weakness or paralysis of the legs.

Massage Consideration/s—In the less severe forms, general massage can be done, but local massage in the lumbosacral area is contraindicated because the pressure of massage may cause damage to the tissues. The more severe forms involve neurological complications. In this case, the massage therapist needs to obtain clearance for massage from the client's health care provider. The aim of the massage treatments is to prevent contractures, prevent pressure ulcers, reduce spasticity, and reduce any edema in the legs. Passive stretching and joint mobilizations may be helpful; force should not be used to stretch muscles that are in spasm. Gliding strokes and gentle kneading can also address tight muscles and help lessen edema. Clients with severe spina bifida may be in a wheelchair. The massage therapist will need to assist the client on and off the table, or the massage may need to be performed while the client is in the wheel-

chair. Clients with spina bifida may also be prone to bedsores. The massage therapist should be aware of and avoid bedsores (see Chapter 3) and bring the bedsores to the attention of the client's caregiver.

Spinal Cord Injury

Description—Spinal cord injuries are most often due to trauma and include extensive musculoskeletal involvement. If the injury is severe, the individual is faced with varying degrees of paralysis. Injuries that completely transect the cord cause permanent damage to both sensory and motor neurons below the level of the lesion.

Massage Consideration/s—The massage considerations are the same as for paralysis/quadriplegia.

Stroke (Cerebrovascular Accident, CVA)

L. Brain; Vessel; Happening

Description—A cerebrovascular accident is caused by an occlusion or blockage of cerebral blood vessels by an embolus or thrombus, resulting in cerebrovascular hemorrhage. Muscular weakness or paralysis, an increase or decrease in sensation, speech abnormalities, or death may result. Subsequent damage depends on the location and extent of neurological damage (Figure 5-34).

Massage Consideration/s—Massage can be performed during the rehabilitation process if the massage therapist has obtained clearance from the client's health care provider. The massage therapist should work in conjunction with the client's physical and/or occupational therapist. The goals of massage are to prevent joint stiffness, decrease muscle spasticity, and address postural changes such as scoliosis and kyphosis that can occur because of weak muscles. Massage strokes should be slow, superficial, soothing, and rhythmic. Deep pressure may increase spasticity and is therefore, contraindicated. Joint mobilizations should be done within the client's tolerance. The first few massage treatments should be short (not more than 30 minutes) and only a couple of times per week so as not to overtire the client. Treatments can gradually be increased to 1 hour.

Thoracic Outlet Syndrome (TOS, Brachial Plexus Injury)

Gr. Chest; Opening; Together; Course

Description—Thoracic outlet syndrome refers to the compression or entrapment of one or more of the structures of the neurovascular bundle located from the neck, upper chest, and axilla (Figure 5-35). Entrapment is commonly

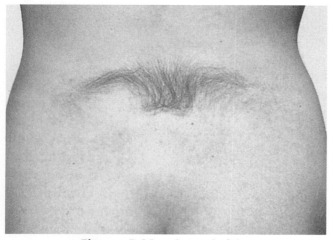

Figure 5-33. Spina bifida.

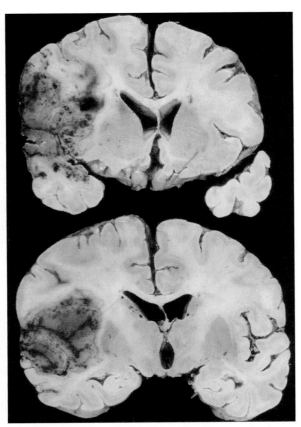

Figure 5-34. Brain damage due to stroke.

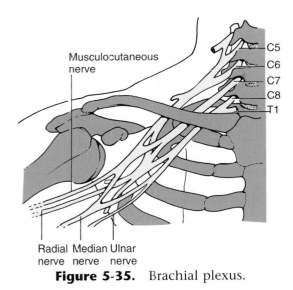

Figure 5-35. Brachial plexus.

caused by tightness of pectoralis minor and scalenes. Compression may be caused when tightness in the muscles causes a reduction of space between the clavicle and first rib. The scalenes pull the ribs upward, reducing the aperture that houses the brachial plexus and related vessels located there,

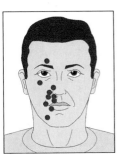

Figure 5-36. Trigger areas of trigeminal neuralgia.

or pectoralis minor may compress the neurovascular bundle into the rib cage. Pain and weakness down the arm are common symptoms. Some people also experience pain in the chest and neck.

Massage Consideration/s—Massage can be performed to reduce muscle tension. Massage treatment should also include the pectoralis minor, the scalenes, and the muscles of the entire shoulder girdle and the arm. Helpful techniques include deep friction, kneading, and ischemic compression on trigger points. The massage therapist needs to communicate with the client about the pressure and effectiveness of techniques.

Trigeminal Neuralgia (Tic Douloureux, Trifacial Neuralgia, Prosopalgia)

(trai·je´·muh·nuhl nu·ral´·gee·uh) (tik´ doh`·luh·roo) (prah`·suh·pal´·gee·uh)

L. Three; Twin; Sinew; Pain

Description—Trigeminal neuralgia is a neurological condition of the trigeminal nerve characterized by excruciating episodic pain in the areas supplied by the trigeminal nerve. Any one or all three of the nerve branches may be affected. First branch involvement results in pain around the eyes and over the forehead; second branch pain involvement results in pain in the upper lip, nose, and cheek; third branch involvement results in pain on the side of the tongue and the lower lip (Figure 5-36). The pain may last from only a few seconds to many hours.

Massage Consideration/s—The massage therapist needs to ask the client about the severity of the symptoms. The massage therapist needs to obtain clearance for massage from the client's health care provider if symptoms are severe. Local massage may be contraindicated because of severe pain; general massage is indicated using light gliding strokes over the affected area as long as it is within the client's tolerance.

MENTAL/EMOTIONAL DISORDERS

Acute or Generalized Anxiety Disorders (Panic Attack, Panic Disorders, Posttraumatic Stress Disorders, Phobias)

L. Sharp; Anxiety; Fr. Join

Description—Acute or generalized anxiety disorders are episodes of intense anxiety and panic, with symptoms ranging from tachycardia, chest pains, nausea and vertigo, to faintness, profuse sweating, trembling, chills or hot flashes, and shortness of breath with feelings of choking or smothering. Attacks typically have a sudden onset, lasting from a few seconds to an hour, and vary in frequency from several times a day to once a month.

Massage Consideration/s—Massage helps reduce stress and may calm the client. By stimulating the parasympathetic nervous system, massage can decrease muscle tension, lower blood pressure, and decrease heart rate. The massage therapist should obtain the name and phone number of a contact person and the client's health care provider in case a panic attack occurs during a massage treatment. Clients with anxiety disorders are often on prescription medications to treat symptoms. See Table 5-1 for more information on medications.

Anorexia Nervosa (a`·nuh·rek´·see·uh ner·voh´·suh)

Gr. Without Appetite; Nerve

Description—See Chapter 9.

Bipolar Disorder

L. Twice; Poles

Description—Bipolar disorder is a mood disorder in which both depressive and manic episodes occur. One or the other phase may be predominate. Characteristics of the depressive phase are underactivity, fatigue, increased need for sleep, apathy, feelings of deep loneliness, sadness, guilt, and reduced self-esteem. Characteristics of the manic phase are limitless energy; hyperactivity; extreme emotional outbursts; an inability to concentrate; decreased need for sleep; feelings of excitement; euphoria, and elation; and delusions of grandeur.

Massage Consideration/s—Massage considerations are the same as for acute anxiety attack.

Bulimia

Gr. Hunger

Description—See Chapter 9.

Dementia

L. To Make Insane

Description—A cognitive disorder, dementia is characterized by personality disintegration, disorientation, and a general loss of cognitive abilities, including impairment of memory and abstract thinking. The most common cause is Alzheimer's disease. Other causes include cerebrovascular disease, CNS infections, brain trauma and tumors, vitamin deficiencies, certain metabolic conditions and endocrine conditions, immune disorders, multiple sclerosis, Huntington's chorea, and Parkinson's disease.

Massage Consideration/s—The massage therapist needs to obtain clearance for massage from the client's health care provider. Massage needs to be tailored to the client's condition if dementia is caused by a specific disorder. If the client is unable to speak for himself or herself, the massage therapist needs to ascertain from the client's caregiver the client's vitality before each massage treatment. Massage considerations are the same as for Alzheimer's disease. Shorter massage sessions may be necessary if the client cannot tolerate longer ones.

Depression (Major Depressive Episode, Clinical Depression, Seasonal Affective Disorder, Dysthymia, Unipolar Disorder, Postpartum Depression)

L. A Pressing Down

Description—Depression is a mood disorder characterized by feelings of deep sadness, despair, pessimism, low self-esteem, withdrawal from personal contact, decreased energy, and sleep and eating disturbances. It can also include feelings of anxiety and irritability, foreboding, guilt, self-reproach, occasional delusions, hallucinations, and preoccupation with death. This disorder, which spans most ages (childhood, adolescence, and adulthood), may develop slowly or suddenly and may last a few days, weeks, or months. Episodes may occur singly or in clusters and be separated by months or even years. Women are more affected by depression than men.

Massage Consideration/s—Massage can be performed on clients with depression, as massage can give a client a sense of well-being. The massage therapist needs to ask the client about energy levels and whether the levels cycle throughout the day. If the client is debilitated, the massage should be more gentle and relaxing so as not to overtire the client. Massage treatments can be scheduled during high-energy times to help in relaxing the client. Or massage treatments could be scheduled during low-energy times to help rejuvenate the client. The massage therapist also needs to ask the client about his or her vitality and sensitivity to pressure. If the client is vital, then vigorous massage can be performed, within the client's tolerance. Clients with depressive disorders are often on prescription medications. See Table 5-1 for more information on medications. Chapter 6 has an entry for seasonal affective disorder.

Obsessive Compulsive Disorder (OCD)

L. To Haunt; To Impel

Description—OCD is an anxiety disorder characterized by emotionally constricted mannerisms that are overly conventional and rigid. There is a preoccupation with trivial details, rules and restrictions, order and organization, schedules, and lists. There is also a tendency to perform repetitive acts, usually as a means of releasing built-up tension or relieving excessive anxiety.

Massage Consideration/s—Massage considerations are the same as for anxiety disorders. Massage can help reduce stress and have a calming effect. It is also important for the massage therapist to have the address and phone number of a contact person if the client has an anxiety attack during a massage session.

Substance Abuse

Description—Substance abuse is classified as the use of a mood or behavior-altering substance that results in distress or impairment. Problems can range from failure to fulfill social or occupational obligations or recurrent use in situations in which it is physically dangerous to do so or that end in legal problems. Substances often abused are alcohol and narcotics.

Massage Consideration/s—Massage therapy may be part of the recovery process for clients with addictions because it is effective for relieving stress during periods of chemical withdrawals, which often produce anxiety. Deep pressure should be avoided during the early stages of withdrawal because it may intensify the release of toxins into the body, which may already be overburdened during the detoxification process. During episodes of recidivism (relapse into a previous condition), massage can be used for both its psychological and physiological benefits.

Although massage can assist the recovering addict through relaxation and increased body awareness, education and support are probably the best tools for overcoming this disorder. Most massage therapists are not licensed to provide counseling services, but can offer these special clients acceptance and moral support as a part of their recovery. If the client is participating in a recovery program, the massage therapist should encourage the client to continue; if not, the massage therapist can recommend a program that deals with his particular addiction issues or refer the client to a professional counselor.

NEUROLOGICAL SYMPTOMS

This section examines various neurological symptoms that some clients commonly experience. These symptoms include hyperesthesia, insomnia, and vertigo. The symptoms themselves may be indicators of other, often more serious, conditions. Please refer to individual entries for more information.

Hyperesthesia (hai`·puhr·es·thee´·zhee·uh)

Gr. Above or Excessive; Sensation

Description—Hyperesthesia is an increased sensitivity to touch, often perceiving touch as painful. This hypersensitivity to touch may be caused by emotional stress, chronic pain, shingles, or nerve compression.

Massage Consideration/s—The massage therapist needs to obtain clearance from the client's health care provider before performing massage. The client and massage therapist need to know the exact cause of the hyperesthesia to make an informed decision as to whether or not massage is appropriate.

Insomnia

L. Not Sleep

Description—Also called wakefulness or sleeplessness, insomnia is the chronic inability to sleep or to remain asleep throughout the night.

Massage Consideration/s—Massage can be performed on clients with insomnia. However, if the insomnia is due to pain from a condition that is a contraindication for massage, massage should not be performed.

Vertigo

L. A Turning Around

Description—Vertigo, or dizziness, is the illusion that either the environment or one's own body is revolving. The sensation of faintness or weakness and mental confusion often accompany vertigo. Vertigo may result from diseases of the inner ear or may be due to disturbances in the CNS.

Massage Consideration/s—The massage therapist needs to obtain clearance for massage from the client's health care provider. The client and the massage therapist need to know the exact cause of the vertigo to make an informed decision as to whether or not massage is appropriate.

SUMMARY

The nervous system is regarded as the master control center of the body. It gathers sensory input from stimuli arising both inside and outside the body, interprets the information, and provides a motor output response by stimulating muscular contractions or glandular secretions. The nervous system is also responsible for mental processes, memory, and emotional responses.

The nervous system is divided into two main sections: the central nervous system (CNS) and the peripheral nervous system (PNS). The organs of the CNS are the brain, spinal cord, cerebrospinal fluid, and meninges. The PNS is an intricate network of many branching nerve fibers—sensory nerves and motor nerves. The sensory nerves conduct stimuli from the sensory receptors to the brain. The motor nerves send output from the CNS to muscles and glands, directing them to respond to the sensory stimuli.

A further division of the PNS is the autonomic nervous system. The autonomic nervous system is also divided into two parts: the sympathetic nervous system and the parasympathetic nervous system.

Pathologies of the nervous system include Alzheimer's disease, carpal tunnel syndrome, cataracts, conjunctivitis, detached retina, encephalitis, glaucoma, Guillain-Barré disease, head injury, Huntington's chorea, Lou Gehrig's disease, macular degeneration, meningitis, multiple sclerosis, myasthenia gravis, neuropathy, nerve compressions and entrapments, palsy, paralysis, Parkinson's disease, poliomyelitis, postpolio syndrome, rabies, radiculopathy, sciatica, seizure disorders, spina bifida, spinal cord injury, stroke, thoracic outlet syndrome, and trigeminal neuralgia.

The nervous system houses the emotional and mental processes, which are subject to another group of disorders. These conditions may be related to age, genetics, adaptation, and chemical imbalances. Mental and emotional disorders of the nervous system include anxiety disorders, anorexia nervosa, bipolar disorder, bulimia, dementia, depression, obsessive compulsive disorder, and substance abuse.

Nervous system pathologies may be suspected when symptoms include sensory impairment; paralysis; loss of coordination; loss of joint range of motion; loss of muscle strength; persistent headaches; acute, persistent, or progressive pain; unexplained arm or leg pain; loss of mental abilities; and sensations of numbness, coldness, tingling, or itching that may or may not be accompanied by loss of motor control. The massage therapist needs to refer the client to a physician immediately when these symptoms are present. Other signs to look for during assessment include affected gait and movement patterns, changes in speech or hearing, breathing patterns, depression, fatigue, insomnia, and medications for mental/emotional disorders.

Resources

Al Anon Family Group Headquarters
1600 Corporate Landing Parkway
Virginia Beach, VA 23454-5617
800-356-9996
www.al-anon.alateen.org

ALS Association National Office
27001 Agoura Road, Suite 150
Calabasas Hills, CA 91301-5104
818-880-9007
www.alsa.org

Alateen
888-425-2666
www.al-anon.alateen.org

Alcoholics Anonymous, General Services
475 Riverside Drive
New York, NY 10018
212-870-3003
www.alcoholics-anonymous.org

Alzheimer's Association
919 North Michigan Avenue, Suite 1000
Chicago, IL 60611-1671
800-272-3900
www.alz.org

American Association of Suicidology
4201 Connecticut Avenue, Suite 310
Washington, DC 20008
202-237-2280
www.suicidology.org

American Paralysis Association
500 Morris Avenue
Springfield, NJ 07081
800-225-0292
www.paralysis.org

American Paralysis/Spinal Cord Hotline
2200 Kernan Drive
Baltimore, MD 21207
800-526-3456

American Parkinson Disease Association
1250 Hylan Boulevard, Suite 4-B
Staten Island, NY 10305
800-223-2132

American Psychiatric Association
1400 K Street NW
Washington, DC 20005
202-682-6000
apa@psych.org

Amyotrophic Lateral Sclerosis Association
27001 Agoura Road, Suite 150
Calabasas Hills, CA 91301-5104
800-782-4747
www.alsa-national.org

Epilepsy Foundation of America
4351 Garden City Drive
Landover, MD 20785
800-EFA-1000
www.efa.org

Foundation for Glaucoma Research
490 Post Street
San Francisco, CA 94102

Guillain-Barré Syndrome Foundation International
PO Box 262
Wynnewood, PA 19096
215-667-0131
www.webmast.com/gbs

International MS Support Foundation
PO Box 90154
Tucson, AZ 85752-0154

Myasthenia Gravis Foundation
222 South Riverside, Suite 1540
Chicago, IL 60606
800-541-5454

National Alliance for Research on Schizophrenia and Depression
60 Cutter Mill Road, Suite 404
Great Neck, NY 11021
516-829-0091
www.mhsource.com/narsad.html

National Alliance for the Mentally Ill
200 North Glebe Road, Suite 1015
Arlington, VA 22203-3754
800-950-NAMI

National Clearinghouse for Alcohol and Drug Information
PO Box 2345
Rockville, MD 20847-2345
800-NCADI64 (800-622-3464)
www.health.org

National Foundation for Depressive Illness
PO Box 2257
New York, NY 10116
800-239-1265
www.depression.org

National Institute of Mental Health
6001 Executive Boulevard, Room 8184, MSC 9663
Bethesda, MD 20892-9663
301-443-4513
nimhinfo@nih.gov

National Mental Health Association
1021 Prince Street
Alexandria, VA 22314-2971
800-969-6642

National Multiple Sclerosis Society
733 Third Avenue
New York, NY 10077
www.info@nmss.org

National Parkinson Foundation
1501 NW 9th Avenue
Miami, FL 33136
800-327-4545
800-433-7022 (in Florida)

National Spinal Cord Injury Association
545 Concord Avenue, Suite 29
Cambridge, MA 02138-1122
800-962-9629
800-638-1733 (in Maryland)

National Stroke Association
96 Inverness Drive East, Suite 1
Englewood, CA 80112-5112
800-STR-OKES

Parkinson's Disease Foundation
Columbia University Medical Center
710 West 168th Street
New York, NY 10032
800-457-6676

Primary Immunodeficiency Association
www.pia.org.uk

Spina Bifida Association of America
4590 Macarthur Boulevard NW, Suite 250
Washington, DC 20007-4226
800-621-3141

United Cerebral Palsy Association
800-872-1827 (Fax)

SELF-TEST

List the letter of the answer to the term or phrase that best describes it.

A. Alzheimer's disease
B. Bipolar disorder
C. Carpal tunnel syndrome
D. Dementia
E. Depression
F. Guillain-Barré syndrome
G. Lou Gehrig's disease
H. Multiple sclerosis
I. Myasthenia gravis
J. Nerve compression
K. Nerve entrapment
L. Neuropathy
M. Obsessive compulsive disorder
N. Paraplegia
O. Parkinson's disease
P. Poliomyelitis
Q. Quadriplegia
R. Sciatica
S. Seizure disorders
T. Spina bifida
U. Stroke
V. Substance abuse
W. Thoracic outlet syndrome
X. Trigeminal neuralgia

_____ 1. Characterized by muscle weakness and fatigue, this is an autoimmune disorder resulting in a loss of acetylcholine receptors at the junction between the neuron and muscle cell.

_____ 2. Compression or entrapment of one or more of the structures of the neurovascular bundle located in the neck, upper chest, and axilla.

_____ 3. A rapidly progressive peripheral nerve paralysis; many cases follow a viral infection.

_____ 4. Caused by an occlusion or blockage of cerebral blood vessels by an embolus or thrombus, resulting in cerebrovascular hemorrhage.

_____ 5. A cognitive disorder characterized by personality disintegration, disorientation, and a general loss of cognitive abilities, including impairment of memory and abstract thinking.

_____ 6. Paralysis of the lower extremities and trunk.

_____ 7. A degeneration of motor neurons characterized by weakness and muscle atrophy of the hands, forearms, and legs, spreading to involve most of the body.

_____ 8. A painful repetitive strain injury of the hand and wrist.

_____ 9. The presence of abnormal and irregular discharges of cerebral electrical activity; a "lightning storm in the brain."

_____ 10. An infectious disease caused by the poliovirus.

_____ 11. Classified as the use of a mood or behavior-altering substance that results in distress or impairment.

_____ 12. Paralysis of the arms and legs.

_____ 13. Caused by pressure against the nerve due to contact with hard tissues such as bone or cartilage.

_____ 14. A progressive, degenerative, neurological disorder marked by the destruction of the dopamine-producing neurons in the brain resulting in depletion of the neurotransmitter dopamine.

_____ 15. An inflammation or degeneration of the peripheral nervous system with numbness or varied sensations.

_____ 16. A mood disorder in which both depressive and manic episodes occur; one or the other phase may be predominate.

_____ 17. An autoimmune disorder in which there is a progressive destruction of myelin sheaths in the central nervous system.

_____ 18. Characterized by confusion, memory failure, disorientation, restlessness, delusions, speech disturbances, and an inability to carry out purposeful movements.

_____ 19. Inflammation of the sciatic nerve.

_____ 20. A mood disorder characterized by feelings of deep sadness, despair, pessimism, low self-esteem, withdrawal from personal contact, decreased energy, sleep and eating disturbances.

_____ 21. Condition resulting from pressure against the nerves from adjacent soft tissues such as muscle, tendon, fascia, and ligaments.

_____ 22. A neurological condition of the trigeminal nerve; any one or all three of the nerve branches may be affected.

_____ 23. An anxiety disorder characterized by emotionally constricted mannerisms that are overly conventional and rigid.

_____ 24. A congenital defect characterized by a lack of bone development in the lamina (posterior vertebral arch), usually in the lumbar spine.

6 Endocrine Pathologies

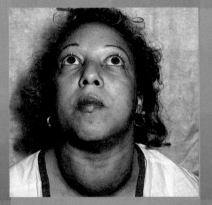

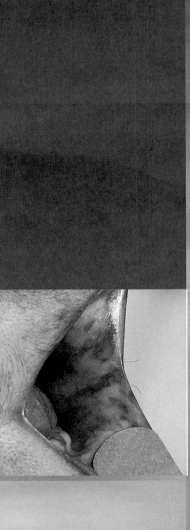

ENDOCRINE SYSTEM OVERVIEW

Because the endocrine system is one of the regulatory systems of the body, it is responsible for helping maintain homeostasis. As such, massage therapists need to have an understanding of what comprises the endocrine system, and how this system works. Massage can also be an adjunct to maintaining homeostasis by affecting the actions of the endocrine system. For example, some of the chemicals released by endocrine glands are responsible for stress responses in the body. By decreasing stress through relaxation, massage can indirectly lower the levels of these hormones and bring about a sense of well-being in a client.

The endocrine system works along with the nervous system to coordinate the functioning of all body systems. While the nervous system uses nerve impulses to communicate, the endocrine system uses chemicals called *hormones*. Most hormones are released in one part of the body and travel through the bloodstream, affecting cells in other parts of the body. Some hormones do not enter the bloodstream but instead work on neighboring cells.

The nervous system takes less time than the endocrine system to respond. Although some hormones can have an effect within seconds, most take a few minutes or longer. The effects of the endocrine system are longer lasting than the effects of the nervous system. The nervous system causes muscles to contract and relax and glands to increase or decrease their secretions. The endocrine system, by contrast, has a more widespread effect—it regulates all types of body cells.

The overall effects of the endocrine system include regulating the activity of smooth muscle, cardiac muscle, and some glands; altering metabolism; regulating the chemical composition and volume of body fluids and fluids inside cells; regulating growth and development; helping regulate reproductive processes; and participating in circadian rhythms. A circadian rhythm is the body's 24-hour cycle. The functions of every hormone in the body fall under at least one of these categories.

The body contains two kinds of glands, *exocrine* and *endocrine*. Exocrine glands secrete their products into ducts that empty into body cavities, the hollow center of an organ, or onto the surface of the body. Examples of exocrine glands are sudoriferous (secretes perspiration), sebaceous (secretes oil), and ceruminous (secretes ear wax). These glands are discussed in Chapter 3. Other examples of exocrine glands are digestive glands, which secrete digestive enzymes into the gastrointestinal tract, and mucous glands, which secrete mucus in a variety of areas of the body.

Endocrine glands secrete their hormones into surrounding interstitial fluid, and then, as stated previously, the hormones move into the blood or affect nearby cells. Endocrine glands include the pituitary, pineal, thyroid, parathyroid, and adrenal glands (Figure 6-1). Some organs and tissues are not endocrine glands but do contain cells that secrete hormones. These include the hypothalamus, thymus, pancreas, ovaries, testes, kidneys, stomach, liver, small intestine, skin, heart, adipose tissue, and placenta.

Generally, negative feedback systems, other hormones, and the nervous system regulate hormonal secretions. An example of negative feedback system control of hormonal secretion involves thyroid hormone from the thyroid gland. Thyroid hormones regulate metabolism. When metabolic needs are low, fewer thyroid hormones are secreted; when metabolic needs are higher, more thyroid hormones are secreted.

An example of hormones controlling the secretion of other hormones is the way the hypothalamus communicates with the pituitary gland. The pituitary gland consists of two parts, an anterior and posterior portion. The anterior portion secretes hormones in response to hormones that the hypothalamus secretes. Some of the hypothalamus hormones cause an increase in the secretion of anterior pituitary hormones; other hypothalamus hormones cause a decrease in the secretion of these hormones.

How the hypothalamus communicates with the posterior pituitary gland is a demonstration of nerve impulses controlling release of hormones. The posterior pituitary gland does not synthesize any hormones. Instead, it stores two hormones (antidiuretic hormone and oxytocin) made by the hypothalamus. Nerve impulses from the hypothalamus cause the posterior pituitary gland to release these hormones. Table 6-1 lists the major hormones and their effects in the body.

THERAPEUTIC ASSESSMENT OF THE ENDOCRINE SYSTEM

The following questions are asked to evaluate the endocrine system. Any of these may indicate hormonal imbalance. Findings need to be documented.

Questions to ask the client in the premassage interview:

- *If the client is currently under care of a health care provider, are there any restrictions on activity?* This can be an indicator of a host of

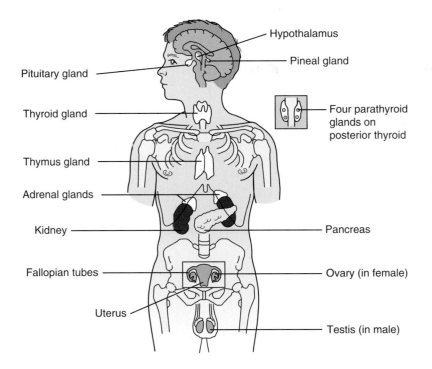

- Hypothalamus
- Pineal gland
- Pituitary gland
- Four parathyroid glands on posterior thyroid
- Thyroid gland
- Thymus gland
- Adrenal glands
- Kidney
- Pancreas
- Fallopian tubes
- Ovary (in female)
- Uterus
- Testis (in male)

Figure 6-1. Location of various endocrine glands.

metabolic disorders. The massage therapist needs to ask the client what the restrictions of activity are, and what the causes are.

- *If the client has diabetes, when was the client's last dose of medication? When was the client's last meal eaten? When was the client's last glucose check? Was the check within normal limits? Does the client have any sugar if it is needed?* The therapist may need to make accommodations for the client's medication administration or food intake during the treatment. See Table 6-2 for more information on diabetes medication including possible side effects.
- *Does the client have any lesions? Are they healing properly?* If the client does not heal reasonably fast, this may indicate diabetes or a diabetic complication.
- *Does the client have any vision problems?* This can be another indication of diabetes or diabetic complications.
- *Does the client have any neurovascular changes such as reduced sensation?* Sometimes neuropathy is a diabetic complication.
- *If the client is an adolescent or a premenopausal adult female, is her menstrual cycle regular? Is her menstrual flow light, medium, or heavy? Is the discomfort associated with menses minimal or excessive?* Problems associated with

reproductive organs are often linked to the endocrine system.

Observations and palpations to make during the premassage interview and during the massage treatment:

- *While assessing the skin, does the client appear to be dehydrated? Retaining fluid? Any abnormal skin pigmentations?* The recommendations outlined in Chapter 2 can be used for this assessment.
- *Do the client's skin, hair, and nails appear to be in good condition? Are there any fungal infections?* When a client's metabolism is not working optimally, it can be apparent in the client's appearance.
- *Does the client appear overanxious? Overly fatigued?* Changes in a client's mood or energy level may indicate endocrine dysfunction.

GENERAL MANIFESTATIONS OF ENDOCRINE DISEASE

If a client has any of the following, the massage therapist needs to refer the client to the client's health care provider for diagnosis and treatment. See Table 6-3 for a list of endocrine pathologies by gland.

Table **6-1** MAJOR HORMONES AND THEIR EFFECTS IN THE BODY

HORMONE	GLAND	PRIMARY ACTION/S
Adrenocorticotropic hormone (ACTH)	Pituitary (anterior lobe)	Regulates endocrine activity of the adrenal cortex
Aldosterone	Adrenals (cortex)	Stimulates reabsorption of sodium and water in kidney filtrate to increase blood volume and increase blood pressure
Androgen	Adrenals (cortex)	Maintains male sex characteristics
Antidiuretic hormone (ADH)	Hypothalamus	Decreases urine output to increase blood volume and increase blood pressure
Calcitonin (CT)	Thyroid	Decreases blood calcium and phosphorus levels by causing them to be stored in the bones
Cortisol	Adrenals (cortex)	Produces antiinflammatory responses and affects carbohydrate, protein, and fat metabolism during periods of long-term stress; also called the "stress hormone"
Epinephrine	Adrenals (medulla)	Helps maintain body responses to stress such as increasing heart rate and force of contraction, dilating airways, mobilizing nutrients for energy, and moving blood to more active tissues such as skeletal muscle and the heart
Estrogen	Ovaries	Prepares the uterus for fertilization and implantation of embryo
Follicle stimulating hormone (FSH)	Pituitary (anterior lobe)	Stimulates ovum (egg) development and estrogen production; stimulates sperm production in testes
Glucagon	Pancreas	Increases blood glucose levels by causing the release of glucose from storage and by converting other nutrients into glucose
Human growth hormone (HGH)	Pituitary (anterior lobe)	Stimulates protein synthesis for muscle and bone growth and maintenance and for tissue repair
Insulin	Pancreas	Decreases blood glucose levels by causing it to enter cells where it is used for energy production
Luteinizing hormone (LH)	Pituitary (anterior lobe)	Stimulates ovulation and production of estrogen and progesterone in ovaries; stimulates testosterone secretion in testes
Melanocyte stimulating hormone (MSH)	Pituitary (anterior lobe)	Stimulates distribution of melanin, increasing skin pigmentation
Melatonin	Pineal	Controls circadian rhythms
Norepinephrine	Adrenals (medulla)	Helps maintain body responses to stress such as increasing heart rate and force of contraction, dilating airways, mobilizing nutrients for energy, and moving blood to more active tissues such as skeletal muscle and the heart
Oxytocin	Hypothalamus	Initiates and strengthens uterine contractions during birth; involved in milk ejection from the mammary glands

Table **6-1** **MAJOR HORMONES AND THEIR EFFECTS IN THE BODY—CONT'D**

HORMONE	GLAND	PRIMARY ACTION/S
Parathyroid hormone (PTH)	Parathyroid	Increases blood calcium levels by releasing it from storage in the bones
Progesterone	Ovaries	Prepares the endometrium (uterine lining) for pregnancy
Prolactin (PRL)	Pituitary (anterior lobe)	Stimulates milk production by the mammary glands
Relaxin	Ovaries	Softens a pregnant woman's connective tissues, especially in the pubic symphysis, in preparation for delivery of the baby
Testosterone	Testes	Promotes secondary male sex characteristics, libido, and sperm production
Thymosin	Thymus	Plays a role in the maturation of lymphocytes, which are involved in the body's immune response
Thyroid-stimulating hormone (TSH)	Pituitary (anterior lobe)	Stimulates the thyroid gland to secrete triiodothyronine and thyroxine
Thyroxine (T_4)	Thyroid	Regulates growth and development and influences mental, physical, and metabolical activities
Triiodothyronine (T_3)	Thyroid	Regulates growth and development and influences mental, physical, and metabolical activities

Table **6-2** **MEDICATIONS USED FOR MANAGING DIABETES**

MEDICATION CLASSIFICATION	MEDICATION NAME	POSSIBLE SIDE EFFECTS THAT MAY AFFECT TREATMENT
Alpha-glucosidase inhibitors (starch blockers)	Acarbose (Precose), miglitol (Glyset)	Abdominal pain, diarrhea, flatulence, skin rash
Biguanides	Metformin (Glucophage)	Abdominal discomfort, diarrhea, nausea and vomiting
Insulin	Nonapplicable	Allergic reactions, changes in subcutaneous fat at injection sites, hypoglycemia
Sulfonylureas	Chlorpropamide (Diabinese), glipizide (Glucotrol), acetohexamide (Dymelor), tolazamide (Tolinase), tolbutamide (Orinase), glimepiride (Amaryl), glyburide (DiaBeta, Micronase)	Constipation and diarrhea, disorientation, gastrointestinal irritation, hypoglycemia, joint pain, lethargy, muscle pain, skin rash, vertigo
Thiazolidinediones (TZDs)	Pioglitazone (Actos), rosiglitazone (Avandia),	Anemia, edema, headaches, upper respiratory tract infection

Table **6-3** **ENDOCRINE PATHOLOGIES BY GLAND**

GLAND	DISEASE
Pituitary	Acromegaly, diabetes insipidus, hypopituitarism, hyperpituitarism
Adrenals	Addison's disease, Cushing's disease
Thyroid	Cretinism, goiter, Graves' disease, hyperthyroidism, hypothyroidism, myxedema
Pancreas	Diabetes mellitus, hypoglycemia
Parathyroid	Hyperparathyroidism, hypoparathyroidism

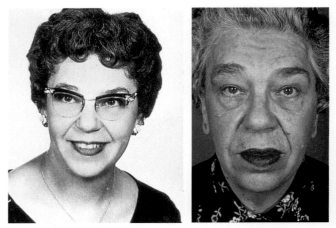

Figure 6-2. Woman with acromegaly.

- Glandular dysfunction in the skin (overproduction or underproduction of sweat, sebum)
- Lumps, nodules, or masses of the anterior neck
- Neuropathy (numbness or tingling)
- Changes in skin pigmentation
- Longstanding skin lesions (wounds that do not heal)
- Tachycardia (heart rate over 100 beats per minute)
- Nervousness and tremors (especially of the hands)
- Unexplained weight loss or weight gain
- Painless foot lesions
- Extreme thirst or urination
- Recurrent or progressive infections
- Sharp changes in energy level

ENDOCRINE PATHOLOGIES

Acromegaly (Acromegalia) (a`·kroh·me´·guh·lee) (a·kroh·me`·guh·lee´·uh)

Gr. Extremity; Big

Description—Acromegaly is a type of hyperpituitarism caused by the overproduction of growth hormone during the adult years. It is characterized by elongation and enlargement of the bones of the extremities, face, and jaw (Figure 6-2). The condition is most common in middle-aged and older persons.

Massage Consideration/s—The massage therapist needs to obtain clearance for massage from the client's health care provider. With the enlargement of the bones and associated muscles, the client may experience a great deal of pain because of the stress of the larger, heavier structures on the joints. The massage therapist should ask how much pain the client is experiencing, and the quality of that pain. The goals of the massage should be to decrease pain and provide as much relaxation as possible. Gentle gliding strokes and kneading are helpful. The massage therapist would need to ask the client's health care provider if joint mobilizations could be performed on the client. Joint mobilizations may be contraindicated because they may damage the joints. The massage therapist needs to communicate with the client about the pressure of massage and effectiveness of techniques.

Addison's Disease (Hypoadrenalism)

(hai`·poh·uh·dree´·nuh·li·zuhm)

Thomas Addison, English Physician; 1793-1860

Description—Addison's disease is caused by failure of adrenal functions, often resulting from an autoimmune disease, local or general infection, or adrenal hemorrhage. The disease is characterized by general weakness and an increase in pigmentation of the skin and mucous membranes (called bronzing) (Figures 6-3 and 6-4). Loss of appetite, nausea and vomiting, depression, and other emotional disturbances often accompany this disease (Figure 6-5).

Massage Consideration/s—The massage therapist needs to obtain clearance for massage from the client's health care provider if symptoms are severe. The massage therapist must ask the client about energy levels and pressure tolerance. If the client is debilitated, a gentle massage of shorter duration is indicated. A more vigorous massage could exhaust the client.

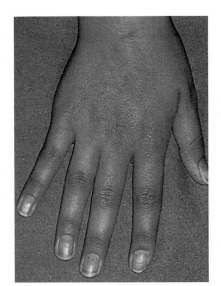

Figure 6-3. Hyperpigmentation seen in Addison's disease.

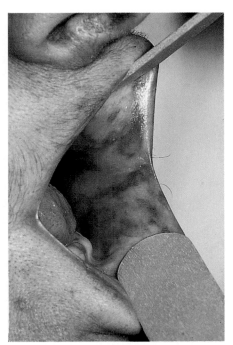

Figure 6-4. Buccal pigmentation of Addison's disease.

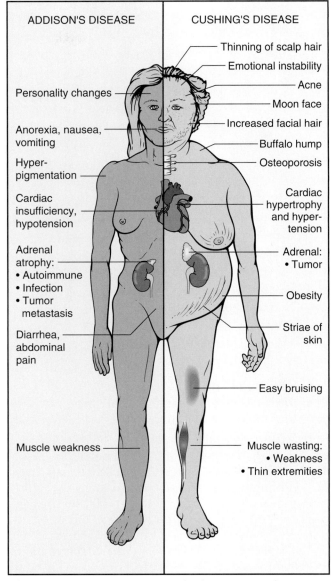

Figure 6-5. Comparison of adrenocortical hyperfunction (Cushing's disease) and hypofunction (Addison's disease).

Cretinism (kree´·tuh·ni·zuhm)

Fr. Idiot

Description—A congenital deficiency in the secretion of thyroid hormones, cretinism is characterized by arrested physical and mental development (Figure 6-6). This condition can result in severe mental retardation if left untreated. Oral thyroid hormone treatment must be started soon after birth and continued through life. This condition is typical in countries where the diet is deficient in iodine and where goiters are common. (See entry in this chapter for goiters.) The addition of iodized salt reduces the occurrence of cretinism.

Massage Consideration/s—The massage therapist needs to obtain clearance for massage from the client's health care provider. A relaxing, gentle massage may be performed, avoiding the neck/throat region.

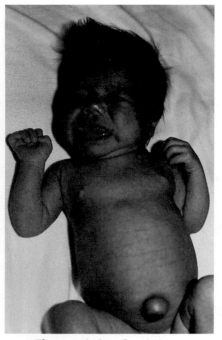

Figure 6-6.   Cretinism.

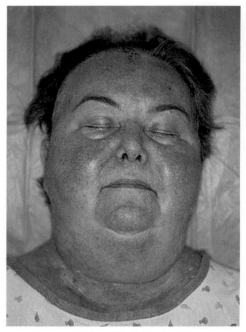

Figure 6-7.   Cushing's disease.

Cushing's Disease (Hyperadrenalism)
(hai·puhr·uh·dree´·nuh·li·zuhm)

Harvey Cushing; American Surgeon; 1869-1939

Description—Classified as a metabolic disorder, Cushing's disease is caused by an overproduction of adrenocortical steroids, which causes an accumulation of fluids and fat on the face, neck, and upper back (buffalo hump). Other conditions that may develop are muscle weakness, striae on the skin, acne, osteoporosis, and diabetes mellitus (Figure 6-7). The person bruises easily, and wound healing is poor. Refer to Figure 6-5 for more information on adrenocortical hyperfunction.

Massage Consideration/s—The massage therapist needs to obtain clearance for massage from the client's health care provider if symptoms are severe. The massage therapist must ask the client about tolerance to pressure and how easily the client bruises. A relaxing massage with gentle pressure is indicated.

Diabetes Insipidus (dai`·uh·bee´·teez in·si´·pi·duhs)

Gr. Passing Through; L. Savory

Description—Diabetes insipidus is caused by a posterior pituitary gland dysfunction that results in deficient production of antidiuretic hormone (ADH). Diabetes insipidus has nothing to do with insulin production or pancreatic dysfunction, but like diabetes mellitus, it results in polyuria (excessive excretion of urine), thus reducing fluid volume in the body and polydipsia (increasing thirst).

Massage Consideration/s—The massage therapist needs to ask about the client's vitality and hydration, and how much pressure the client can tolerate. If the client is not well hydrated, water can be offered to help maintain body fluid levels. If the client is vital, a more vigorous massage can be performed. If the client is debilitated, a gentle massage is indicated so as not to overtire the client. It is important that the client have the necessary medication (ADH) handy during the massage treatment.

Diabetes Mellitus (dai`·uh·bee´·teez me´·luh·tuhs)

Gr. Passing Through; Sweet

Description—Diabetes mellitus is a group of disorders that lead to elevated blood glucose levels (hyperglycemia). Glucose appears in the urine and is accompanied by polyuria (excessive urination), polyphagia (excessive eating), polydipsia (excessive thirst), and peripheral neuropathy. In *type 1* diabetes, there is a deficiency of insulin and regular injections of insulin are needed (Figure 6-8). It is thought to be an autoimmune disease because the beta cells of the pancreas, which produce insulin, are destroyed. *Type 2* diabetes accounts for more than 90% of all diabetic cases. The person makes enough insulin, but the body cells are no longer sensitive to it, so glucose does not enter the cells. Type 2 diabetes usually occurs later in life and can be controlled by diet, exercise, and weight loss.

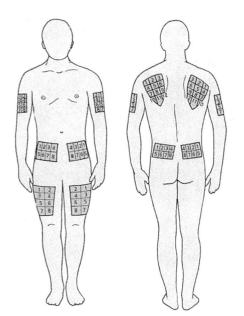

Figure 6-8. Insulin injection sites.

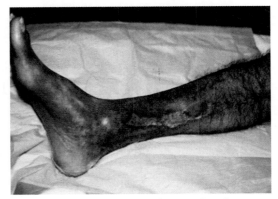

Figure 6-9. Peripheral vascular disease.

Long-term complications such as peripheral vascular disease (decreased circulation in the hands and feet that could lead to gangrene) (Figure 6-9) and neuropathy (decrease/change in sensation in hands and feet) may develop as the disease progresses. Other complications are atherosclerosis, high blood pressure, cataracts and blindness, stroke, and scarred kidneys (Figure 6-10). Many fungi thrive in an environment rich in sugar, so persons with type 2 diabetes easily contract infections such as thrush, jock itch, athlete's foot, and ringworm. Table 6-4 compares type 1 and type 2 diabetes.

Massage Consideration/s—The massage therapist needs to ask when the client took the last dose of medication, when the client last ate, and when the client last checked the glucose level and whether it was within normal limits. The therapist may need to make accommodations for the client's medication

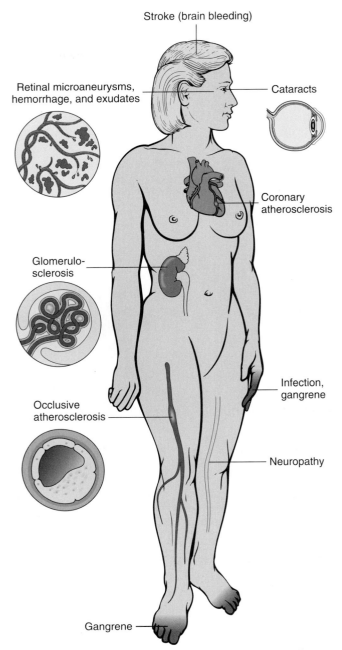

Figure 6-10. Complications of diabetes mellitus.

administration or food intake during treatment. A relaxing and gentle massage is indicated for a client with diabetes mellitus. Sometimes the client cannot give accurate feedback about pressure because of accompanying neuropathy, so lighter pressure is necessary. See Chapter 5 for more information on neuropathy. The massage therapist needs to inform the client of any bruises or breaks in the client's skin, especially on the feet. If the client is taking insulin, massage should not be done for at least 10 days on or around the injection site. Because massage can

Table 6-4   GENERAL COMPARISON OF TYPE 1 AND TYPE 2 DIABETES

CHARACTERISTIC	TYPE 1	TYPE 2
Age of onset (years)	Usually <30	Usually >30
Speed of onset	Sudden	Gradual
Body build	Normal	Obese (90%)
Family history	<20%	60%
Histology of islets	Loss of beta cells	Normal
Treatment	Insulin	Diet
		Oral hypoglycemics or insulin

Damjanov I: Pathology for the health-related professions, *ed 2, Philadelphia, 2000, WB Saunders.*

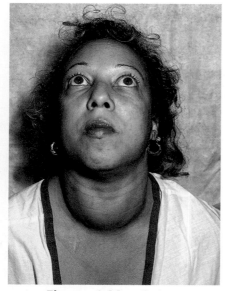

Figure 6-11.   Goiter.

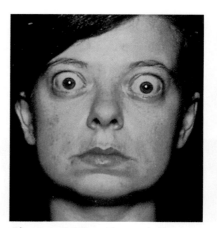

Figure 6-12.   Graves' disease.

Goiters are more prevalent in countries where dietary iodine intake is inadequate. Iodized salt reduces the occurrence of goiters.

Massage Consideration/s—General massage may be performed on clients with a goiter. The massage therapist needs to ask the client about his or her vitality. If the client is vital, then vigorous massage can be performed within the client's tolerance. If the client is debilitated, the massage should be more gentle and relaxing so as not to overtire the client. The neck and throat region should be avoided because the pressure of massage may damage the area.

Graves' Disease

Robert J. Graves; Irish Physician; 1797-1853

Description—Graves' disease is characterized by hyperthyroidism and associated anxiety, fatigue, tremors of the hands, loss of appetite, and increased metabolic rate (Figure 6-12). An enlarged thyroid or goiter and enlarged lymph nodes often accompany this condition, as well as an unusual protrusion of the eyeballs. This disease is thought to be an autoimmune disorder.

increase local blood flow, the insulin may enter the blood more rapidly than it is supposed to and cause a low blood sugar reaction. Also, injection sites are sensitive, and the pressure of massage could cause pain and damage to the area. Vigorous massage, especially percussion and vibration, must be carefully administered because it can damage already compromised blood vessels. Vigorous massage increases local circulation; the increased circulation may also speed up insulin absorption. It is important that the client have the necessary medications (e.g., insulin) when the client comes for treatment in the event of a diabetes-related emergency.

Goiter

L. Throat

Description—An enlarged thyroid gland, or goiter, may be associated with hyperthyroidism, hypothyroidism, inflammation, infection, or lack of iodine in the diet (Figure 6-11).

Massage Consideration/s—General massage may be performed on clients with a goiter. The massage therapist needs to ask the client about his or her vitality. If the client is vital, then vigorous massage can be performed, within the client's tolerance. If the client is debilitated, the massage should be more gentle and relaxing so as not to overtire the client. Gentle massage may help relieve anxiety and reduce fatigue. The neck and throat region, and any enlarged lymph nodes, should be avoided because the pressure of massage may damage the area.

Hyperparathyroidism
(hai`·puhr·pa`·ruh·thai´·roi·di`·zuhm)

Gr. Above; Beside; Shield; Condition

Description—An overproduction of parathyroid hormone results in hyperparathyroidism. It is characterized by increased reabsorption of calcium from the bones and increased absorption of calcium by the kidneys and gastrointestinal tract. The client may experience pain and tenderness and even spontaneous fractures. Gastrointestinal symptoms such as loss of appetite, nausea, vomiting, and abdominal pains may also be experienced.

Massage Consideration/s—The massage therapist needs to obtain clearance for massage from the client's health care provider if symptoms are severe. The massage therapist should ask the client how fragile his or her bones are to determine how vigorous the massage can be performed. This will help determine what regions of the body may need to be avoided during the massage because of fractures or pain in those areas. Gentle gliding strokes and gentle kneading can be performed to help with any muscle tension the client may have. Carefully administer or avoid joint mobilizations and stretches.

Hyperpituitarism (hai`·puhr·pi·too`·uh·tar´·ee·izm)

Gr. Above; L. Phlegm; Gr. Condition

Description—Hyperpituitarism with overproduction of growth hormone causes acromegaly. Acromegaly occurs during the adult years. It is characterized by elongation and enlargement of the bones of the extremities, face, and jaw (see page 176). Gigantism results from overproduction of growth hormone during childhood and puberty (Figure 6-13). Hyperpituitarism may also lead to Cushing's disease (see page 178).

Massage Consideration/s—The massage therapist needs to obtain clearance for massage from the client's health care provider if symptoms are severe. With the enlargement of the bones and associated muscles, the client may experience a great deal of pain because of the stress of the larger, heavier structures on the joints. The massage therapist needs to ask the client how much pain he or she is experiencing, and the quality of that pain. The goals of the massage should be to decrease pain and provide as much relaxation as possible. Gentle gliding strokes and kneading would be helpful. The massage therapist needs to ask the client's health care provider if joint mobilizations and stretches can be performed on the client; if these maneuvers are approved, they should be applied carefully. Joint mobilizations may be contraindicated because they may damage the joints. The massage therapist needs to communicate with the client about the pressure of massage and effectiveness of techniques.

Hyperthyroidism (hai`·puhr·thai´·roi·di`·zuhm)

Gr. Above; Shield; Condition

Description—Hyperactivity of the thyroid gland, hyperthyroidism is characterized by an enlarged thyroid or goiter (see page 180), nervousness and tremor, heat intolerance, increased appetite with weight loss, rapid, forceful pulse, and increased respiration rate (Figure 6-14). This condition can lead to Graves' disease (see page 180).

Massage Consideration/s—The massage therapist needs to obtain clearance for massage from the client's health care provider if symptoms are severe. The massage therapist should ask the client about his or her vitality. If the client is vital, then vigorous massage can be performed, within the client's tolerance. If the client is debilitated, the massage should be more gentle and relaxing so as not to overtire the client. Gentle massage may help relieve anxiety and reduce fatigue. The massage therapist must communicate with the client about the pressure and effectiveness of techniques. When massaging the throat area, perform a tissue release by gently lifting the skin from the superficial fascia over the thyroid cartilate. Manual traction of the cervical vertebrae and light nerve strokes are often helpful.

Hypoglycemia (hai`·poh·glai`·see´·mee·uh)

Gr. Under; Sweet; Blood

Description—Hypoglycemia is almost the opposite of diabetes mellitus, although it can also be related to pancreatic dysfunction. Hypoglycemia refers to an excessive decrease in blood glucose levels that can result in a variety of symptoms including weakness, light-headedness, headaches, excessive hunger, visual disturbances, anxiety, and sudden changes in personality. If

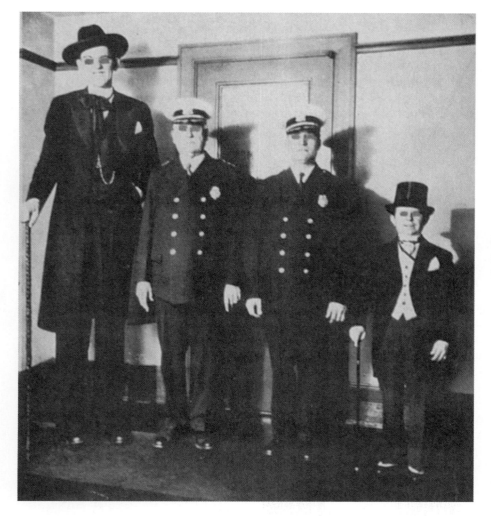

Figure 6-13. Gigantism (man on the far left) and dwarfism (man on the far right).

hypoglycemia is left untreated, the result may be delirium, diabetic coma, and death. Causes of hypoglycemia can be an overdose of prescribed insulin, an excessive level of insulin production by the pancreas, or extreme dietary deficiencies. An overdose of prescribed insulin can result in insulin shock, which may occur in clients with type 1 diabetes mellitus. Immediate medical intervention is necessary, as death can occur quickly unless blood glucose levels are raised (Table 6-5).

Massage Consideration/s—Massage can be performed on clients with hypoglycemia. The massage therapist needs to ask the client about his or her vitality and sensitivity to pressure. If the client is vital, then vigorous massage can be performed, within the client's tolerance. If the client is debilitated, the massage should be more gentle and relaxing so as not to overtire the client. The massage therapist needs to communicate with the client about the pressure and effectiveness of techniques. The therapist needs to be aware that the client may experience light-headedness when getting up from the massage table; be ready to assist.

Hypoparathyroidism
(hi`·poh·pa`·ruh·thai´·roi·di`·zuhm)
Gr. Under; Beside; Shield; Condition

Description—Hypoparathyroidism is a condition that results from diminished function of the parathyroid gland. It is caused by either surgical removal of the glands, an autoimmune disease, or genetic factors. With a fall in calcium levels, the client may experience muscle pain. Other symptoms include tingling in the

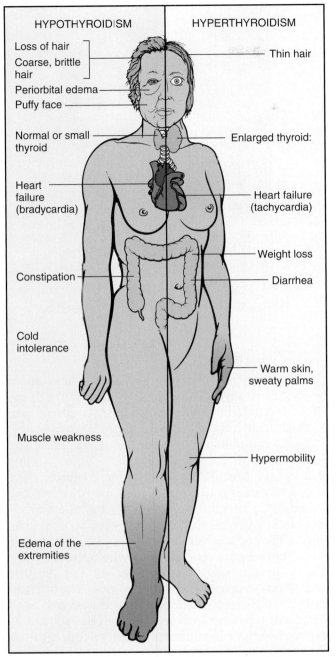

HYPOTHYROIDISM | HYPERTHYROIDISM

Loss of hair
Coarse, brittle hair

Thin hair

Periorbital edema
Puffy face

Normal or small thyroid

Enlarged thyroid:

Heart failure (bradycardia)

Heart failure (tachycardia)

Weight loss

Constipation

Diarrhea

Cold intolerance

Warm skin, sweaty palms

Muscle weakness

Hypermobility

Edema of the extremities

Figure 6-14. Comparison of hyperthyroidism and hypothyroidism.

Table 6-5 SYMPTOMS OF HYPERGLYCEMIA AND HYPOGLYCEMIA	
HYPERGLYCEMIA (CAN LEAD TO DIABETIC COMA)	HYPOGLYCEMIA (CAN LEAD TO INSULIN SHOCK)
Abdominal pain	Abdominal pain
Loss of appetite and weight loss	Anxiousness
Thirst	Shallow breathing
Rapid respiration rate	Hunger
Dry and flushed skin	Lethargy
Frequent urination	Tachycardia
Headaches	Moist and pale skin
Nausea and vomiting	Disorientation
Metallic breath and taste in mouth	Profuse sweating
Constipation	Convulsion

muscles. If the client is vital, then vigorous massage can be performed, within the client's tolerance. If the client is debilitated, the massage should be more gentle and relaxing so as not to overtire the client. Gliding strokes and kneading can help relieve muscle pain. If the client has tingling in the hands and/or feet, the pressure of massage over these areas needs to be gentle because the client may not be able to give accurate feedback. Joint mobilizations and stretching can help the client maintain flexibility. The massage therapist must communicate with the client about the pressure and effectiveness of techniques. Lubricants may alleviate the client's dry skin. The client may experience light-headedness when getting up from the massage table; be ready to assist.

Hypopituitarism
(hai`·poh·pi·too`·uh·tar´·ee·izm)

Gr. Under; L. Phlegm; Gr. Condition

Description—Hypopituitarism is a decrease in the secretion of hormones by the pituitary gland. If it occurs during childhood, it results in dwarfism (see Figure 6-13). If it occurs during adulthood, it can result in infertility, lethargy, dry, thick skin, hypoglycemia, loss of appetite, hypotension, abdominal pain, and intolerance to cold.

Massage Consideration/s—The massage therapist needs to obtain clearance for massage from the client's health care provider if symptoms are severe. The massage therapist should ask the client about his or her vitality and sensitivity to pressure. If the

hands and feet, dry, scaly skin, and a rapid, irregular heartbeat.

Massage Consideration/s—The massage therapist needs to obtain clearance for massage from the client's health care provider if symptoms are severe. The massage therapist should ask the client about his or her vitality, sensitivity to pressure, whether there is muscle tension, and, if so, in which

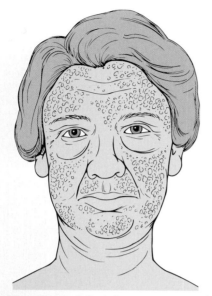

Figure 6-15. Typical facial appearance of myxedematous female.

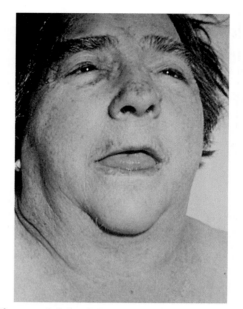

Figure 6-16. Woman with myxedema.

client is vital, then vigorous massage can be performed, within the client's tolerance. If the client is debilitated, the massage should be more gentle and relaxing so as not to overtire the client. Gliding strokes and kneading can help relieve muscle pain. The massage therapist must communicate with the client about the pressure and effectiveness of techniques. If the client chills easily, make sure the client is properly covered at all times with a sheet and a blanket. The therapist needs to be aware that the client may experience light-headedness when getting up from the massage table; be ready to assist.

Hypothyroidism (hai`·poh·thai´·roi·di`·zuhm)

Gr. Under; Shield; Condition

Description—A deficiency of thyroid hormone secretion, hypothyroidism in the adult years is called myxedema. It is marked by fatigue and lethargy, weight gain, slowed mental processes, skin dryness, and slow digestive, heart, and respiration rates. Other symptoms include waxy swelling of the skin, and excessive swelling of the face, hands, and feet. The edema is nonpitting and there are distinctive facial changes such as a bulbous nose and swollen lips (Figure 6-15). This condition is more common in women (Figure 6-16). Congenital hypothyroidism (cretinism) occurs at birth.

Massage Consideration/s—The massage therapist needs to obtain clearance for massage from the client's health care provider if symptoms are severe.

The massage therapist should ask the client about his or her vitality and sensitivity to pressure. If the client is vital, then vigorous massage can be performed, within the client's tolerance. If the client is debilitated, the massage should be more gentle and relaxing so as not to overtire the client. Gliding strokes and kneading can help relieve muscle pain. When massaging the throat area, perform a tissue release by gently lifting the skin from the superficial fascia over the thyroid cartilage. Manual traction of the cervical vertebrae and light nerve strokes are often helpful. The massage therapist needs to communicate with the client about the pressure and effectiveness of techniques. If the client chills easily, make sure the client is properly covered at all times with a sheet and a blanket. The client may experience light-headedness when getting up from the massage table; be ready to assist.

Myxedema (mik`·suh·dee´·muh)

Gr. Mucus; Swelling

Description—See entry for hypothyroidism in this chapter.

Seasonal Affective Disorder (SAD)

Description—SAD is a type of depression that affects some people during winter months, when day length is shorter than in summer months. Overproduction of melanin occurs and is thought to be at least a partial cause of the depression. Doses of exposure to full-spectrum bright light can provide some relief.

Massage Consideration/s—Massage can be performed on clients with SAD and may help relieve some of the symptoms of depression, as massage can give a client a sense of well-being. The massage therapist needs to ask the client about energy levels, and whether the levels cycle throughout the day. If the client is debilitated, the massage should be more gentle and relaxing so as not to overtire the client. Massage treatments can be scheduled during high-energy times to help in relaxing the client. Or, massage treatments could be scheduled during low-energy times to help rejuvenate the client. The massage therapist also needs to ask the client about his or her vitality and sensitivity to pressure. If the client is vital, then vigorous massage can be performed, within the client's tolerance. The therapist needs to communicate with the client about the pressure and effectiveness of the techniques.

SUMMARY

The endocrine system is a key player in maintaining homeostasis in the body. The main function of the endocrine system is to produce and secrete hormones, which in turn regulate growth and development, metabolism, and fluid balance; maintain homeostasis; and contribute to the reproductive process.

Hormones are the chemical messengers of the body. They may act directly on physiological activities, or they may act as a catalyst and stimulate a physiological reaction from another organ, tissue, or cell.

Endocrine glands are ductless and secrete their products directly into the bloodstream. Endocrine glands include the pituitary, pineal, thyroid, parathyroid, and adrenal glands. Some organs and tissues are not endocrine glands but do contain cells that secrete hormones. These include the hypothalamus, thymus, pancreas, ovaries, testes, kidneys, stomach, liver, small intestine, skin, heart, adipose tissue, and placenta. Common pathologies of these glands include acromegaly, Addison's disease, cretinism, Cushing's disease, diabetes insipidus, diabetes mellitus, goiter, Graves' disease, hyperparathyroidism, hyperpituitarism, hyperthyroidism, hypoglycemia, hypoparathyroidism, hypopituitarism, hypothyroidism, and myxedema.

Endocrine pathologies may be suspected when symptoms include glandular dysfunction; lumps, nodules, or masses of the anterior throat; neuropathy; changes in skin pigmentation and condition; longstanding skin lesions; tachycardia; nervousness; tremors; unexplained weight loss or weight gain; painless foot lesions; extreme thirst or urination; and recurrent or progressive infections. The massage therapist needs to refer the client to a physician immediately when these symptoms are present. Other signs to look for during assessment include dehydration, lymphedema, slow healing, anxiety, vision problems, diabetic medications, and menstrual cycle problems.

Resources

American Diabetes Association
800.ADA-DISC
703-549-1500 (In Virginia and Washington, DC)
www.diabetes.org

American Thyroid Association
Mayo Clinic
200 First Street NW
Rochester, MN 55905
www.thyroid.org
and
www.thyroid.com

Endocrine Society
9650 Rockville Pike
Bethesda, MD 20814
www.endo-society.org

National Diabetes Information Clearinghouse
PO Box NDIC
Bethesda, MD 20892
301-468-2162
www.niddk.nih.gov

SELF-TEST

List the letter of the answer to the term or phrase that best describes it.

A. Acromegaly
B. Addison's disease
C. Cretinism
D. Cushing's disease
E. Diabetes insipidus
F. Diabetes mellitus
G. Graves' disease
H. Hyperparathyroidism
I. Hyperpituitarism
J. Hyperthyroidism
K. Hypoglycemia
L. Hypoparathyroidism
M. Hypopituitarism
N. Hypothyroidism

_____ 1. An overproduction of parathyroid hormone resulting in an increased reabsorption of calcium from the bones and an increased absorption of calcium by the kidneys and gastrointestinal tract.

_____ 2. Also called hypoadrenalism, this condition is characterized by general weakness, decreased tolerance, and an increase in pigmentation of the skin and mucous membranes (called bronzing).

_____ 3. This disease is due to an increase in growth hormone and causes acromegaly during adulthood or gigantism during childhood and puberty.

_____ 4. A condition resulting from diminished function of the parathyroid gland.

_____ 5. Also called hyperadrenalism, this metabolic disorder is caused by an overproduction of adrenocortical steroids, resulting in an accumulation of fluids and fat on the face, neck, and upper back.

_____ 6. This disease is characterized by hyperactivity and an enlarged thyroid; nervous-ness and tremor; heat intolerance; increased appetite with weight loss; rapid, forceful pulse; and increased respiration rate.

_____ 7. This type of hyperpituitarism is characterized by elongation and enlargement of the bones of the extremities, face, and jaw.

_____ 8. This group of disorders leads to elevated blood glucose levels; kinds are type 1 and type 2.

_____ 9. A disease resulting in a decrease in blood glucose levels that can lead to a variety of symptoms including weakness, light-headedness, headaches, excessive hunger, visual disturbances, anxiety, and sudden changes in personality; if left untreated, the result may be delirium, diabetic coma, and death.

_____ 10. A disease characterized by hyperthyroidism and associated anxiety, fatigue, tremors of the hands, loss of appetite, increased metabolic rate, enlarged thyroid, enlarged lymph nodes, as well as an unusual protrusion of the eyeballs.

_____ 11. A deficiency of thyroid hormone secretion marked by fatigue and lethargy; weight gain; slowed mental processes; skin dryness; and slow digestive, heart, and respiration rates.

_____ 12. A congenital deficiency in the secretion of thyroid hormones characterized by arrested physical and mental development.

_____ 13. A decrease in secretion of pituitary hormones. If it occurs during childhood, it results in dwarfism. If it occurs during adulthood, it can result in infertility; lethargy; dry, thick skin; hypoglycemia; loss of appetite; hypotension; abdominal pain; and intolerance to cold.

_____ 14. Caused by a posterior pituitary gland dysfunction that results in deficient production of ADH. Symptoms are similar to diabetes mellitus.

7

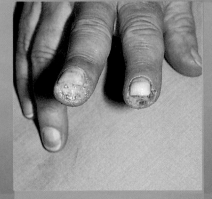

Cardiovascular and Lymphatic/Immune Pathologies

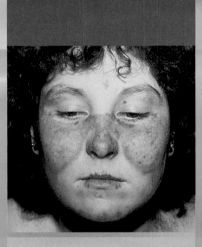

Heart disease and other cardiovascular disorders are the most prevalent diseases in industrialized countries. There is no question that massage therapists will encounter clients with all manners of pathologies of the blood, heart, and blood vessels. Therefore it is extremely important for massage therapists to have a good understanding of the anatomy and physiology of the cardiovascular system. With this understanding, massage therapists will then be able to understand cardiovascular pathologies and develop appropriate massage treatment plans for clients with these diseases.

The lymphatic/immune system is one of the major protectors from disease. It is amazing how many disease-producing organisms are nearby; what is more amazing is that humans do not get sick more often than they do. They have their lymphatic/immune system to thank for that. With all the diseases that modern medicine has been able to eliminate or control, there are still quite a few that can attack the body. It is important for massage therapists to understand the anatomy and physiology of the lymphatic/immune system so that they can also understand the pathologies of this system. Massage therapists will then be able to know the best approaches for massaging clients with particular lymphatic/immune pathologies. More important, they will also know when massage is inappropriate and the client needs to be referred to his or her health care provider.

The cardiovascular and lymphatic/immune systems play major roles in maintaining homeostasis. Most of the body's cells are embedded in tissues and thus are stationary. They cannot move around and obtain oxygen and nutrients; nor can they remove carbon dioxide, heat, and other wastes they produce or move away from changes in pH. Instead, three fluids interact to service these stationary cells: the blood (part of the cardiovascular system), interstitial fluid (discussed next), and lymph (part of the lymphatic/immune system).

Blood transports oxygen from the lungs and nutrients from the digestive tract to the body's cells. Interstitial fluid not only surrounds and bathes the cells and tissues, it also functions as a medium for exchange between the blood and the tissues; oxygen and nutrients move from the blood through the interstitial fluid into tissues. Carbon dioxide, wastes, heat, and cellular products such as enzymes and hormones move from the tissues through the interstitial fluid, and they and some of the interstitial fluid then enter the blood, which carries them away from the tissues.

Some of the interstitial fluid continually drains into lymphatic vessels and becomes lymph. After undergoing a sophisticated filtering process to remove pathogens and cellular debris, lymph returns to and becomes part of blood.

The body's homeostasis depends on the continual movements of blood, interstitial fluid, and lymph, and of having the right amount of each of these fluids. If not enough interstitial fluid enters the blood or drains into lymphatic vessels, the excess interstitial fluid around the tissues is called edema.

Because the cardiovascular and lymphatic/immune systems are responsible for fluid movement and maintenance, they may be collectively referred to as the circulatory system. In this discussion, however, the two divisions are discussed separately.

The main components of the cardiovascular system are the blood, heart, and blood vessels. Blood consists of a liquid portion called plasma and blood cells (corpuscles) (Figure 7-1). There are three types of blood cells (Figure 7-2). Erythrocytes, or red blood cells, are biconcave disks containing hemoglobin. Hemoglobin is responsible for carrying oxygen in the blood. Leukocytes are white blood cells. There are many types of leukocytes; they all function to protect the body against pathogens. Thrombocytes, or platelets, are responsible for clotting mechanisms that occur to prevent excessive blood loss, called hemorrhage, when vessels are damaged. Blood also contains plasma proteins, which provide a variety of functions. Some are transporters, some help with blood coagulation, some are part of the lymphatic/immune system, and some are enzymes and hormones.

In addition to transporting oxygen, nutrients, carbon dioxide, heat, ions wastes, enzymes, and hormones, blood has other functions. It helps regulate pH because it contains buffers. Buffers are

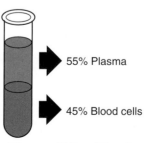

55% Plasma

45% Blood cells

Figure 7-1. Blood.

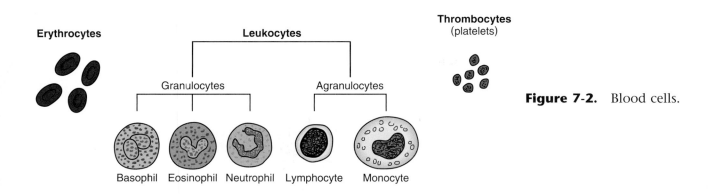

Figure 7-2. Blood cells.

chemicals that help neutralize acids and bases; these are produced as cellular by-products of the cell's metabolic activities. Blood also helps adjust body temperature. Blood is made mainly of water, which can absorb heat produced from cellular metabolism. As blood flows through the skin, excess heat can then be lost to the external environment. Blood can clot, which, as stated previously, protects against its excessive loss as a result of injury. Plasma proteins called antibodies and the leukocytes protect the body from disease.

The purpose of the heart is to pump the blood through a vast closed network of blood vessels (Figure 7-3). Surrounding and protecting the heart is the pericardium. The outer layer of the pericardium is composed of tough, fibrous, connective tissue. The inner layer of the pericardium consists of two layers of membrane with serous fluid in between to decrease friction as the heart beats.

The heart itself is mainly thick myocardium. The myocardium is cardiac muscle, which is responsible for the pumping action of the heart. The inner layer of the heart is called the endocardium, and the outer layer is called the epiordium.

The heart is divided into four chambers: two superior chambers called the atria (atrium is singular), and two inferior chambers called the ventricles. Between the right atrium and the right ventricle is the tricuspid valve. Between the left atrium and the left ventricle is the mitral (bicuspid) valve.

The major blood vessels associated with the heart are the superior vena cava, the inferior vena cava, the pulmonary trunk (which splits into right and left pulmonary arteries and pulmonary veins), aorta, the coronary sinus, and coronary arteries. The pulmonary trunk connects with the right ventricle. The valve between the right ventricle and the pulmonary trunk is the pulmonary semilunar valve. The aorta connects with the left ventricle. The valve between the left ventricle and the aorta is called the aortic semilunar valve. All the valves associated with the heart and major blood vessels help regulate blood flow through and out of the heart.

The right atrium receives deoxygenated blood from the entire body via the superior vena cava, the inferior vena cava, and the coronary sinus. All the veins of the body eventually empty their deoxygenated blood into one of these three veins. The flow of blood from the heart to the lungs and back is called pulmonary circulation (Figure 7-4). The deoxygenated blood pushes open the tricuspid valve and enters the right ventricle. The right ventricle contracts, the blood pushes open the pulmonary semilunar valve, and the blood enters the pulmonary trunk. The deoxygenated blood is then carried by the right and left pulmonary arteries (the only arteries in the body to carry deoxygenated blood) to each of the lungs. In the lungs, blood picks up oxygen and gives up carbon dioxide. The blood, which is now oxygenated, returns to the heart through pulmonary veins (the only veins in the body to carry oxygenated blood). The pulmonary veins empty the blood into the left atrium. The oxygenated blood pushes open the bicuspid valve and enters the left ventricle. The left ventricle contracts, and blood pushes open the aortic semilunar valve; the blood then enters the aorta, which carries the oxygenated blood out to the entire body.

It is important to note that blood enters both the right and left atria at the same time; it goes from the atria into the right and left ventricles at the same time; and both ventricles contract at the same time, ejecting blood into the pulmonary trunk and the aorta at the same time. Thus the heart is actually two pumps—the right ventricle pumps blood to the lungs at the same time that the left ventricle pumps blood into the aorta and on into the systemic circulation.

The heart has its own blood supply, which is called coronary circulation. The coronary arteries branch off the aorta. The coronary arteries continue to branch, supplying the thick wall of the heart by

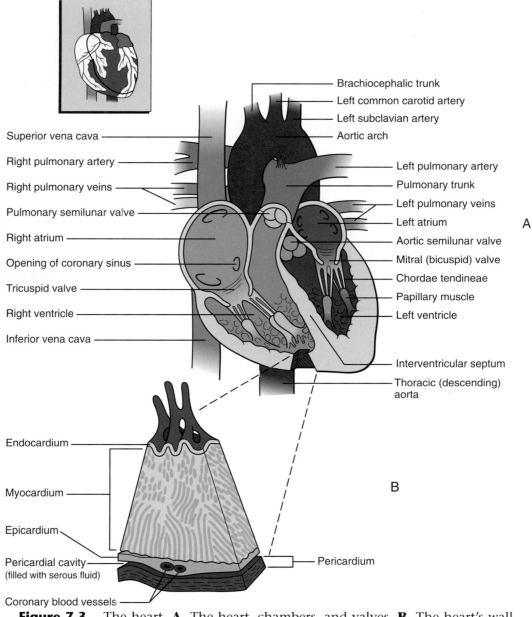

Brachiocephalic trunk
Left common carotid artery
Left subclavian artery
Aortic arch
Superior vena cava
Right pulmonary artery
Right pulmonary veins
Pulmonary semilunar valve
Right atrium
Opening of coronary sinus
Tricuspid valve
Right ventricle
Inferior vena cava
Left pulmonary artery
Pulmonary trunk
Left pulmonary veins
Left atrium
Aortic semilunar valve
Mitral (bicuspid) valve
Chordae tendineae
Papillary muscle
Left ventricle
Interventricular septum
Thoracic (descending) aorta
A

Endocardium
Myocardium
Epicardium
Pericardial cavity (filled with serous fluid)
Coronary blood vessels
Pericardium
B

Figure 7-3. The heart. **A,** The heart, chambers, and valves. **B,** The heart's wall.

winnowing into its tissues. After exchange occurs, coronary veins drain the deoxygenated blood into the coronary sinus, which drains into the right atrium. Coronary artery disease is the number 1 killer of men and women in the United States, causing 750,000 deaths a year.

The pumping action of the heart occurs as a result of its conduction system (Figure 7-5).

The heart has a property called autorhythmicity; it is able to repeatedly generate its own electrical impulses. Outside innervation is not necessary to make the heartbeat. The impulses the heart generates travel through a specific pathway in the heart,

the conduction system, which ensures a regular, coordinated heartbeat.

The nerve impulse is generated in the sinoatrial (SA) node, which is also called the pacemaker, because it "sets the pace" for the rest of the heart to beat. The nerve impulse from the SA node travels through the atria. This impulse causes both atria to contract at the same time. While the atria are contracting, the ventricles are relaxing.

When the impulse reaches the inferior part of the right atrium, it contacts the atrioventricular (AV) node. The AV node then sends the impulse to the AV bundle or the bundle of His located in the inter-

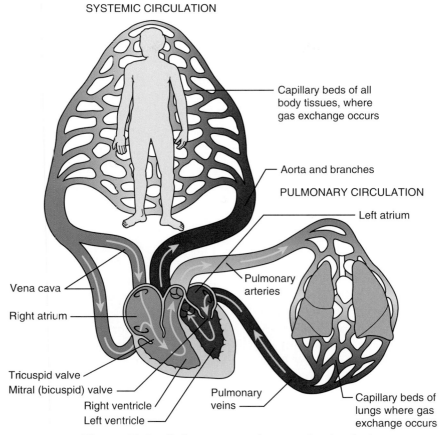

SYSTEMIC CIRCULATION

Capillary beds of all body tissues, where gas exchange occurs

Aorta and branches

PULMONARY CIRCULATION

Left atrium

Vena cava

Pulmonary arteries

Right atrium

Tricuspid valve

Mitral (bicuspid) valve

Right ventricle

Left ventricle

Pulmonary veins

Capillary beds of lungs where gas exchange occurs

Figure 7-4. Pulmonary and systemic circulations.

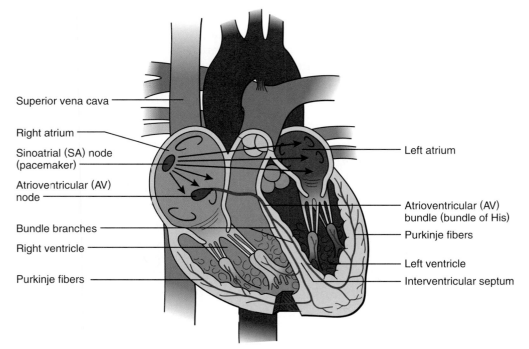

Superior vena cava

Right atrium

Sinoatrial (SA) node (pacemaker)

Atrioventricular (AV) node

Bundle branches

Right ventricle

Purkinje fibers

Left atrium

Atrioventricular (AV) bundle (bundle of His)

Purkinje fibers

Left ventricle

Interventricular septum

Figure 7-5. The heart's conduction system.

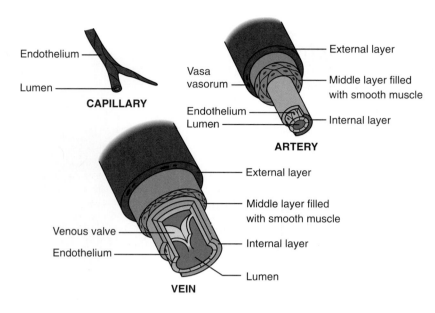

Figure 7-6. Blood vessels.

ventricular septum. The AV bundle splits into right and left bundle branches. These branches send the impulse to the right and left ventricles via the Purkinje fibers. The right and left ventricles then contract, and at this point the atria relax.

Although the heart does not need outside innervation to beat, heart rate and force of contraction can be influenced by hormones and other nerves. For instance, the hormone epinephrine (adrenaline) and nerve impulses from the sympathetic division of the autonomic nervous system increase heart rate and the force of contraction. Nerve impulses from the parasympathetic division of the autonomic nervous system decrease heart rate.

The blood vessels are a closed system of tubes the blood travels through. In systemic circulation, arteries carry blood away from the heart (see Figure 7-4), so they carry oxygenated blood. The only exceptions are the pulmonary arteries, discussed previously; they carry deoxygenated blood, but they carry it away from the heart to the lungs. Arteries have thick walls with lots of smooth muscle tissue and elastic tissue (Figure 7-6). The elastic tissue allows the arteries to stretch and accommodate the surge of blood coming out of the heart. Elastic recoil then moves the blood farther along. The smooth muscle tissue contracts and relaxes, regulating blood pressure.

Arteries branch off the aorta to distribute blood to various regions of the body (Figure 7-7). Arteries continue to branch, becoming smaller and smaller, until they become arterioles. Arterioles do not have the thick walls that arteries have. They have a single layer of tissue covered by some smooth muscle.

Arterioles enter the tissues and become narrower vessels called capillaries. Exchange between the blood and interstitial fluid occurs at the capillary level. Capillaries have just a single layer of epithelial tissue, which makes it easier for substances to move through. Capillaries join into venules; venules exit the tissues.

Venules also have a single layer of tissue and some smooth muscle. They drain deoxygenated blood into veins, moving deoxygenated blood back to the heart. The only exceptions are the pulmonary veins, discussed previously; they carry oxygenated blood from the lungs to the heart. Veins are made of smooth muscle and elastic tissue, but their walls are much thinner than arterial walls. Blood also moves much more slowly in veins than in arteries because the force of the heartbeat is no longer driving blood flow. Skeletal muscles help move blood through the veins by contracting and squeezing the veins in a pumping action. Also, veins have valves in their walls to prevent backflow of blood (Figure 7-8).

The lymphatic/immune system is composed of lymph, lymphatic vessels, structures and organs containing lymphatic tissue (lymph nodes, lymphatic nodules, thymus gland, and spleen), lymphocytes (specialized leukocytes), and red bone marrow (Figure 7-9). There are three primary functions of the lymphatic/immune system.

The first function is to drain excess interstitial fluid. As stated previously, the interstitial fluid enters lymphatic vessels, specifically lymphatic capillaries. Lymphatic capillaries have a structure similar to blood capillaries except that they have

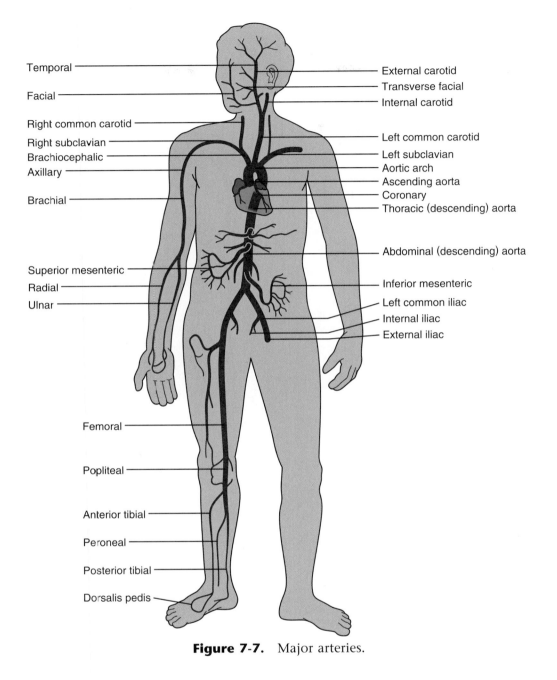

Temporal

Facial

Right common carotid

Right subclavian

Brachiocephalic

Axillary

Brachial

Superior mesenteric

Radial

Ulnar

External carotid

Transverse facial

Internal carotid

Left common carotid

Left subclavian

Aortic arch

Ascending aorta

Coronary

Thoracic (descending) aorta

Abdominal (descending) aorta

Inferior mesenteric

Left common iliac

Internal iliac

External iliac

Femoral

Popliteal

Anterior tibial

Peroneal

Posterior tibial

Dorsalis pedis

Figure 7-7. Major arteries.

larger diameters and fluid only flows into them, not into and out of them as with blood capillaries. Lymphatic capillaries drain lymph into larger lymphatic vessels, which have lymph nodes situated along their path. Lymph nodes contain lymphatic tissue that filters out pathogens and cellular debris.

The lymphatic vessels drain lymph into larger and larger vessels, eventually draining lymph into two large veins near the neck—the right and left subclavian veins. In contrast to the circuit formed by the cardiovascular system, the lymphatic system is a one-way system of drainage (Figure 7-10). Like venous blood flow, lymphatic flow is maintained by contraction of skeletal muscles.

The second function of the lymphatic/immune system is to transport dietary lipids and lipid-soluble vitamins (A, D, E, and K) from the digestive tract to the blood. Lipids and lipid-soluble vitamins are large molecules that cannot fit into blood capillaries. Thus when they are absorbed from the digestive tract, they move into the larger-diameter lymphatic capillaries instead, entering the blood when lymph drains back into the bloodstream.

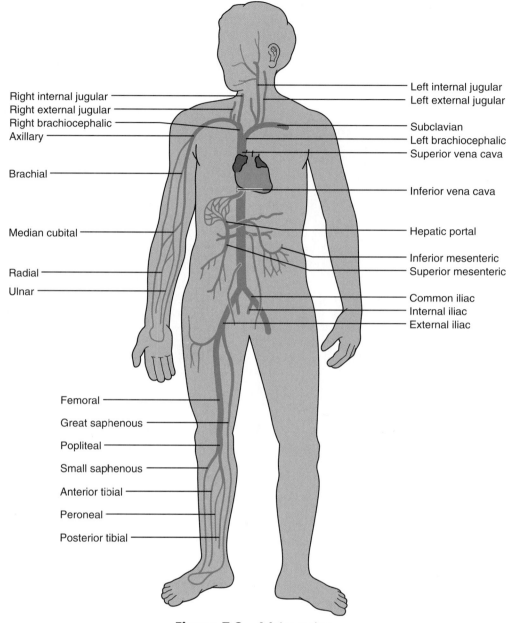

Right internal jugular
Right external jugular
Right brachiocephalic
Axillary

Brachial

Median cubital

Radial

Ulnar

Femoral

Great saphenous

Popliteal

Small saphenous

Anterior tibial

Peroneal

Posterior tibial

Left internal jugular
Left external jugular

Subclavian
Left brachiocephalic
Superior vena cava

Inferior vena cava

Hepatic portal

Inferior mesenteric
Superior mesenteric

Common iliac
Internal iliac
External iliac

Figure 7-8.   Major veins.

The third function of the lymphatic/immune system is carrying out immune functions. The body has two major categories of defenses. The first is natural immunity. These are the body's first and second lines of defense, and they protect against a wide range of pathogens. A person is born with these defenses. They include skin and mucous membranes, stomach acid (gastric juice), inflammation, fever, and several antimicrobial proteins made by the body.

If pathogens penetrate the first and second lines of defense, the lymphatic system becomes acti-

vated. This process is referred to as acquired immunity and it involves lymphocytes.

All types of blood cells, including lymphocytes, are formed in the red bone marrow. Two main types of lymphocytes are created: T cells and B cells. To be able to recognize and attack pathogens, the T and B cells need to undergo a further maturing process. B cells continue to mature in the red bone marrow. T cells go to the thymus gland to complete their maturing process (Figure 7-11).

Once the T and B cells are mature, they travel to areas of lymphatic tissues. These include lymph

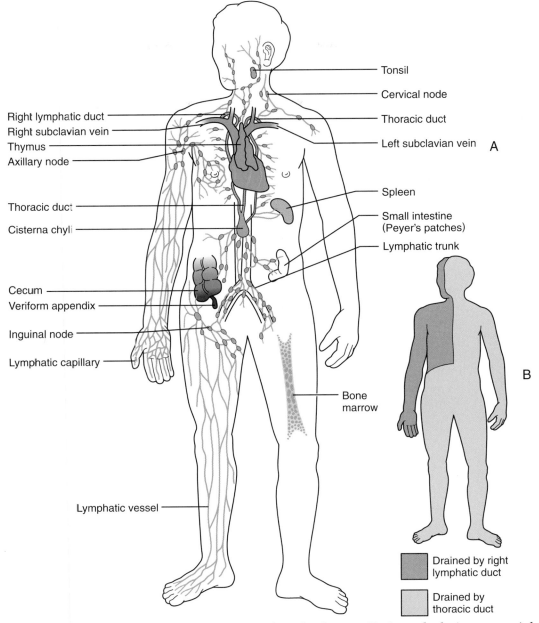

Tonsil

Cervical node

Right lymphatic duct

Right subclavian vein

Thymus

Axillary node

Thoracic duct

Left subclavian vein   A

Thoracic duct

Cisterna chyli

Spleen

Small intestine
(Peyer's patches)

Lymphatic trunk

Cecum

Veriform appendix

Inguinal node

Lymphatic capillary

Bone
marrow

B

Lymphatic vessel

Drained by right
lymphatic duct

Drained by
thoracic duct

Figure 7-9. The lymphatic organs. **A,** Lymph ducts and node clusters. **B,** Lymph drainage on right and left sides of body.

nodes, the lymphatic tissue inside the spleen, and lymphatic nodules, which are clusters of lymphatic tissue embedded in the mucous membranes of the respiratory, digestive, urinary, and reproductive tracts. Examples of lymphatic nodules are the tonsils, which form a ring at the back of the throat, Peyer's patches found in the small intestine, and lymphatic nodules found inside the appendix.

For T and B cells to mount an immune response, they need to come in contact and interact with

a pathogen. This contact and interaction can occur in three main ways: (1) the pathogen can travel through the lymph to a lymph node, (2) the pathogen can travel through the blood to the lymphatic tissue in the spleen, and (3) the pathogen can penetrate mucous membranes and come in contact with the embedded lymphatic nodules.

Once the T and B cells contact the pathogen, they are activated for that specific pathogen. The T

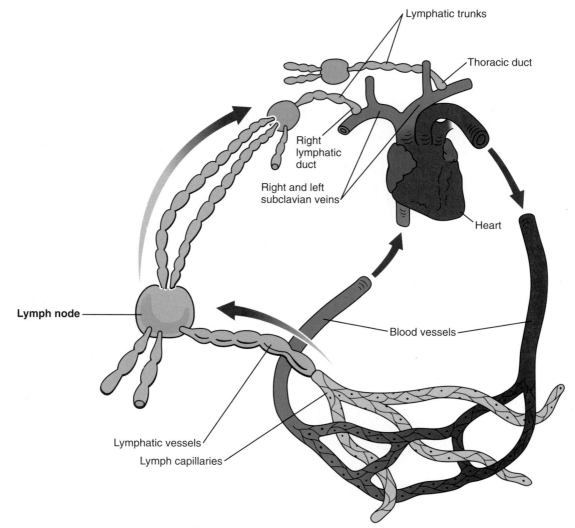

Figure 7-10. Lymph circulation.

and B cells clone themselves by the thousands, which accounts for the swelling of lymph nodes during infection. The T cells leave the lymphatic tissue and kill the pathogen as they come across it. The B cells produce antibodies that leave the lymphatic tissue and circulate in body fluids, like the blood. The antibodies inactivate pathogens as they come across them.

In autoimmune diseases, T and B cells are unable to distinguish the body's own tissues from something that is foreign to the body. They then attack the tissues. For instance, in rheumatoid arthritis, the immune system attacks the synovial lining of joints (Chapter 4); in multiple sclerosis, the immune system attacks the myelin sheath around neurons in the central nervous system (Chapter 5); in type 1 diabetes mellitus, the immune system attacks the insulin-producing cells of the pancreas (Chapter 6).

THERAPEUTIC ASSESSMENT OF THE CARDIOVASCULAR AND LYMPHATIC/IMMUNE SYSTEMS

The following list of pertinent questions serves as a review of how to evaluate the cardiovascular and lymphatic/immune systems. Findings need to be documented.

Questions to ask the client in the premassage interview:

- *Does the client have any cardiovascular conditions? Does the client have any lymphatic/immune system conditions?* These should include both current and previous conditions. For example, massage considerations for a client who experienced a heart attack 6 months before the massage are different from massage considerations for a heart attack 5 years before the massage.

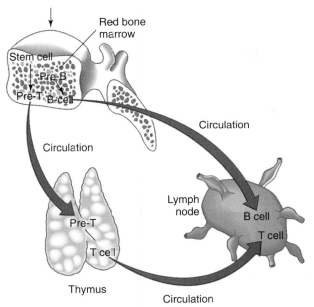

Figure 7-11. Development of B and T cells.

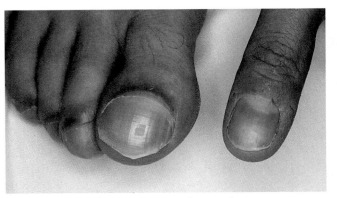

Figure 7-12. Cyanosis.

A client who has had a recent heart attack is still healing and benefits more from gentle, relaxing techniques. Deep pressure is contraindicated because it may cause the client pain, during which his heart may try to beat harder and faster. It puts an unnecessary load on the healing heart. A client who has recovered from a heart attack experienced several years before the massage and who has made lifestyle changes to maintain health can have more vigorous techniques and deeper pressure (within the client's tolerance) performed on him.

- *If the client has any cardiovascular disorders, is it being managed by medication? If nitroglycerine is being used, is it nearby if needed?* Table 7-1 has more information including possible side effects.
- *Does the client have a pacemaker, an implantable cardioverter defibrillator (ICD), or central venous catheter?* The massage therapist needs to be prepared to use the modified supine position, side-lying position, or seated position if needed. Pillows and bolsters may provide extra comfort and support. Boxes 7-1, 7-2, and 7-3 have additional information.
- *Does the client experience shortness of breath? Are there any positions that help or make it worse?* The massage therapist needs to be prepared to use the modified supine position, side-lying position, or seated position if needed.

- *Does the client complain of fatigue, anxiety, insomnia, or headaches?* These may be indicators of cardiovascular disease or medication side effects. The massage therapist needs to discuss these symptoms with the client, and may need to refer the client to the client's health care provider for evaluation or clearance before proceeding with massage.
- *Does the client have any hives or rashes on the skin?* These areas need to be avoided during the massage.

Observations and palpations to make during the premassage interview and during the massage treatment:

- *What is the condition of the client's skin?* It should be assessed for color (bruising, pallor, flushing, jaundice, cyanosis, superficial varicosities) and temperature (client may be cold or hot or may feel cold/hot to the touch) (Figure 7-12).
- *Are the client's nail bed color and shape in good condition?* Chapter 2 has a discussion of nail clubbing and spooning.
- *Are there any signs of edema (e.g., pitting edema or molted skin)?* If so, caution is advised. The massage therapist needs to ascertain the cause of the edema from the client, and clearance may need to be obtained from the client's health care provider before massage therapy can be performed. If the edema is not due to a serious condition such as congestive heart failure or renal failure, massage can be performed. If indicated, the massage therapist should elevate the affected area during treatment to promote drainage and perform lymphatic drainage techniques.
- *Can any swollen lymph nodes be palpated?* This often indicates local or systemic

Table **7-1** MEDICATIONS USED TO MANAGE CARDIOVASCULAR DISEASE

MEDICATION CLASSIFICATION	MEDICATION NAME	POSSIBLE SIDE EFFECTS THAT MAY AFFECT TREATMENT
Alpha receptor drugs	Doxazosin (Cardura), prazosin (Minipress), tamsulosin (Flomax), terazosin (Hytrin)	Abdominal discomfort, anxiety, constipation and diarrhea, edema, hypertension, irregular heartbeat, joint pain, nausea and vomiting, skin rashes, vertigo
Angiotensin-converting enzyme inhibitors (ACE inhibitors)	Benazepril (Lotensin), captopril (Capoten), enalapril (Vasotec), fosinopril (Monopril), lisinopril (Prinivil, Zestril), moexipril (Univasc), perindopril (Aceon), quinapril (Accupril), ramipril (Altace), trandolapril (Mavik)	Anxiety, chest pain, diarrhea, dry mouth, edema, fever, gastrointestinal irritation, headaches, hypotension, insomnia, joint pain, lethargy, nausea and vomiting, vertigo
Hematological agents*	Acetylsalicylic acid (aspirin), dipyridamole (Persantine), heparin, streptokinase, warfarin (Coumadin), clopidogrel (Plavix)	Abdominal pain, gastric irritation, hemorrhage, nausea, skin rashes
Beta blockers	Acebutolol (Sectral), atenolol (Tenormin), bisoprolol (Zebeta), carteolol (Cartrol), carvedilol (Coreg), labetolol (Trandate), metoprolol (Lopressor, Toprol-XL), nadolol (Corgard), pindolol, propranolol (Inderal), sotalol (Betapace), timolol (Blocadren)	Abdominal pain, anxiety, bruising, chest pain, chills, constipation and diarrhea, disorientation, drowsiness, dry mouth, edema, fever, headaches, hypotension, insomnia, irregular heartbeat, joint pain, lethargy, nausea and vomiting, shortness of breath, skin rashes, vertigo
Calcium channel blockers	Amlodipine (Norvasc), bepridil (Vascor), Diltiazem (Cardizem, Cartia-XT, Dilacor-XR, Diltia-XT, Tiazac), Felodipine (Plendil), Isradipine (Dynacirc), Nicardipine (Cardene), Nimodipine (Nimotop), Nifedipine (Adalat, Procardia), Nisoldipine (Sular), Verapamil (Calan, Covera-HS, Isoptin, Verelan)	Allergic reaction, anxiety, chest pain, drowsiness, dry mouth, fever, headaches, hypotension, insomnia, irregular heartbeat, joint pain, lethargy, nausea, shortness of breath, skin rashes, vertigo
Cardiac glycosides	Digitalis compounds (digoxin, Lanoxin)	Allergic reactions, diarrhea, disorientation, hallucinations, irregular heartbeat, nausea and vomiting

Table 7-1 MEDICATIONS USED TO MANAGE CARDIOVASCULAR DISEASE—CONT'D

MEDICATION CLASSIFICATION	MEDICATION NAME	POSSIBLE SIDE EFFECTS THAT MAY AFFECT TREATMENT
Diuretics	Amiloride (Midamor), bumetanide (Bumex), chlorothiazide (Diuril), hydrochlorothiazide (Esidrix, Oretic) spironolactone (Aldactone), triamterene (Dyrenium, Dyazide, Maxzide) furosemide (Lasix), torsemide (Demadex)	Diarrhea, disorientation, dry mouth, gastrointestinal irritation, headaches, hyperglycemia, lethargy, muscle cramps/spasms, nausea and vomiting, shortness of breath, vertigo
Lipid-lowering drugs	Bile acid sequestrants [cholestyramine (Questran), colesevelam (Welchol), colestipol (Colestid)] Fibric acid derivatives [clofibrate, fenofibrate (Tricor), gemfibrozil (Lopid)] HMG Co A reductase inhibitors [atorvastatin (Lipitor), fluvastatin (Lescol), lovastatin (Mevacor), pravastatin (Pravachol), simvastatin (Zocor)] Nicotinic acid [niacin (Nicolar)]	Abdominal cramps, allergic reactions, bruising, chest pain, constipation, disorientation, drowsiness, dry mouth, fever, flushing, gastrointestinal irritation, gout, hypoglycemia, hypertension and hypotension, insomnia, irregular heartbeat, joint pain, lethargy, nausea and vomiting, shortness of breath, vertigo
Vasodilators	Nitroglycerin	Anxiety, disorientation, edema, headaches, hypotension, irregular heartbeat, joint pain, nausea, skin rashes, vertigo

When clients are taking anticoagulants and platelet inhibitors, massage techniques such as deep effleurage (e.g., ironing); deep petrissage; ischemic compression; and deep, specific frictions (e.g., crossfiber, chucking, circular) should be carefully monitored or avoided. These specific techniques often produce a mild inflammatory response that is usually resolved within 48 hours. Performing these techniques when a client is taking these medications may result in internal bleeding (bruising) and excessive inflammatory response.

infection. Massage may be contraindicated if the client has an infection.

GENERAL MANIFESTATIONS OF THE CARDIOVASCULAR AND LYMPHATIC/IMMUNE DISEASES

If a client has any of the following, the massage therapist needs to refer the client to the client's health care provider for diagnosis and treatment.

- Bradycardia (lower than normal heart rate) or tachycardia (higher than normal heart rate)
- Difficulty or rapid breathing
- Skin discolorations (pallor, redness, jaundice, cyanosis)
- Unexplained bruising or skin pigmentation
- Presence of rashes, hives, or scaliness (with or without itching)
- Unexplained chest or calf pain
- Swollen lymph nodes
- Edema as evidenced by pitting edema, molted skin, or limbs of unequal circumference
- Limbs unequal in temperature
- History of chronic fatigue
- Failure to gain or maintain weight
- Unexplained weight loss

Box **7-1**

Artificial Pacemaker

An artificial pacemaker is a surgically implanted device that sends out small electrical currents to stimulate the heart to contract. Newer pacemakers are activity-adjusted pacemakers that automatically speed up the heartbeat during exercise. The artificial pacemaker is implanted under the skin with wires going directly to the sinoatrial node or the atrioventricular node.

Because the site is usually very sensitive, local massage is contraindicated. The primary concern is to make sure the incision from the surgery has completely healed. While the client is prone, a soft pillow to be placed under the chest should be offered. This will provide added comfort for the client during the massage.

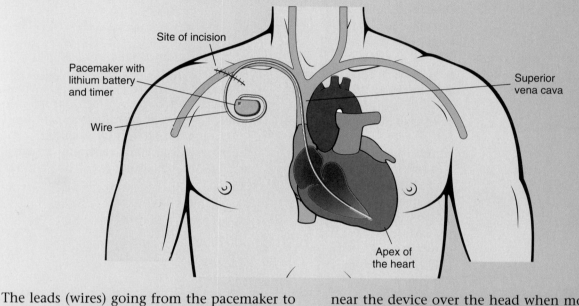

Site of incision

Pacemaker with lithium battery and timer

Wire

Superior vena cava

Apex of the heart

The leads (wires) going from the pacemaker to the heart often travel up over the clavicle and down into the chest cavity. For this reason, the massage therapist should avoid moving the arm near the device over the head when mobilizing the shoulder joint, as it may disturb the lead connections.

CARDIOVASCULAR PATHOLOGIES

Anemia

Gr. Without; Blood

Description—Anemia is a reduction of the oxygen-carrying capacity of the blood, a decrease in erythrocytes, or a reduced amount of functional hemoglobin in the blood. It is usually a sign of other disorders. Characteristics of anemia include fatigue, dizziness, headaches, insomnia, paleness, and intolerance to cold. There are many types of anemia. The most common type is iron-deficiency anemia resulting from insufficient iron intake or blood loss. Other types of anemia include pernicious, hemolytic, and hemorrhagic. Vitamin B_{12} is needed for healthy red blood cell production. Pernicious anemia occurs when the stomach is unable to manufacture intrinsic factor, a substance needed for absorption of vitamin B_{12} from the digestive tract (Figure 7-13).

Treatment of pernicious anemia involves injections of vitamin B_{12}. In hemolytic anemia, the cell membranes of erythrocytes rupture prematurely. The liberated hemoglobin spills into the plasma and can damage the kidneys. Hemolytic anemia can be due to genetics (causing abnormal red blood cell enzymes) or from agents such as parasites, toxins, or antibodies from incompatible blood transfusions. Hemorrhagic anemia results when there is excessive loss of erythrocytes through bleeding, which could be due to wounds, stomach ulcers, or very heavy menstruation.

Massage Consideration/s—If a client indicates that he or she has anemia, the massage therapist needs to ask the client the type. Massage should be

Box 7-2

Implantable Cardioverter Defibrillator

The implantable cardioverter defibrillator is a device used to treat dangerously fast heart rates in the ventricles (see Box 7-6). It can detect heart rhythms and, when necessary, delivers an electrical shock to restore normal heart rate and rhythm. Much like a pacemaker, the defibrillator is implanted under the skin near the clavicle. It is attached to one or more leads positioned in the right ventricle, and right atrium when necessary. The electrical shock is painful to the client. The shock may be felt by the massage therapist if the client is touching the patient when the device discharges. It may feel like a tingling sensation, if felt at all, and is generally not harmful to the massage therapist. Massage should be discontinued if the device delivers a shock during treatment. The client then needs to seek immediate medical attention.

performed only when the client feels up to it. If the client is debilitated, the massage may, in fact, make the client feel worse and, therefore, should not be done. Massage techniques such as gliding strokes, kneading, and friction can help oxygenate an anemic client. If the anemia is due to a bleeding disorder, however, lighter pressure should be used, since the client may bruise easily.

Aneurysm

Gr. A Widening

Description—An aneurysm is a weakened section of a blood vessel wall that bulges outward (Figure 7-14). Common causes are atherosclerosis, hypertension, and trauma, but it can also be due to a congenital vascular weakness. The most common areas for aneurysms are the aorta and blood vessels in the brain, but they can occur in the extremities. Aneurysms may burst, causing hemorrhage and possibly death.

Massage Consideration/s—If a client has a history of hypertension or atherosclerosis, the massage therapist must consult the client's health care provider before performing deep pressure massage. If a client has been diagnosed with an abdominal aortic aneurysm, abdominal massage is contraindicated.

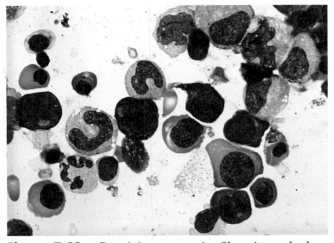

Figure 7-13. Pernicious anemia. Showing a lack of functional red blood cells in the blood.

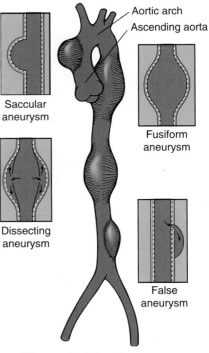

Figure 7-14. Aneurysms.

Box **7-3**

Central Venous Catheter

A central venous catheter, or central line, is a flexible tube that is inserted and sewn into a large vein (usually the right subclavian vein in the upper chest) and left in place for an extended period. This type of catheter is used to keep a vein open for dialysis, blood withdrawal, chemotherapy, and frequent administration of medications, which must be taken regularly and cannot be taken orally. The three common types of central venous catheters are Hickman catheters, Quinton catheters, and Groshong catheters. Another style of central venous catheter inserted under the skin of the chest wall, a port-a-cath, does not have an external opening.

The use of these catheters makes it difficult or impossible for the client to lie prone comfortably. The massage therapist should use bolsters, pillows, or other positional modifications such as a side-lying position for the client's comfort. Sometimes a small towel or washcloth over the area is all that is needed. The catheter is usually sutured to fascia and muscle. During the massage, the massage therapist should take precautions not to dislodge the catheter by exerting tension or excessive movement on nearby skin tissues. Avoid traction near the area or on joints near the area where

the device is located so as not to damage the device or the surrounding tissues. Avoid traction near the area or on joints near the area where the device is located so as not to damage the device or the surrounding tissues. Massage lubricant should not come into contact with the catheter dressing or sutures. If a catheter is placed in the arm, the area below the catheter should not be massaged because these tissues may be sensitive. Pressure from massage can also possibly damage the tissues. Massage work above the catheter in these extremities should be gentle. Avoid shoulder joint mobilizations near the device.

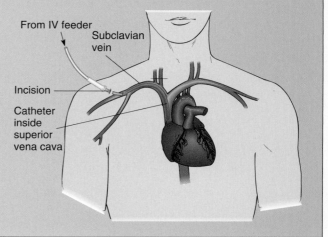

From IV feeder
Subclavian vein
Incision
Catheter inside superior vena cava

Angina Pectoris

L. To Choke; Chest

Description—Often felt as chest pain, angina pectoris is frequently caused by constriction of coronary arteries and myocardial anoxia (lack of oxygen in the heart muscle). The pain originates from the chest and may radiate down the inner side of the left arm and upper back or to the neck and throat. The pain travels in this pattern because of dermatomes and referred pain. Dermatomes are defined as the area of skin that provides sensory input into the central nervous system via a pair of spinal nerves or cranial nerve V. Referred pain in this instance is pain felt in the surface of the body distal to the stimulated organ. The organ involved and the area to where the pain is referred are served by the same segment of the spinal cord. The sensory nerves from the heart, the skin over the heart, and the skin up to the chin, down along the inner side

of the arm and upper back, enter the same spinal cord segments. That is why the pain of angina pectoris and a heart attack (myocardial infarction) is usually felt in the skin over the heart and along the left arm (Figure 7-15). The pain disappears with rest, and there is no lasting tissue damage. Angina pectoris is often associated with physical overexertion, when the heart needs more oxygen. Emotional stress and exposure to intense cold can also trigger angina pectoris.

Massage Consideration/s—Massage can help clients by reducing stress. Massage also decreases the effects of the sympathetic nervous system, which is partially responsible for coronary artery vasoconstriction. It is important that clients have with them their necessary medications (e.g., nitroglycerin) when they come for treatment, in the case of a medical emergency. Because sudden exposure to extreme cold or heat can bring on an attack, the massage therapist needs to keep the client warm during treatment but should avoid using heat or cold packs. If a client has an attack during a massage treatment, assist him or her in taking any necessary medications. If nitroglycerin is taken by the client while the client is in the office, make sure the client sits or lies down for at least an hour, as nitrates cause vasodilation and could induce fainting.

Arteriosclerosis (ahr·tee`·ree·oh·skluh·roh´·sis)

Gr. Air Pipe; Hardening

Description—Arteriosclerosis is a group of arterial diseases characterized by a thickening and loss of elasticity that leads to a hardening of the arterial walls. This can result in high blood

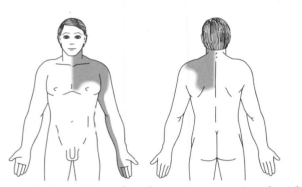

Figure 7-15. Pain referral patterns associated with angina.

pressure and/or a decrease in blood supply, especially to the brain, heart, or lower extremities. The patient is usually given a prescription of adequate rest, moderate exercise, and avoidance of stress.

Massage Consideration/s—It is recommended that the massage therapist obtain clearance from the client's health care provider. A gentle, relaxing massage can help the client with stress management. Deep pressure massage may cause pain, which can cause the client's blood pressure to increase.

Atherosclerosis (a`·thuh·roh`·skluh·roh´·sis)

Gr. Porridge; Hardening

Description—A type of arteriosclerosis, atherosclerosis is the narrowing and hardening of arteries caused by the accumulation of lipid plaques in their walls (Figure 7-16). Atherosclerosis is often associated with obesity, hypertension, and diabetes. The narrowed arteries reduce blood flow, especially to the heart and brain. Because the plaque has a rough surface, platelets can snag on it and rupture, forming clots, which can further impede blood flow (Figure 7-17).

Massage Consideration/s—Consulting the client's health care provider is recommended. A client who has atherosclerosis may be prone to thrombosis (blood clot) formation. Deep pressure massage may dislodge the thrombus that could travel as an embolus and lodge in smaller blood vessels in the lungs, heart, or brain, leading to dif-

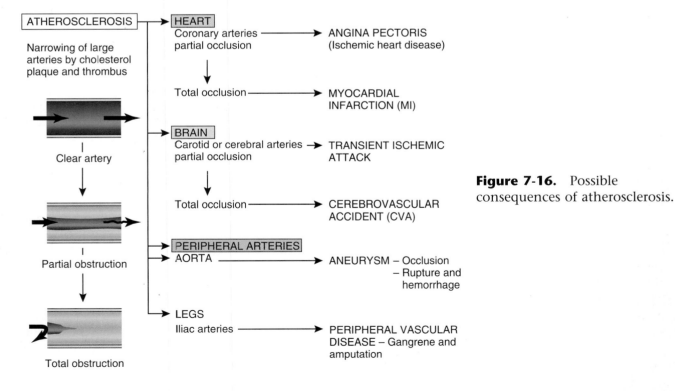

Figure 7-16. Possible consequences of atherosclerosis.

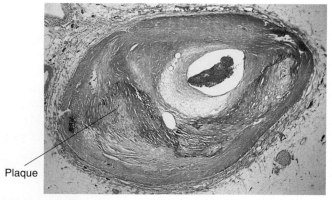

Figure 7-17. Atherosclerosis. Note the plaque that narrows the lumen of the coronary artery.

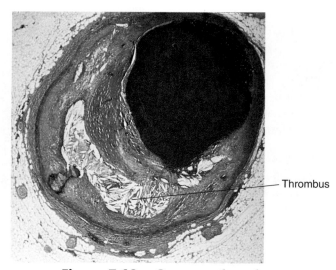

Figure 7-18. Coronary thrombus.

ficulty breathing, heart attack, or stroke. Consulting the client's health care provider is recommended. If clearance is given, a lighter massage is indicated. Avoid the use of electric massagers; such massagers jar the tissue and may dislodge blood clots.

Cardiac Arrest

Gr. Heart; L. To Withstand

Description—A cardiac arrest is the sudden and complete cessation of the heartbeat, stopping all cardiac output, including pulmonary and systemic circulation. Once a cardiac arrest occurs, vascular delivery of oxygen and nutrients, as well as removal of carbon dioxide and waste products, is interrupted. Anaerobic metabolism begins and, if measures are not taken to stimulate the pumping action of the heart, damage to the brain, kidneys, heart, and lungs can occur. Death may result.

Massage Consideration/s—If the client has a history of cardiac arrest, massage considerations are the same as for myocardial infarction, listed later in this chapter.

Cerebrovascular Accident (CVA, Stroke)

L. Brain; Vessel; Happening

Description—A CVA occurs when blood flow to the brain is reduced or when there is hemorrhage in the brain. This reduction in flow may be caused by an occlusion (blockage) in the cerebral blood vessels because of an embolus or thrombus (Figure 7-18). Muscular weakness or paralysis, an increase or decrease in sensation, speech abnormalities, or even death may occur. Subsequent problems resulting from CVA depend on the location and extent of neurological damage.

Massage Consideration/s—Massage considerations for CVA can be found in the section Stroke, Nervous System Pathologies.

Cluster Headaches

See entry on Migraine Headaches in this chapter.

Congestive Heart Failure (CHF)

L. To Heap Together; AS. Heart; L. To Deceive

Description—In CHF, the heart is a slowly failing pump. Causes include coronary artery disease, long-term hypertension, and myocardial infarcts (areas of dead heart tissue from previous heart attacks) (Figure 7-19). If the left ventricle fails first, blood backs up in the lungs and can result in pulmonary edema. The client may experience shortness of breath on exertion and fatigue. If the right ventricle fails first, blood backs up in peripheral blood vessels and can result in edema in the extremities, most noticeably the feet and ankles. See Figure 7-20 for other signs of congestive heart failure.

Massage Consideration/s—Massage should be performed only after obtaining clearance from the client's health care provider. A light massage of shorter duration is indicated because vigorous massage stimulates the return of fluid to the blood, and the increased blood volume may tax an already debilitated heart. Also, if the client has edema in the extremities from CHF, lymphatic massage is contraindicated because lymphatic massage encourages lymph flow and lymph drainage back into the bloodstream. This, too, increases blood volume and can tax an already debilitated heart.

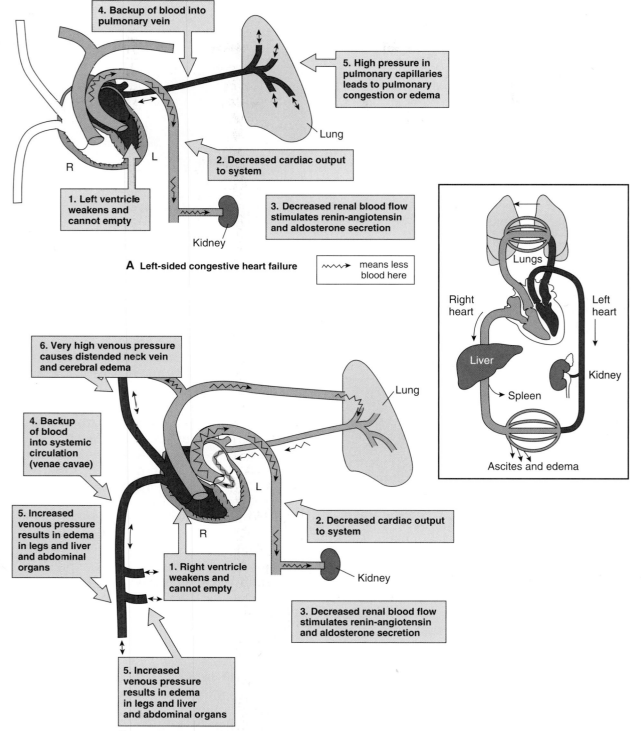

Figure 7-19. Pathophysiological mechanisms of congestive heart failure. **A,** Left-sided heart failure leads to pulmonary edema. **B,** Right-sided ventricular failure causes peripheral edema that is most prominent in the lower extremities. *Inset,* Integration of the pulmonary and systemic circulation. When the heart contracts normally, it pumps blood simultaneously into both loops, but pump failure causes circulatory or pulmonary problems depending on the underlying pathological mechanism.

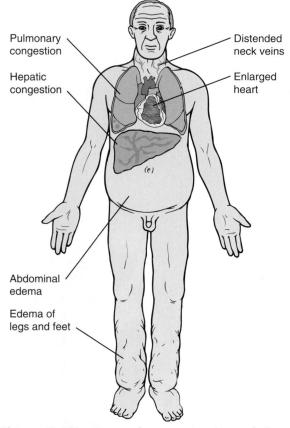

Figure 7-20.   Signs of congestive heart failure.

Coronary Artery Disease (CAD, Ischemic Heart Disease, IHD)

L. Crown; Gr. Air Pipe; Fr. From; Ease

Description—In CAD the coronary arteries are narrowed and there is reduced blood flow to the heart (Figure 7-21). CAD is the leading cause of death in the United States, with symptoms ranging from mild angina to a full-scale heart attack (Table 7-2). Symptoms usually start when about 60% to 75% of a coronary artery is blocked. The main cause is atherosclerosis (see page 205).

Massage Consideration/s—A client who has CAD may be prone to thrombosis (blood clot) formation. Deep pressure massage may dislodge the thrombus, which could float as an embolus in the bloodstream and lodge in smaller blood vessels in the lungs, heart, or brain, leading to difficulty breathing, heart attack, or stroke. Consulting with the client's health care provider is recommended. A lighter massage is indicated. Avoid the use of electric massagers; such massagers jar the tissue and may dislodge blood clots.

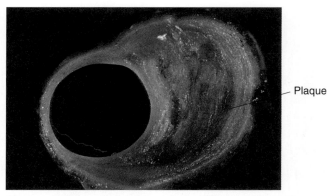

Figure 7-21.   Coronary artery disease. Note the plaque in the cross section.

Embolism

Gr. A Plug

Description—An embolus is a blood clot, bubble of air, or any piece of debris transported by the bloodstream (Figure 7-22). When an embolus becomes lodged in a vessel and cuts off circulation, it is then called an embolism. An embolus can lodge in the lungs, brain, heart, or extremities, causing serious injury or death (Figure 7-23).

Massage Consideration/s—A client who is prone to clotting is at high risk for developing emboli. Therefore it is important for the massage therapist to obtain clearance from the client's health care provider before performing massage. Deep, vigorous massage is contraindicated because of the danger of dislodging the clot. If a client is taking anticoagulants to prevent blood clots, clearance from the client's health care provider is still necessary and a lighter massage is indicated, since clients taking anticoagulants tend to bruise easily.

Endocarditis (en`·doh·kahr`·dai´·tuhs)

Gr. Within; Heart; Inflammation

Description—The inside of the heart is lined with epithelial tissue called endocardium. When the lining of the heart's chambers becomes infected or is interrupted by abnormal growths, it is called endocarditis (Figure 7-24). The heart's valves, which are folds of the endocardium, are often affected. Endocarditis may occur as a primary disorder or as a complication of another disease. Left untreated, endocarditis is often fatal.

Massage Consideration/s—Endocarditis is a debilitating disorder that requires medical attention. Massage is contraindicated.

Table 7-2 CORONARY ARTERY DISEASE RISK FACTORS

MODIFIABLE RISK FACTORS			NONMODIFIABLE RISK FACTORS	NEW PREDICTORS OF RISK FACTORS
RISK FACTORS FOR WHICH INTERVENTION HAS BEEN SHOWN TO REDUCE INCIDENCE OF *CAD*	RISK FACTORS FOR WHICH INTERVENTION IS LIKELY TO REDUCE INCIDENCE OF *CAD*	RISK FACTORS FOR WHICH INTERVENTION MIGHT REDUCE INCIDENCE OF *CAD*		RISK FACTORS UNDER INVESTIGATION
Cigarette smoking	Obesity	Psychological factors and emotional response to stress	Age >55 yr (women) >45 yr (men)	Elevated homocysteine (>15 micromoles/L)
Elevated total serum cholesterol level	Physical inactivity	Discriminatory medicine[†]	Male gender	C-reactive protein
Elevated LDL cholesterol	Diabetes or impaired glucose tolerance; insulin resistance	Oxidative stress	Family history; genetic determinants	Fibrinogen
Hypertension	Low HDL <40 mg/dl (men) <50 mg/dl (women)	Excessive alcohol consumption or complete abstinence	Ethnicity	Lipoprotein (a); Lp(a) (>30 mg/dl)[‡]
Poor nutrition	Hormonal status; oral contraceptives; hysterectomy or oophorectomy; menopause without hormone replacement (especially before age 40 yr)	Elevated triglycerides	Infection (viral, bacterial)	Troponin T
Thombogenic factors*		Sleep-disordered breathing		Plasminogen activator inhibitor (PAI; marker for recurrence of MI) D-dimer (fibrin) Dermatological indicators Male pattern baldness Graying of the hair Earlobe creases Male impotence Ankle/brachial blood pressure index (ABI)

CAD, coronary artery disease; LDL, low-density lipoprotein; HDL, high-density lipoprotein; MI, myocardial infarction.
* *Individual is not receiving antiplatelet or anticoagulant therapy and/or after age 50 yr, the association of total cholesterol levels with CAD declines and increased levels of fibrinogen and factor VII seem to be markers of a prethrombotic tendency and increased risk for CAD.*
[†] *Discriminatory medicine is not technically a risk factor for CAD but rather results in a different natural history for some individuals.*
[‡] *Applies to whites and Asians but not to blacks.*
From Goodman CC, Boissonnault WG, Fuller KS: Pathology: implications for the physical therapist, ed 2, Philadelphia, 2003, WB Saunders.

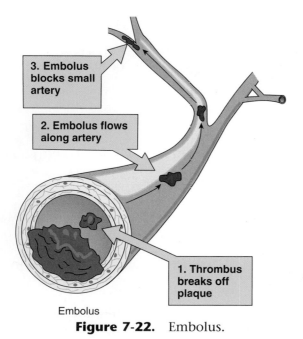

3. Embolus blocks small artery

2. Embolus flows along artery

1. Thrombus breaks off plaque

Embolus

Figure 7-22. Embolus.

Heart Murmur (Cardiac Murmur)

AS, Heart; L. A Humming

Description—Heart murmurs are abnormal heart sounds resulting from turbulence of blood through the heart. These usually are a result of valvular abnormalities. They are diagnosed by the sound they create, hence the name murmur. Murmurs are graded from 1 to 6 on the basis of increasing loudness. The most common heart murmur is a mitral valve prolapse in which the mitral valve is pushed backward (prolapses) into the left atrium during ventricular contraction (Figure 7-25). It affects 10% of the population, women more often than men. Symptoms can range from slight to serious.

Massage Consideration/s—Whether massage is indicated for a client with a heart murmur depends on the severity of the condition. Massage is fine for a client with a slight heart murmur; however, with more severe murmurs, clearance from the client's health care provider is necessary, and a lighter massage is indicated.

Hemangioma (hee`·man`·jee·oh´·muh)

Gr. Blood; Vessel; Tumor

Description—A hemangioma is a benign tumor consisting of a localized mass of dilated blood vessels (Figure 7-26).

Massage Consideration/s—Local massage is contraindicated because pressure over the hemangiomas may cause subcutaneous bleeding.

Hematoma (Blood Blister)

Gr. Blood; Tumor

Description—A hematoma is a localized collection of blood trapped in the tissues of an organ, body space, or the skin (Figure 7-27). It is often the result of trauma or surgery. If the hematoma is near the skin's surface, it can be palpated.

Massage Consideration/s—Local massage is contraindicated because it can cause or worsen pain associated with the hematoma, and there is a danger of disturbing blood clots.

Hemophilia (hee·moh·fee´·lee·uh)

Gr. Blood; To Love

Description—Hemophilia is a genetic disorder that affects the clotting mechanism in the blood. There are three types of hemophilia. In each case, only one clotting factor is missing, making it difficult or impossible for the blood to clot. Large hematomas can develop in the muscles or under the skin, either spontaneously or with mild trauma. There may be bleeding into the joints causing pain, swelling, and permanent joint stiffness. Often referred to as *free bleeders*, people with hemophilia receive transfusions of their missing clotting factor.

Massage Consideration/s—Because of the danger of causing bleeding, massage is contraindicated for moderate to severe hemophilia. For clients with mild cases of hemophilia, the massage therapist needs to obtain clearance from the client's health care provider. Once clearance is received, a lighter massage is indicated. Because of possible damage within the joints from the hemophilia, stretches and joint mobilizations are contraindicated.

Hemorrhage (he´·muh·rij)

Gr. Blood; To Burst Forth

Description—Hemorrhaging is excessive bleeding, either internally (from blood vessels into tissues) or externally (from blood vessels directly to the surface of the body). The blood spillage may come from arteries, veins, or capillaries (Figure 7-28).

Massage Consideration/s—Massage is contraindicated. Excessive blood loss can lead to cardiovascular shock and possibly death. The person needs medical attention.

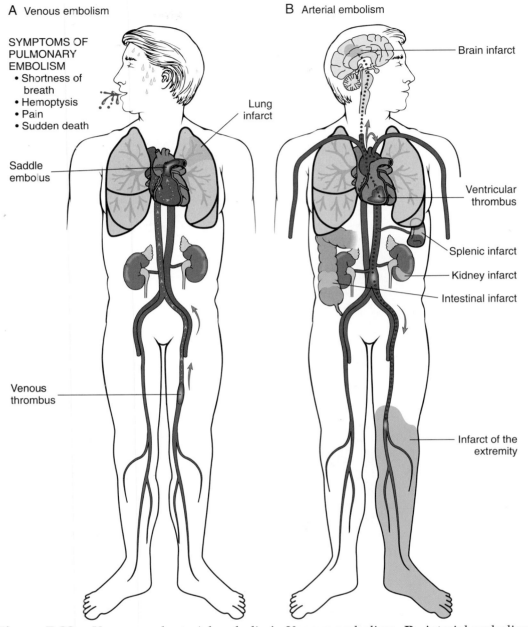

A Venous embolism

SYMPTOMS OF
PULMONARY
EMBOLISM
• Shortness of
  breath
• Hemoptysis
• Pain
• Sudden death

Saddle
embolus

Lung
infarct

Venous
thrombus

B Arterial embolism

Brain infarct

Ventricular
thrombus

Splenic infarct

Kidney infarct

Intestinal infarct

Infarct of the
extremity

Figure 7-23. Venous and arterial emboli. **A,** Venous embolism. **B,** Arterial embolism.

Hypercholesterolemia (High Cholesterol in the Blood) (hai`·puhr·kuh·les`·tuh·ruh·lee´·mee·uh)

Gr. Above; Bile; Solid; Blood

Description—Hypercholesterolemia is a condition in which greater than normal amounts of cholesterol are present in the blood. It can be inherited or acquired through high consumption of saturated fats, which are found in red meats, eggs, and dairy products. High levels of cholesterol and other lipids may often develop into atherosclerosis.

Massage Consideration/s—See entry for Atherosclerosis.

Hypertension (High Blood Pressure, HBP)

Gr. Above; Tension

Description—Hypertension is a common, often asymptomatic disorder of elevated blood pressure: 140/90 mm Hg is regarded as the threshold of hypertension, and 160/95 mm Hg is classified as serious hypertension. With sustained hypertension, arterial walls become inelastic and

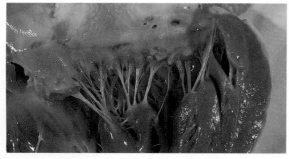

Figure 7-24. Endocarditis.

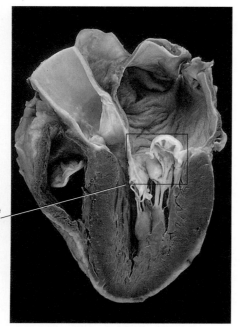

Mitral valve prolapse

Figure 7-25. Mitral valve prolapse.

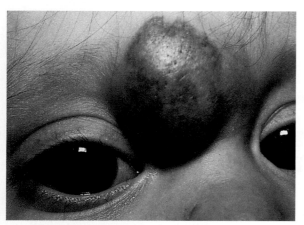

Figure 7-26. Hemangioma.

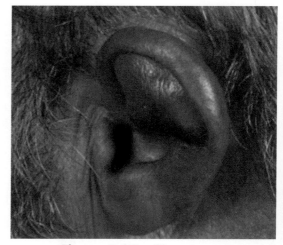

Figure 7-27. Hematoma.

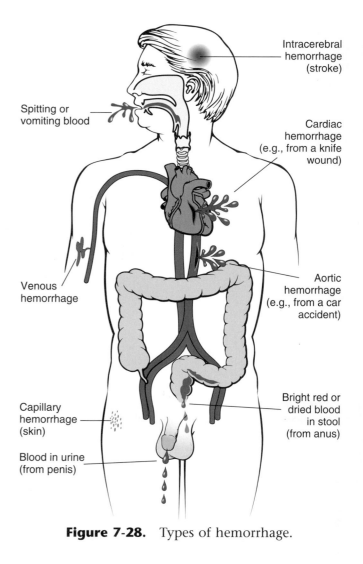

Intracerebral hemorrhage (stroke)

Spitting or vomiting blood

Cardiac hemorrhage (e.g., from a knife wound)

Venous hemorrhage

Aortic hemorrhage (e.g., from a car accident)

Capillary hemorrhage (skin)

Blood in urine (from penis)

Bright red or dried blood in stool (from anus)

Figure 7-28. Types of hemorrhage.

resistant to blood flow and, as a result, the left ventricle may become enlarged to maintain normal circulation. Risk factors for hypertension are cigarette smoking, obesity, lack of exercise, diabetes, and genetic predisposition. Hypertension can be controlled, in some cases, with a low-sodium diet, losing weight, and regular exercise. The use of antihypertensive medications may also be necessary.

Massage Consideration/s—It is important for the massage therapist to ask the client with hypertension how the client controls the condition. Clients whose hypertension is not under control by diet, exercise, and/or medication should not receive massage.

For clients who do have their hypertension under control, massage helps keep blood pressure lowered by reducing both stress and the activity of the sympathetic nervous system. Clients on antihypertensive medications may be prone to postural hypotension (a low blood pressure from the massage treatment). These clients will feel lightheaded, and may need assistance to get up slowly from the table after the massage.

Hypotension (Low Blood Pressure, Orthostatic Hypotension) (ohr`·thuh·sta´·tik hai`·poh·ten´·shuhn)

Gr. Beneath; Tension

Description—Blood pressure that is abnormally low, or hypotension, may cause damage to the body's tissue because of a lack of oxygen. Hypotension may be due to shock, dilated blood vessels, or diminished cardiac output. The client may feel tired, experience dizziness, or have blurred vision. These symptoms may also occur on standing or when standing motionless in a fixed position.

Massage Consideration/s—Because massage tends to lower blood pressure, clients may need assistance getting off the table after the massage. Clients with severe hypotension may need to be massaged in the seated position.

Migraine Headaches and Cluster Headaches

Fr. Half; Skull

Description—Also called vascular headaches, migraines are caused by dilation of extracranial blood vessels. Women are affected more often than men. Migraines may be triggered by foods (carbohydrates, iodine-rich foods, cheese, chocolate), alcohol (red wine), bright lights, loud noises, hormonal changes during the menstrual cycle, or the period of relaxation after physical or emotional stress. The acute phase may be accompanied by nausea, vomiting, chills, sweating, irritability, and extreme fatigue. After an attack the individual often has dull head and neck pains, and a great need for sleep.

Cluster headaches and migraine headaches have similar symptoms, but cluster headaches occur one after the other for several days in a row and affect men more often than women.

Massage Consideration/s—Because of the pain and nausea associated with migraine, it is unlikely that a client experiencing a migraine would want a massage. After the migraine headache, however, massage can lessen the frequency and intensity of migraines between attacks. At this time, a full body relaxation massage is indicated. Craniosacral therapy, biofeedback, and mediation have also been helpful to reduce migraine headaches.

Myocardial Infarction (MI, Heart Attack) (mai·oh·kahr´·dee·uhl in·fahrk´·shuhn)

Gr. Muscle; Heart

Description—A myocardial infarction, or the death (necrosis) of myocardial tissue, is due to interrupted coronary blood supply (Figure 7-29). Blood clots, atherosclerosis, and vascular spasms could lead to a myocardial infarction. Preceding symptoms are a viselike pain in the chest, which may radiate down the left arm, neck, or sternal region (Figure 7-30).

Massage Consideration/s—If a client has a history of MI, it is important for the massage therapist to find out when it occurred and how well recovery is proceeding. If the MI was recent, and the client is still weak and debilitated, clearance from the client's health care provider is essential. If the

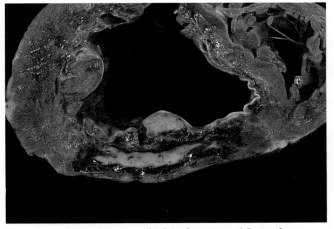

Figure 7-29. Myocardial infarction. Note the yellow necrotic area.

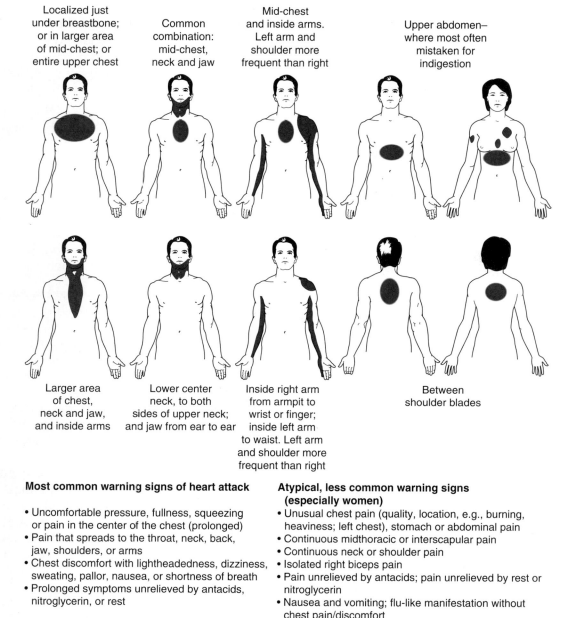

Localized just under breastbone; or in larger area of mid-chest; or entire upper chest

Common combination: mid-chest, neck and jaw

Mid-chest and inside arms. Left arm and shoulder more frequent than right

Upper abdomen— where most often mistaken for indigestion

Larger area of chest, neck and jaw, and inside arms

Lower center neck, to both sides of upper neck; and jaw from ear to ear

Inside right arm from armpit to wrist or finger; inside left arm to waist. Left arm and shoulder more frequent than right

Between shoulder blades

Most common warning signs of heart attack

- Uncomfortable pressure, fullness, squeezing or pain in the center of the chest (prolonged)
- Pain that spreads to the throat, neck, back, jaw, shoulders, or arms
- Chest discomfort with lightheadedness, dizziness, sweating, pallor, nausea, or shortness of breath
- Prolonged symptoms unrelieved by antacids, nitroglycerin, or rest

Atypical, less common warning signs (especially women)

- Unusual chest pain (quality, location, e.g., burning, heaviness; left chest), stomach or abdominal pain
- Continuous midthoracic or interscapular pain
- Continuous neck or shoulder pain
- Isolated right biceps pain
- Pain unrelieved by antacids; pain unrelieved by rest or nitroglycerin
- Nausea and vomiting; flu-like manifestation without chest pain/discomfort
- Unexplained intense anxiety, weakness, or fatigue
- Breathlessness, dizziness

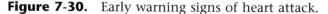

Figure 7-30. Early warning signs of heart attack.

client is cleared for massage, a lighter massage of shorter duration is indicated. The goal of massage is relaxation for the client. If the client is further along in the recovery and has regained most of his or her strength, clearance from the client's health care provider is still necessary, and, if given, a massage with moderate pressure is indicated. Deep pressure may cause pain and an elevated heart rate, which is a danger to a healing heart. If the client has completely recovered and regained all of his or her strength, a more vigorous massage can be per-

formed. The best way the massage therapist can determine the stage of recovery is to ask the client. It is important that clients have with them their necessary medications (e.g., nitroglycerin) when they come for treatment, in the event of a medical emergency.

Massage can help clients by reducing stress. Massage also decreases the effects of the sympathetic nervous system, which is partially responsible for coronary artery vasoconstriction. Because sudden exposure to extreme cold or heat can bring on an attack, the massage therapist should keep the client warm during treatment but avoid using heat or cold packs.

If a client has an attack during a massage treatment, assist him or her in taking medications needed for this medical emergency. Then call 911 or local emergency medical services. If the client takes nitroglycerin while in the office, the massage therapist needs to make sure the client sits or lies down for at least an hour, as nitroglycerin causes vasodilation and may induce fainting.

Myocarditis (mai`·oh·kahr·dai´·tis)

Gr. Muscle; Heart; Inflammation

Description—Inflammation of the muscular walls of the heart, or myocarditis, is often caused by a viral, bacterial, fungal, or chemical agent; rheumatic fever; or as a complication of a collagen disease. Myocarditis often leads to acute heart failure.

Massage Consideration/s—Myocarditis is a debilitating disorder and requires medical attention. Massage is contraindicated.

Pericarditis (pe`·ree·kahr·dai´·tis)

Gr. Around; Heart; Inflammation

Description—Pericarditis is an inflammation of the parietal pericardium, often due to trauma or infectious disease (Figure 7-31).

Massage Consideration/s—Pericarditis is a debilitating disorder and requires medical attention. Massage is contraindicated.

Peripheral Vascular Disease

Gr. Circumference; L. Vessel

Description—Peripheral vascular disease affects both blood and lymphatic vessels. Various metabolic disorders (such as diabetes), obesity, sedentary lifestyles, and cigarette smoking cause or contribute to this disease. Symptoms include numbness, pain and discomfort, and skin discoloration (see Figure 6-9).

Massage Consideration/s—Because accurate feedback about pressure is essential, it is important for the massage therapist to ask the client to describe symptoms and identify which area of the body is involved to determine how to proceed with the massage. Mild symptoms, such as numbness and/or tingling in a small area, indicate light pressure massage. Moderate to severe symptoms, including numbness and pain in large areas, indicate a local contraindication.

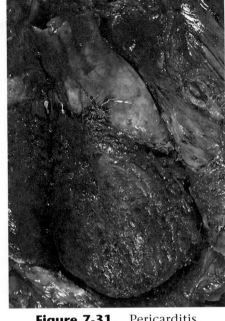

Figure 7-31. Pericarditis.

Phlebitis (fluh·bai´·tuhs)

Gr. Vein; Inflammation

Description—Phlebitis is an inflammation of the veins, frequently accompanied by a thrombus (blood clot). Phlebitis usually occurs after acute or chronic infection, surgery, pregnancy, or childbirth, or prolonged sitting, standing, or immobilization. The affected area is hypersensitive to pressure and swollen and can be either hot or cold to the touch. It generally affects the extremities.

Massage Consideration/s—Local massage is contraindicated because the pressure of massage causes undue pain and may dislodge a clot. The massage can also worsen the accompanying inflammation.

Raynaud's Syndrome (Raynaud's Disease, Raynaud's Phenomenon) (ray·nohs´)

Maurice Raynaud, French Physician; 1834-1881

Description—Raynaud's syndrome is a cycle of periodic vasospasm in blood vessels, usually the most distal parts of the body (i.e., fingers, toes, ears, nose). It is most frequently caused by exposure to cold, by emotional stress, or by smoking (nicotine is a powerful vasoconstrictor). This condition can lead to ischemia, tissue necrosis, and nerve damage (Figure 7-32).

Massage Consideration/s—It is important for the massage therapist to ask the client where he or she is in the cycle of vasospasm and how much pain the client is currently experiencing. With greater pain, a lighter massage is indicated. With less pain, a more vigorous massage may be performed. Massage helps increase local circulation. By reducing stress, massage helps reduce sympathetic stimulation and so relaxes the smooth muscle of blood vessels. Heat and ice packs are contraindicated.

Shock

Description—Shock is the failure of the cardiovascular system to deliver enough oxygen and nutrients to meet the metabolic needs of

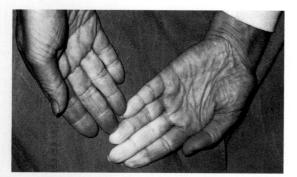

Figure 7-32. Ischemia of Raynaud's syndrome.

the body. There are many causes of shock; all are characterized by an inadequate blood flow to the body's tissues. Types of shock include hypovolemic shock, cardiogenic shock, vascular shock, septic shock, and obstructive shock. Hypovolemic shock occurs as a result of low blood volume. Hemorrhage, or loss of body fluid through excessive sweating, diarrhea, or vomiting can all cause hypovolemic shock. In cardiogenic shock, the heart does not pump effectively. This could be due to a myocardial infarction, heart valve problems, or other problems with the heart. In vascular shock, blood vessels dilate inappropriately, and blood pressure drops. An example of vascular shock is anaphylactic shock in which a severe allergic reaction causes the release of body chemicals (i.e., histamine) that cause blood vessels to dilate. Another example of vascular shock is septic shock in which bacterial toxins cause the dilation of blood vessels. Obstructive shock occurs when blood flow is impeded. The most common cause is a pulmonary embolism. The individual's demeanor ranges from restlessness and anxiety to weakness and lethargy. The person will also have pale, cool, moist skin. As shock progresses, body temperature begins to fall, and respiration rate becomes shallow and rapid (Figure 7-33).

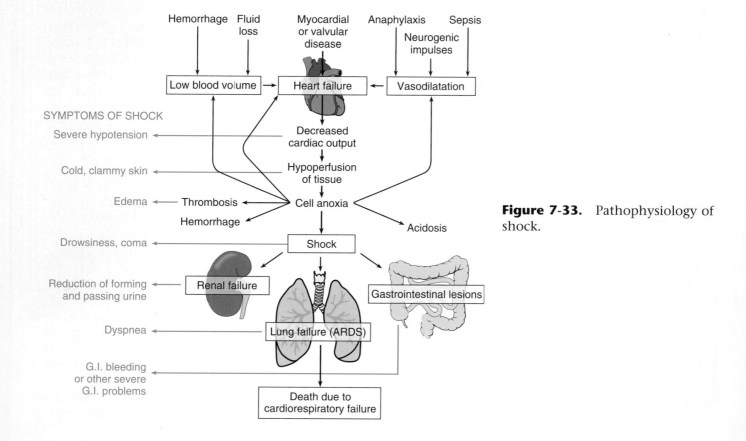

Figure 7-33. Pathophysiology of shock.

Massage Consideration/s—Massage is contraindicated because the person needs immediate medical attention. It is important for the massage therapist to ask the client about any allergies to prevent a reaction to a product ingredient that could lead to shock. This can be done as a question on the intake form or verbally in the premassage interview.

Sickle Cell Disease (Sickle Cell Anemia)

AS. Crescent; L. A Chamber; Fr. From; Ease

Description—Sickle cell disease is a genetic disorder characterized by abnormal hemoglobin, which causes red blood cells to "sickle" (Figure 7-34). This shape greatly reduces the amount of oxygen that can be supplied to the tissues, eventually causing extensive tissue damage. Sickle cell anemia is characterized by lethargy, fatigue, pain in the joints, thrombosis, and headaches. Treatments include analgesics to relieve pain, antibiotics to counter infections, and blood transfusions.

Massage Consideration/s—Clearance from the client's health care provider is needed. Clients with this disorder have periods of remission and flare-ups. Massage is contraindicated during flare-ups because the client will be in pain and debilitated. During periods of remission, a lighter massage of shorter duration, paying close attention to the client's vitality, is indicated. Massage should consist mainly of gliding strokes, which will help the client relax.

Syncope (Fainting) (sing´·kuh·pee)

Gr. Fainting

Description—A temporary suspension of consciousness, or syncope, is often due to reduced blood flow to the brain. It is usually preceded by light-headedness. Once the individual feels faint, collapsing can often be prevented by lying or sitting down with the head between the knees. Syncope may be caused by many different factors, including emotional stress, a change in body temperature, a change in body position, or blood pooling in the legs.

Massage Consideration/s—Massage is contraindicated. The client needs to be referred to the health care provider to find out the cause of the syncope.

Telangiectasia (Spider Capillaries, Spider Nevus, Nevus Araneus)

(te`·lan`·jee·ek·tay´·zhee·uh) (nee´·vuhs uh·ran´·ee·uhs)

Gr. End; Vessel; Dilation

Description—Telangiectasia is permanent dilation of superficial capillaries or small blood vessels (venules and arterioles) (Figure 7-35). The face is the most common region affected. Common causes are rosacea, elevated estrogen levels, and collagen vascular diseases.

Massage Consideration/s—Light massage of the affected area/s is indicated. Deep pressure massage may further damage the blood vessels.

Thromboangiitis Obliterans (Buerger's Disease) (thrahm`·boh·an·jee·ai´·tis uh·bli´·tuh·ranz)

Gr. Clot; Vessel; Inflammation; L. To Remove; Leo Buerger, American Physician; 1879-1943

Description—Occurring most often in young men, thromboangiitis is an inflammatory disease of the blood vessels of the extremities caused by long-term use of smoking tobacco (Figure 7-36). The small and medium-sized blood vessels in the upper and lower extremities are affected;

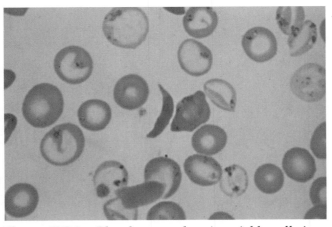

Figure 7-34. Blood smear showing sickle cells in sickle cell anemia.

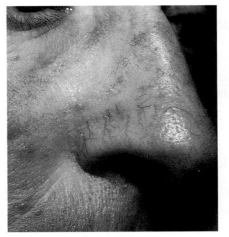

Figure 7-35. Telangiectasia.

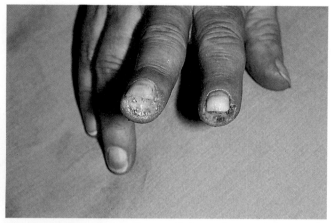

Figure 7-36. Skin ulcers of thromboangiitis obliterans (Buerger's disease).

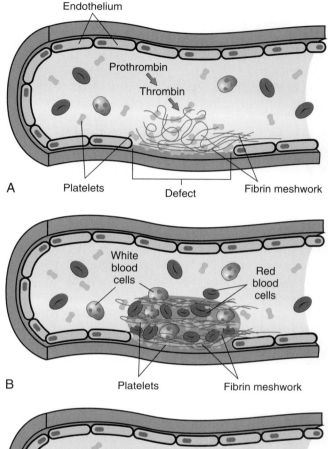

Figure 7-37. Thrombus formation.

however, the lower extremities are most often involved. As the disease advances, chronic inflammation and clot formation may totally occlude major vessels. Pulsation in the limb below the occluded blood vessels may be absent. This condition often leads to ischemia, skin ulcers, phlebitis, and gangrene.

Massage Consideration/s—Because there is a possibility of blood clot formation, the massage therapist should ensure from the client's health care provider that the client has no clots. If the physician indicates the possibility of blood clots, local massage of the affected area is contraindicated. In most cases, massage is beneficial by reducing stress, improving peripheral circulation, and reducing sympathetic impulses. Deep pressure massage is contraindicated due to the presence of blood clots and/or fragile skin. Avoid the use of electric massagers; such massagers jar the tissue and may dislodge blood clots. Heat and cold packs are contraindicated so as not to disturb clots and because heat increases local blood flow and cold decreases local blood flow, thus stressing already debilitated blood vessels.

Thrombophlebitis (Thrombosis, Deep Vein Thrombosis, DVT, Venous Thrombosis)

(thrahm`·boh·fluh·bai´·tis)

Gr. Clot; Vein; Inflammation

Description—Thrombophlebitis is thrombus (blood clot) formation in an unbroken blood vessel, restricting blood flow. Tissue damage can result due to an interrupted blood supply. When the thrombus becomes dislodged and floats in the blood, it is referred to as an embolus (Figures 7-37 and 7-38).

Massage Consideration/s—Local massage is contraindicated. Because of the possibility of clot formation, deep pressure massage should be avoided in the inner thigh, especially in older clients. This area is referred to as the "valley of the clots." The use of electric massagers should be avoided, as these devices jar the tissue and may dislodge blood clots.

Transient Ischemic Attack (TIA)

L. To Go By; Gr. To Hold Back; Blood; Fr. Join

Description—Transient ischemic attack is an event of temporary cerebral dysfunction caused by ischemia or reduced blood flow.

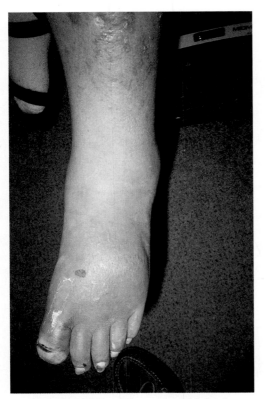

Figure 7-38.   Thrombophlebitis.

TIAs can be characterized by abnormal vision in one or both eyes, vertigo, shortness of breath, general loss of sensation, or unconsciousness. Common causes are occlusion by embolus, thrombus, or atherosclerotic plaque. The attack is typically sudden and brief (lasting only a few minutes), leaving no long-term neurological damage. TIAs are often recurrent and may be a presage to a cardiovascular accident (CVA).

Massage Consideration/s—If a client has a history of TIAs, clearance from the client's health care provider is necessary before massage can be performed. The client who is on anticoagulant therapy may be prone to bruising and bleeding, so a lighter massage is indicated. Because TIAs predispose a client to a stroke, the massage therapist should immediately refer the client to the health care provider if the client experiences tingling, numbness, or loss of movement during or immediately after the massage session.

Varicose Veins

L. Full of Dilated Veins

Description—Varicose veins are dilated veins resulting from incompetent valves. In healthy veins, small valves promote the forward move-

ment of blood and prevent backflow. Veins with incompetent valves do not seal and gravity prevents large amounts of blood from flowing upward. The back pressure overloads the vein and pushes its walls outward. The veins lose elasticity and become stretched and flabby (Figure 7-39).

Thrombi may form in the varicose veins. They are typically caused by a congenital defect or by repeated stress from overloading, such as pregnancy or obesity. This condition may worsen if the client is on his or her feet for a long time.

Massage Consideration/s—Clearance from the client's health care provider is necessary. In the past, varicosities were considered a local contraindication. However, physician research refutes the need for local contraindications of all varicosities, unless blood clots are present. According to Tiffany Field, there has been no research linking massage to increasing varicosities. It is important for the massage therapist to ask the client how painful to the touch the varicosities are and if the client has a history of clot formation. Varicosities that are warm and painful to the touch are contraindicated for massage because massage can cause pain and damage to the tissues and because there is the possibility of dislodging a clot. Less severe varicosities may benefit from massage. Avoid the use of electric massagers; such massagers jar the tissue and may dislodge blood clots. Massage should be geared to reduce edema and prevent venous and lymphatic stasis. These client's legs should be raised above the heart during treatment. Gliding strokes toward the heart help empty veins, aiding circulation.

LYMPHATIC/IMMUNE SYSTEM PATHOLOGIES

Acquired Immunodeficiency Syndrome (AIDS)

L. To Get; Immunity; To Lack; Gr. Together; Course

Description—Acquired immunodeficiency syndrome (AIDS) is a disease caused by the human immunodeficiency virus (HIV) (Figure 7-40). Transmission of the virus occurs through the exchange of bodily fluids such as blood, semen, vaginal secretions, and mother's milk. The average time between infection with the virus and symptom development and diagnosis is 8 to 10 years. The time period from exposure to detection is 90 days. In 90 days, the infected person begins to produce HIV antibodies; the presence of these antibodies determines the diagnosis. Generally, symptoms of primary infection with HIV may include enlarged

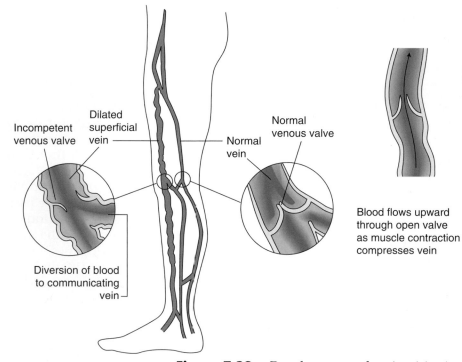

Blood flows upward through open valve as muscle contraction compresses vein

Competent closed valve prevents backflow of blood

Incompetent or "leaky" valve permits blood to flow backward in vein, causing varicosities

Figure 7-39. Development of varicosities in the leg.

lymph nodes, weight loss, fatigue, night sweats, and fever. The CDC estimates that between 800,000 and 900,000 people are living with HIV or AIDS in the United States. Worldwide, approximately 60 million people have been infected since the global epidemic began. Medications are often prescribed to manage AIDS (Table 7-3).

Massage Consideration/s— Massage treatment for a client with AIDS needs to be tailored to that client's vitality; ask the client about his or her vitality before each and every massage. A gentle massage of shorter duration may be indicated if the client is feeling debilitated. However, many people living with AIDS can typically tolerate even a vigorous massage. It is unlikely that the massage therapist will come in contact with client blood or body fluids; however, if this occurs, the therapist should contact a health care provider immediately for testing and counseling. If a massage therapist has open wounds or cuts or scratches on his or her hands, the therapist needs to cover it or not perform any massages until the wound has completely healed. Chapter 1 has information on universal precautions (see Box 1-3). Also, Boxes 7-4 and 7-5 have more information on AIDS.

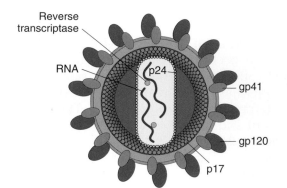

Figure 7-40. Human immunodeficiency virus.

Allergies

Gr. Other; Work

Description—Allergies are also known as hypersensitivities. They are an overreaction of the immune system to otherwise harmless agents (most are environmental or dietary). The person may experience inflammation, a runny nose from excess mucus secretion, or, more seriously, go into anaphylactic shock (see page 216) in which air

Table 7-3 MEDICATION USED TO MANAGE HIV/AIDS

MEDICATION CLASSIFICATION	MEDICATION NAME	POSSIBLE SIDE EFFECTS THAT MAY AFFECT TREATMENT
Non-nucleoside reverse transcriptase inhibitors	Delavirdine (Rescriptor), efavirenz (Sustiva), nevirapine (Viramune)	Abdominal pain, anxiety, chills, diarrhea, drowsiness, fever, gastrointestinal irritation, headaches, insomnia, lethargy, nausea and vomiting, skin rash, vertigo
Nucleoside analogs	Abacavir (Ziagen), acyclovir (Zovirax), didanosine (ddI, Videx), lamivudine (3TC, Epivir), stavudine (d4T, Zerit), zalcitabine (ddC, HIVID), zidovudine (AZT, Retrovir)	Convulsions, diarrhea, drowsiness, fever, gastrointestinal irritation, headaches, hypertension, insomnia, joint pain, lethargy, nausea, pancreatitis, peripheral neuropathy, seizures, skin rashes, vertigo
Protease inhibitors	Amprenavir (Agenerase), indinavir (Crixivan), lopinavir/ritonavir (Kaletra), nelfinavir (Viracept), ritonavir (Norvir), saquinavir (Fortovase)	Abdominal pain, anxiety, convulsions, diarrhea, disorientation, drowsiness, dry mouth, fever, gastrointestinal irritation, hair loss, hypotension and hypertension, insomnia, joint pain, lethargy, nausea and vomiting, numbness, muscle pain, pneumonia, seizures, skin rashes, vertigo

passageways constrict. A local allergic reaction could result in a rash or hives.

Massage Consideration/s—The massage therapist should make sure that the massage products and treatment room do not contain items to which the client is allergic (pet dander, lubricants that contain nut oils, or other possible allergens). For clients with known allergies or hypersensitive skin, the massage therapist needs to ask the client to review the ingredient list before applying massage lubricant on the skin.

Chronic Fatigue Syndrome (CFS)

Gr. Time; L. To Tire; Gr. Together; Course

Description—Chronic fatigue syndrome is characterized by the onset of disabling fatigue, sometimes after a viral infection. CFS is often accompanied by flulike symptoms such as low-grade fevers, sore throat, and headaches. Memory deficits and sleep disturbances are also associated with this condition. As with fibromyalgia, treatment is geared toward relieving symptoms. Counseling is often indicated, as depression is common. Although CFS occasionally resolves spontaneously, it is typically a lifelong condition.

Massage Consideration/s—Massage can be helpful for a client with CFS. It can soothe the nervous system, relieve muscle and joint pain, and give the client a chance to rest. Because the client is fatigued, a shorter duration of treatment may be indicated. Because symptoms vary among clients and within an individual client, and also because symptoms vary from massage to massage, it is important for the massage therapist to ask the client for a list of current symptoms before treatment. It is also helpful to ask the client who has had massages previously how massage and the amount of pressure and vigor of techniques have affected him or her in the past. Adjust the treatment accordingly.

Edema (Lymphedema)

Gr. Swelling

Description—Edema is the abnormal accumulation of interstitial fluid in tissue spaces and is characterized by swelling (Figure 7-41). It is usually not detectable until the volume of the interstitial fluid is 30% above normal. It is caused by inflammation, obstruction of lymph flow (e.g., by tumors), removal of lymph channels, (e.g., as occurs during a mastectomy), or physical trauma. Other causes include high blood pressure, damage

Box **7-4**

Clients Who Are HIV-Positive or Living with AIDS

Considered a chronic illness, acquired immunodeficiency syndrome (AIDS) is a disease that infects T lymphocytes (T cells) and is caused by the human immunodeficiency virus (HIV). People who have the virus are said to be HIV-positive; people who have AIDS are HIV-positive and have three or more opportunistic infections and/or a T-cell count below 200 (a normal T-cell count is 1200). To become infected by the HIV virus, there must be contact with contaminated body fluids.

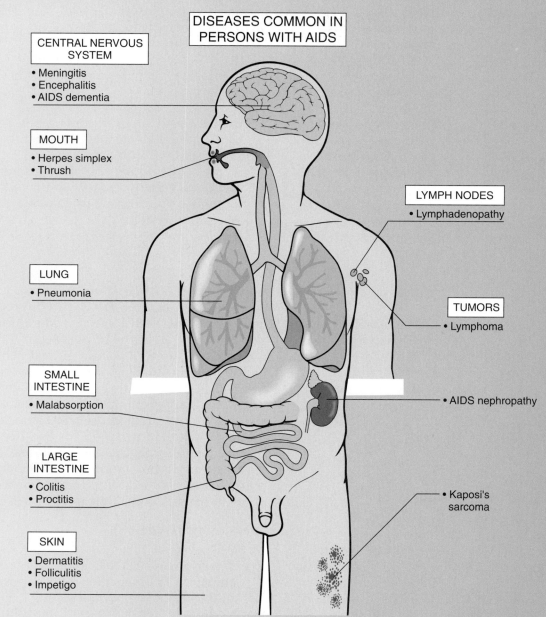

DISEASES COMMON IN PERSONS WITH AIDS

CENTRAL NERVOUS SYSTEM
• Meningitis
• Encephalitis
• AIDS dementia

MOUTH
• Herpes simplex
• Thrush

LUNG
• Pneumonia

SMALL INTESTINE
• Malabsorption

LARGE INTESTINE
• Colitis
• Proctitis

SKIN
• Dermatitis
• Folliculitis
• Impetigo

LYMPH NODES
• Lymphadenopathy

TUMORS
• Lymphoma

• AIDS nephropathy

• Kaposi's sarcoma

The only body fluids that contain high concentrations of the virus are blood, semen, vaginal secretions, and mother's milk. Tears, sweat, and saliva do not appear to contain enough of the virus to cause infection, as there are no known reported cases of transmission by these body fluids. (It has been speculated that it would take 6 to 10 gallons of saliva to have enough concentration for the virus to be transmitted.)

The virus is spread through sexual contact, by sharing needles/syringes with an infected person or, less commonly, through transfusions of infected blood or blood clotting factors. If can also be spread by transplacental route. The HIV virus cannot be transmitted by simple contact with an infected person. Intact skin is adequate protection from the virus.

The massage for an HIV-infected client is not that different from any other client. The massage therapist needs to inquire about the areas that need to be avoided, including the most recent site of blood work. If the HIV-infected client has Kaposi's sarcoma (*Moritz K. Kaposi, Australian Dermatologist, 1837-1902*), deep pressure massage is contraindicated because it can cause internal bleeding. Even light massage may be contraindicated around lesions, which can be extremely painful. Of course, as with any other client, any open lesions should be avoided.

When massaging a client who has AIDS, the therapist may take into consideration the client's

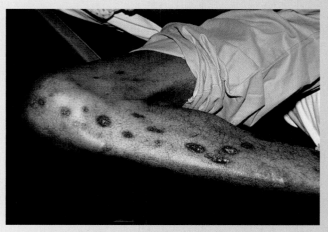

Kaposi's sarcoma

general vitality and any secondary conditions. If and when secondary complications occur, the massage therapist should assess them as a separate and individual condition. The massage therapist may need to limit any joint mobilizations and stretching if the client is bedridden because inactivity affects bone integrity; however, this depends on the individual client. Joint mobilizations are often

beneficial for those bedridden to maintain range of motion. Case-by-case decisions need to be made with input from the client's health care provider. If the massage is given in the hospital, the massage therapist should check with the health care provider about additional information needed to serve the client most effectively. The massage therapist should work carefully around tubes, catheters, needles, monitors, and other medical equipment. Under these circumstances, even a massage that lasts less than an hour can bring comfort to an HIV-infected client.

As true in all cases, if there is any spillage of body fluids while the client is on the massage table, contaminated linens need to be removed using gloved hands and washed separately in hot water with detergent and a quarter cup of chlorine bleach. Linens should be dried with hot air. Because it is not always possible to tell if linens have come in contact with body fluids, some therapists tend to treat all sheets as "hot" or contaminated. If the therapist accidentally comes into contact with body fluids, the therapist should immediately wash the area of contact with a hand soap for 2 minutes. Implements used during the massage (e.g., pressure bars) should be immersed in either a 10% bleach solution or a 70% alcohol solution for 10 minutes.

There have been no known reported cases of a massage therapist contracting the HIV virus from a client while performing massage. There has been only one instance of patients being infected by an HIV-positive health care worker. This involved transmission from an infected dentist to 6 patients. A therapist who believes to have been exposed to HIV should contact the health care provider and/or the local HIV/AIDS foundation for testing, information, and free counseling. The resource list in this chapter has more information.

Sanitation and cleanliness are important for the client *and* the massage therapist. Because the immune system of the HIV-infected client is not fully functional, the client is more susceptible to contacting infections through simple exposure. The massage therapist is a greater health hazard to the HIV-infected client than the infected client is to the massage therapist.

Box **7-5**

Malignancies and Common Opportunistic Infections and Conditions in AIDS

- Kaposi's sarcoma: an aggressive malignancy of the blood vessels that appears as purple or blue patches often on the skin, or in the mouth, but can appear anywhere on the body.
- Lymphoma: cancerous lesions of lymphoid tissues (Hodgkin's and non-Hodgkin's).
- *Pneumocystis carinii* pneumonia (PCP): a lung infection that can progress to be life threatening. It is the most common lung disease in persons with AIDS.
- Tuberculosis: a tumorous infection of the lungs or other organs.
- Herpes simplex: painful blisterlike lesions of the mouth, genitalia, or anus, caused by the herpesvirus.
- Herpes zoster (shingles): characterized by clusters of red, blisterlike skin lesions that follow an inflamed nerve path.
- Thrush: a fungal infection of the mucous membranes of the mouth, genitalia, or skin.

- Toxoplasmosis: an infection caused by protozoan intracellular parasites. There can be a rash and lymphadenopathy, and the central nervous system, heart, or lungs can be involved.
- Neurological complications: examples are inflammation of nerves, peripheral neuropathy, neoplasms, and AIDS dementia.
- Diarrhea: symptom of a host of bacterial and viral infections of the gastrointestinal tract, liver, or gallbladder.
- *Cytomegalovirus:* a type of herpes virus, it usually results in a retinal infection, causing blindness or gastrointestinal infection.
- Cryptococcal meningitis: an infectious disease caused by a fungus. The lungs are a primary site of infection. It can spread to the meninges and cause headache, blurred vision, and difficulty speaking.

Modified from Frazier MS, Drzmykowski JW: Essentials of human diseases and conditions, *ed 2, Philadelphia, 2000, WB Saunders.*

to blood vessels by chemicals, bacteria, preeclampsia, heat or physical trauma, liver disease, kidney disease, or heart disease. Edema can be aggravated by prolonged standing, pregnancy, and obesity.

Massage Consideration/s—It is important for the massage therapist to ascertain the cause of the edema. Massage is contraindicated in clients with a history of heart or kidney disease. As massage moves fluid into the blood, the heart or kidneys, which are already debilitated, can become overloaded. For clients without a history of these diseases, light friction and gliding strokes can be most effective. Massage can help lymphatic drainage by moving excess fluid into lymphatic vessels. The client's edematous limb should be supported and elevated. Elevation will promote dependent drainage (lymph drainage assisted by gravity). Proximal areas should be worked first to help clear the path for lymph from distal areas.

Fever

L. Fever

Description—Fever is an abnormal elevation of the body's temperature above 37° C (98.6° F). Infection, neurological disease, malignancy,

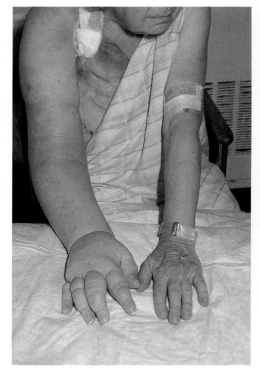

Figure 7-41. Lymphedema.

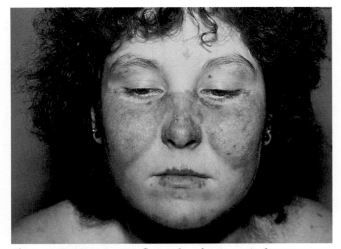

Figure 7-42. Butterfly rash of systemic lupus erythematosus.

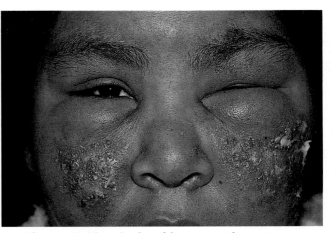

Figure 7-43. Scale of lupus erythematosus.

anemia, thrombotic or embolic disease, tachycardia, congestive heart failure, injury or trauma, and certain medications may cause the development of fever. Exercise, anxiety, and dehydration may cause fever in healthy people.

Massage Consideration/s—Massage is contraindicated. Fever has system-wide effects on the body. Massage will worsen the symptoms. Also, fever may indicate tissue damage, usually from an infection, in which massage will only make the condition worse.

Lupus (Lupus Erythematosus)

L. Wolf

Description—Lupus is an autoimmune, inflammatory disease of the connective tissues. It is not contagious. The cause of lupus is unknown, and its onset may be abrupt or gradual, but it primarily affects women 20 to 40 years old. A rash develops around the nose and check, resembling a wolf (also called a butterfly rash) (Figure 7-42). Symptoms include painful joints, scales (Figure 7-43), fever, fatigue, weight loss, enlarged lymph nodes and spleen, and sensitivity to light. There are periods of remission and exacerbation. Triggers for exacerbation include certain drugs, exposure to excessive sunlight, injury, and stress. Serious complications of the disease involve inflammation of the kidneys, liver, spleen, lungs, heart, and central nervous system. There are three main types of lupus: discoid, systemic, and drug-induced.

Discoid

Discoid lupus erythematosus (DLE) is a skin disease characterized by the presence of skin rash showing

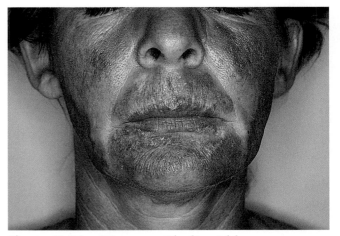

Figure 7-44. Woman with discoid lupus erythematous.

varying degrees of edema, redness, and scaliness (Figure 7-44).

Systemic

Systemic lupus erythematosus (SLE) is the most serious type of lupus. The body attacks connective tissue in joints, skin, and organs. This is a chronic, remitting, relapsing, inflammatory process; it is typically a multisystemic disorder. The client is often photosensitive (Figure 7-45).

Drug-Induced

Medications used to treat hypertension and irregular heartbeat (arrhythmia) can cause the onset of lupus, which usually resolves after the medication is withdrawn (Box 7-6).

Massage Consideration/s—Massage is contraindicated when clients have a flare-up. During

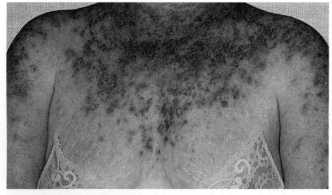

Figure 7-45. Typical photosensitive rash of systemic lupus erythematosus.

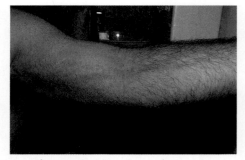

Figure 7-46. Lymphangitis.

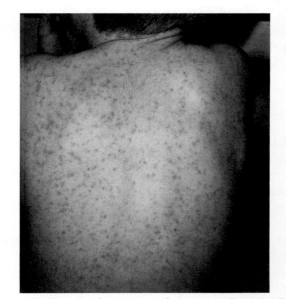

Figure 7-47. Rash commonly seen in Epstein-Barr virus.

periods of remission, a gentle full body massage is indicated, with special care taken of joints during stretches and joint mobilizations. Clients may be taking corticosteroids and antiinflammatory drugs, and thus may be more susceptible to bruising. See Chapter 4 for information on these medications. Clients could also be on immunosuppressants, so care should be taken not to expose the clients to any form of infection. It is important to ask each client for a list of his or her symptoms and plan massage accordingly.

Lymphangitis (Angioleukitis, Angiolymphitis)
(lim`·fuhn·jai´·tis) (an`·jee·oh`·loo·kai´·tis)
(an`·jee·oh`·lim·fai´·tis)

L. Water; Gr. Inflammation

Description—Lymphangitis is inflammation of one or more lymphatic vessels, usually resulting from an acute streptococcal infection in the extremities. It manifests itself by painful, subcutaneous red streaks extending from the infected area to the axilla or groin, and by fever, chills, and headaches (Figure 7-46).

Massage Consideration/s—Massage is contraindicated because of the subsequent pain and swelling; massage only worsens these conditions. Additionally, a client with lymphangitis will more than likely feel too sick to receive a massage.

Mononucleosis (mah`·noh·noo`·klee·oh´·sis)

Gr. Single; Kernel; Condition

Description—Infectious mononucleosis is an acute viral infection that results from the Epstein-Barr virus (EBV). Symptoms are a

slight to high fever, sore throat, red throat and soft palate, stiff neck, enlarged lymph nodes, coughing, and fatigue. Sometimes a rash is present (Figure 7-47). It is highly contagious and is transmitted by droplets that contain the virus. There is no cure; treatment is letting the disease run its course while treating any complications.

Massage Consideration/s—Massage is contraindicated until the client has recovered and is released by his or her physician. Once the client receives permission, a gentle massage is indicated, especially on the abdominal region, as the spleen may be enlarged. Heat packs may help relieve persistent body ache.

Box **7-6**

Cardiac Arrhythmias

Arrhythmia (Dysrhythmia) (uh·rith´·mee·uh) (dis·rith´·mee·uh)

Gr. Without; Rhythm

Description—Any deviation from a normal cardiac rhythm is considered an arrhythmia. The abnormality may be of the heart rate, the regularity of the heart rhythm, the sinoatrial node, or other components of the heart's conduction system. This general term encompasses abnormally fast yet regular rhythms, irregular rhythms, and loss of rhythm.

Bradycardia

Gr. Slow; Heart

Description—A type of arrhythmia, bradycardia is an abnormally slow heartbeat, to less than 60 beats per minute. Bradycardia is normal in well-trained endurance athletes. Also, heart rate normally slows during sleep. Pathological bradycardia may be symptomatic of a myxedema, a brain tumor, or other conditions. When cardiac output is decreased, the person may experience faintness, dizziness, chest pain, syncope, and circulatory collapse.

Flutter

AS. To Fly About

Description—A flutter is an abnormally rapid heartbeat. Atrial flutter means the atria are contracting up to 240 to 360 beats per minute. However, the atria still contract in a synchronized fashion. Atrial flutter is caused by coronary artery disease, congenital heart disease, and other heart diseases.

Fibrillation

L. Little Fiber; Process

Description—Fibrillation occurs when the chambers of the heart contract asynchronously, and thus stop pumping blood. It can be caused by a myocardial infarction and other heart diseases. Atrial fibrillation decreases the pumping effectiveness of the heart by only 20% to 30% in a strong heart. Ventricular fibrillation, however, can result in death, as blood is no longer ejected from the heart. Defibrillation, a procedure in which a brief, strong electrical current is passed through the heart, often stops ventricular fibrillation. See Box 7-2 for more information.

Heart Blocks

Description—A heart block is an impairment of the conduction activity in the heart. Heart blocks are further defined according to the location and type of block. One example is a first-degree atrioventricular block. In this type of block, atrial impulses do reach the ventricles, but are delayed by a fraction of a second. A heart block can occur in the sinoatrial node, atrioventricular node, bundle of His, atria, or in a combination of these. An artificial pacemaker is a device that is often surgically implanted. See Box 7-1 for more information.

Tachycardia (ta`·kee·kahr´·dee·uh)

Gr. Swift; Heart

Description—A type of arrhythmia, tachycardia is an excessively rapid heartbeat, as evidenced by the pulse rate being over 100 beats per minute in an adult. Heart rate normally accelerates in response to fever, during and immediately after exercise, or during periods of anxiety and excitement. Pathological tachycardia may be symptomatic of anemia, congestive heart failure, hemorrhage, or shock. Tachycardia increases the blood flow and amount of oxygen available to the body's tissues.

SUMMARY

The two main fluid transport systems of the body are the cardiovascular and lymphvascular systems. Together these two systems deliver oxygen and nutrition to body tissues while removing toxins and waste products. They also fight disease and provide for the body's immune system response.

The organs of the cardiovascular system are the blood, heart, and blood vessels. There are two main circuits of the cardiovascular system: the pulmonary and the systemic. Significant pathologies of the cardiovascular system include a legion of disorders: angina, anemia, aneurysm, cardiac arrest, congestive heart failure, cerebrovascular accident, embolism, endocarditis, heart murmur, hemangioma, hematoma, hemophilia, hemorrhage, hypertension, hypotension, migraine headache, cluster headache, myocardial infarction, Raynaud's syndrome, shock, sickle cell disease, fainting, and transient ischemic attack.

The lymphvascular system is composed of lymph fluid, lymph vessels, and specialized tissues such as bone marrow, thymus, spleen, lymph nodes, and lymphatic nodules. The lymphvascular system does not have a central pump like the heart. Instead, lymph is moved along the lymph channels by the muscular contraction of surrounding tissues. These two channels drain into two large veins near the neck, returning interstitial fluid back to the cardiovascular system. Lymphvascular pathologies include acquired immunodeficiency syndrome, allergies, chronic fatigue syndrome, edema, fever, lupus, lymphangitis, and mononucleosis.

Cardiovascular and lymphvascular pathologies may be suspected when symptoms include bradycardia, tachycardia, hypertension, skin discolorations (pallor, redness, jaundice, cyanosis), unexplained bruising or skin pigmentation, rashes, hives, scaliness (with or without itching), unexplained chest or calf pain, swollen lymph nodes, lymphedema, chronic fatigue, and unexplained weight loss. The massage therapist needs to refer the client to a physician immediately when any of these symptoms are present. Other signs to look for during assessment include skin condition, nail condition, edema, fatigue, anxiety, insomnia, headaches, and shortness of breath.

Resources

American Heart Association
7272 Greenville Avenue
Dallas, TX 75231
800-AHA-USA1
www.amhrt.org

American Lupus Society
23751 Madison Street
Torrance, CA 90503
213-373-1335

Cooley's Anemia Foundation
129-09 26th Street, Suite 203
Flushing, NY 11354
800-522-7222
ncaf@aol.com

Family AIDS Network
678 Front Street NW
Grand Rapids, MI 49504

Lupus Foundation of America
800-558-0121
301-670-9292 (in Maryland)

National AIDS Hotline
PO Box 13827
RTP, NC 27709
800-342-AIDS (24 hours a day)
www.hivmail@cdc.gov

National Heart Attack Alert Program
PO Box 30105
Bethesda, MD 20824-0105
301-251-1272

National Hemophilia Foundation
116 West 32nd Street
New York, NY 10001
www.hemophilia.org

National Lupus Erythematosus Foundation
5430 Van Nys Boulevard, Suite 206
Van Nys, CA 91401
213-885-8787

National Patient Organization for Primary Immunodeficiencies
www.ipopi.org/

National STD Hotline
800-227-8922

Sickle Cell Disease Association of America
200 Corporate Point, Suite 495
Culver, CA 90230-7633
800-421-8453
www.sicklecelldisease.org

SELF-TEST

List the letter of the answer to the term or phrase that best describes it.

A. Acquired immunodeficiency syndrome
B. Allergy
C. Anemia
D. Aneurysm
E. Arteriosclerosis
F. Chronic fatigue syndrome
G. Congestive heart failure
H. Edema
I. Embolus
J. Fever
K. Hemangioma
L. Hematoma
M. Hemophilia
N. Hypertension
O. Hypotension
P. Lupus
Q. Migraine headaches
R. Mononucleosis
S. Myocarditis
T. Pericarditis
U. Peripheral vascular disease
V. Phlebitis
W. Raynaud's syndrome
X. Sickle cell disease
Y. Telangiectasia
Z. Varicose veins

_____ 1. A genetic disorder affecting the blood's clotting mechanism.

_____ 2. Inflammation of the parietal pericardium.

_____ 3. A weakened section of a blood vessel wall.

_____ 4. A syndrome characterized by cycles of vasospasm in blood vessels, usually the most distal parts of the body (i.e., fingers, toes, ears, nose).

_____ 5. A blood clot, bubble of air, or any piece of debris transported by the bloodstream.

_____ 6. Abnormal accumulation of interstitial fluid in tissue spaces; characterized by swelling.

_____ 7. A group of arterial diseases characterized by a thickening and loss of elasticity, which leads to a hardening of the arterial walls.

_____ 8. Dilated veins resulting from incompetent valves; these veins lose elasticity and become stretched and flabby.

_____ 9. An autoimmune, inflammatory disease of the connective tissues.

_____ 10. A genetic disorder characterized by abnormal hemoglobin, which causes red blood cells to "sickle."

_____ 11. An infectious acute viral infection that results from the Epstein-Barr virus.

_____ 12. A permanent dilation of superficial capillaries or small blood vessels commonly affecting the face.

_____ 13. A common, often asymptomatic disorder of elevated blood pressure.

_____ 14. Also called vascular headaches, these headaches are caused by dilation of extracranial blood vessels.

_____ 15. Inflammation of the veins; generally affecting the extremities.

_____ 16. In this condition, the heart becomes a slowly failing pump.

_____ 17. This condition is a reduction of the oxygen-carrying capacity of the blood, a decrease in erythrocytes, or a reduced amount of functional hemoglobin in the blood.

_____ 18. Abnormal elevation of the body's temperature; above 37° C (98.6° F).

_____ 19. A vascular disease that affects both blood and lymphatic vessels. Symptoms include numbness, pain and discomfort, skin discoloration, and elevated blood pressure.

_____ 20. A disease caused by the human immunodeficiency virus (HIV).

_____ 21. A benign tumor consisting of a localized mass of dilated blood vessels.

_____ 22. A condition characterized by disabling fatigue, often accompanied by flulike symptoms.

_____ 23. Inflammation of the muscular walls of the heart.

_____ 24. Also known as hypersensitivity, this is an overreaction of the immune system to otherwise harmless agents (most are environmental or dietary).

_____ 25. Low blood pressure.

_____ 26. A localized collection of blood trapped in the tissues of an organ, body space, or the skin.

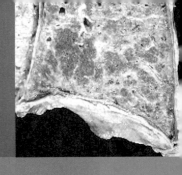

8   **Respiratory Pathologies**

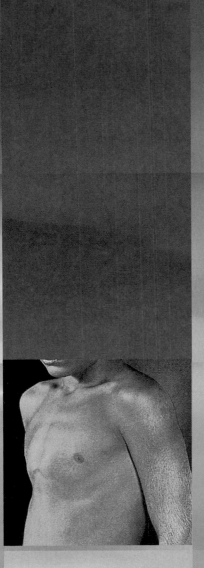

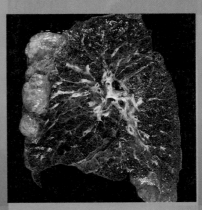

Breath and the breathing process are synonymous with life itself. Breathing is the most easily observable of the body's vital signs. One way a massage therapist can assess a client is to observe the client's breathing. Is the client holding his or her breath while massage techniques are being performed? That may mean the pressure is too deep. Does the client breathe shallowly and rapidly? That could indicate an anxious client.

Massage therapy also directly affects the respiratory system. By massaging the muscles of respiration, the massage therapist can perhaps ease a client's breathing. When a client receives a relaxing, nurturing massage the client will breathe more deeply and slowly, and become more oxygenated. By encouraging a client to take deep, slow breaths during deep pressure application, the client is less likely to tense up while the work is being done.

Cells continually use oxygen for the metabolic reactions that release energy from nutrient molecules. The released energy is used throughout the entire body for processes such as protein synthesis, nerve impulse conduction, and muscle contraction. A by-product of oxygen use in metabolism is carbon dioxide. An excessive amount of carbon dioxide produces acids that can be toxic to cells. Excess carbon dioxide must be eliminated quickly and efficiently.

The two body systems that cooperate to supply oxygen and eliminate carbon dioxide are the cardiovascular and respiratory systems. The respiratory system is responsible for gas exchange (intake of oxygen and elimination of carbon dioxide); the cardiovascular system transports the blood containing the gases between the lungs and the body cells. Failure of either system has the same effect on the body—namely disruption of homeostasis and rapid cell death from oxygen deprivation and buildup of wastes.

Besides the function of gas exchange, the respiratory system also helps regulate blood pH (by eliminating carbon dioxide and thus decreasing acidity). The respiratory system contains olfactory receptors (for sense of smell), filters incoming air, produces sounds, and eliminates some water and heat in exhaled air.

Air movement and gas exchange are accomplished by the anatomical structures of the respiratory system. These include the nose and nasal cavity, pharynx (throat), larynx (voice box), trachea (windpipe), bronchial tree, and lungs (Figure 8-1).

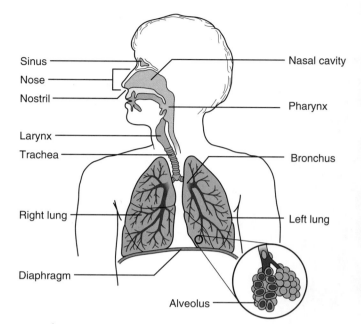

Figure 8-1. General respiratory structures.

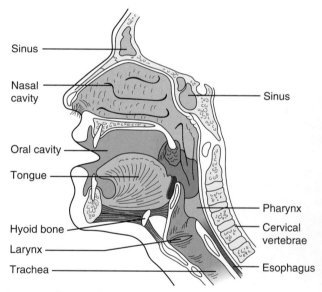

Figure 8-2. Upper respiratory tract.

Inhaled air is first affected in the nasal cavity. The entire respiratory tract is lined with mucous membrane. In the nasal cavity, the sticky mucus traps particles, and the air is moistened and warmed.

The air proceeds down through the pharynx and larynx and into the trachea (Figure 8-2). The trachea consists of 16 to 20 incomplete rings of cartilage stacked on top of each other. They form a semirigid support that keeps that part of the airway open. At about the level of the fifth thoracic vertebra, the

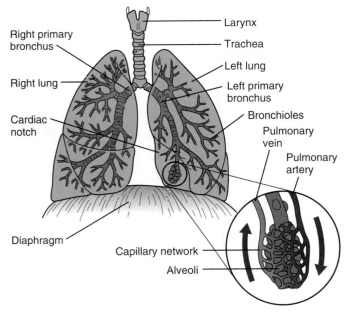

Figure 8-3. Lower respiratory tract.

trachea divides in right and left primary bronchi, which enter each lung.

The lungs are in the thoracic cavity and rest on the diaphragm (Figure 8-3). Each lung is a separate organ. If one were to collapse, the other would continue to function. The pleural membrane (pleura) surrounds and protects each lung. This is a double-layered membrane with a space in between the layers that contains a thin film of fluid. This fluid decreases friction as the lungs move with each inhalation and exhalation.

The right lung has three lobes and is thicker and broader than the left lung because the liver, a large organ, is underneath the diaphragm on the right side. The left lung has two lobes and an indentation called the cardiac notch. The heart, whose inferior portion tilts to the left, fits into this notch.

Inside each lung the primary bronchi branch into smaller secondary bronchi, which then branch into smaller tertiary bronchi. The tertiary bronchi branch further into even smaller bronchioles. This extensive branching of airways from the trachea resembles an inverted tree and is referred to as the bronchial tree. As the branching becomes more extensive, there is less and less cartilage in the walls of the airways, and more and more smooth muscle until the bronchioles have no cartilage at all. The smooth muscle allows the airways and lung tissue to stretch to accommodate incoming air. Because there is no cartilage to keep the airways open, however, during an acute asthma attack, the walls of the bronchioles can spasm and cut off air flow.

Eventually, the bronchioles branch into alveoli (alveolus is singular). Alveoli are the air sacs in the lungs. They have very thin walls that contain a lot of elastic tissue. Alveoli stretch as they fill with air, like little balloons. An alveolar sac consists of two or more alveoli that share a common opening. The pulmonary capillary network surrounds the alveoli and is fused to the outer wall of the alveoli. The structure resembles basketballs in a net. The pulmonary capillaries are derived from pulmonary arteries, which transport deoxygenated blood from the heart to the lungs.

Between the wall of the pulmonary capillaries and the walls of the alveoli is the respiratory membrane. The respiratory membrane is the site of gas exchange: oxygen diffuses from air in the alveoli across the respiratory membrane into blood in the pulmonary capillaries. Carbon dioxide diffuses from the blood in the pulmonary capillaries to the air in the alveoli.

After the blood in the pulmonary capillaries becomes oxygenated, it flows into pulmonary veins that carry it back to the heart so that it can be pumped to all the tissues of the body. At the tissue level, the oxygen diffuses from the blood into the cells, and carbon dioxide from the cells diffuses into the blood. The deoxygenated blood then travels back to the heart so that it can be pumped to the lungs to become oxygenated again.

Air movement into and out of the lungs is called pulmonary ventilation, and it consists of inspiration (inhalation) and expiration (exhalation). Pulmonary ventilation is controlled by the respiratory center in the brainstem (medulla oblongata) of the brain. It automatically controls the rate and depth of breathing. However, the respiratory center can be overridden, and a person can voluntarily alter the pattern of breathing. Examples include holding the breath and consciously breathing more deeply during activities such as exercise and yoga.

Pulmonary ventilation is a mechanical process because it involves muscular contraction, muscular relaxation, and elastic recoil of the alveoli. Air moves from high pressure to low pressure. Just before each inhalation, atmospheric air pressure equals air pressure in the lungs. To move air into the lungs, the air pressure in the lungs needs to become lower than atmospheric pressure. This is accomplished by enlarging the thoracic cavity.

The diaphragm is the main muscle of inhalation. When it contracts, it descends and enlarges the thoracic cavity. The external intercostal muscles also assist in inhalation by lifting the ribs. Air pressure in the lungs drops, air is drawn in, and normal, quiet inhalation occurs; this is an active process. The alveoli fill up with air. Normal, quiet exhalation occurs when the diaphragm relaxes and descends, and elastic recoil of the alveoli pushes air out; this is a passive process.

During deep, forceful inhalation, secondary muscles of respiration are used. These include the scalenes, which lift ribs one and two; sternocleidomastoid, which lifts the sternum and the clavicle; pectoralis minor, which lifts ribs three, four, and five; and serratus posterior superior, which lifts ribs five, six, and seven. All of these contract to greatly increase the size of the thoracic cavity and to assist in drawing in air.

During deep, forceful exhalation, secondary muscles of respiration will also be used. These include the abdominal muscles, which assist in pushing the diaphragm upward; internal intercostals, which depress the ribs; and serratus posterior inferior, which depresses ribs nine, ten, eleven, and twelve. All of these contract to greatly decrease the size of the thoracic cavity and assist in pushing out air.

THERAPEUTIC ASSESSMENT OF THE RESPIRATORY SYSTEM

The following list of pertinent questions serves as a review of how to evaluate the respiratory system. Findings need to be documented.

Questions to ask the client in the premassage interview:

* *Is the client taking any medication/s for respiratory illness?* Table 8-1 has more information on medications including possible side effects.

Table **8-1** MEDICATIONS USED TO MANAGE RESPIRATORY DISORDERS

MEDICATION CLASSIFICATION	MEDICATION NAME	POSSIBLE SIDE EFFECTS THAT MAY AFFECT TREATMENT
Antihistamine	Chlorpheniramine (Chlor-Tripolon), diphenhydramine (Benadryl)	Anxiety, chills, constipation and diarrhea, disorientation, drowsiness, dry mouth, headaches, insomnia, nausea and vomiting, shortness of breath, skin rashes, vertigo, wheezing
Antitussives	Antihistamines, benzonatate (Tessalon), dextromethorphan hydrobromide (the DM in cough and cold medicine)	Gastrointestinal irritation, sedation
Bronchodilators	Albuterol (Ventolin), epinephrine HCl (Primatene Mist), fenoterol hydrobromide (Berotec) [fenoterol is not available in US], formoterol (Foradil), isoproterenol (Isuprel), levalbuterol (Xopenex), metaproterenol (Alupent), pirbuterol (Maxair), salmeterol (Serevent), terbutaline (Brethine), oxtriphylline (Choledyl), theophylline (Slo-bid, Theo-Dur)	Anxiety, drowsiness, dry mouth, headaches, hypertension, insomnia, irregular heartbeat, nausea and vomiting
Decongestants	Oxymetazoline (Afrin, Coricidin), pseudoephedrine (Sudafed)	Hallucinations, headaches, hypertension, irregular heartbeat
Expectorants	Guaifenesin, potassium iodide	Fever, nausea and vomiting, skin rashes
Mast cell stabilizers	Cromolyn sodium (Crolom, Intal Inhaler, Intal, Nasalcrom, Opticum), nedocromil sodium (Alocril, Tilade)	Dizziness, irregular heartbeat, nausea and vomiting

- *If the client has any known allergies or asthma, does the client know what his or her triggers are?* The massage therapist needs to be prepared to make adjustments to the massage environment.
- *Does the client use an inhaler?* If so, it should be handy during the massage treatment.
- *If the client has sleep apnea, what positions are most comfortable?* The massage therapist needs to be prepared to use pillows or bolsters to increase client comfort.
- *Are there any positions that make breathing easier or more difficult?* The massage therapist needs to be prepared to use pillows or bolsters to increase client comfort.

Observations and palpations to make during the premassage interview and during the massage treatment:

- *What is the condition of the client's skin?* The massage therapist should assess both color and temperature, and look for signs of pallor and cyanosis, particularly on the fingertips or lips. This indicates possible hypoxia or reduced blood oxygenation.
- *Are there signs of edema?* If so, caution is advised. The massage therapist needs to ascertain the cause of the edema from the client and clearance may need to be obtained from the client's health care provider before massage therapy can be performed. If the edema is not due to a serious condition such as congestive heart failure or renal failure, massage can be performed. If indicated, the massage therapist should elevate the affected areas during treatment to promote drainage and use lymphatic drainage techniques.
- *Are the client's nail bed color and shape in good condition?* These are signs of hypoxia. Chapter 2 has a discussion of nail clubbing.
- *Are cervical and axillary lymph nodes swollen?* These may be indicators of respiratory infection.
- *What is the client's respiration rate?* Normal adult respiration is about 16 breaths (one inhale and one exhale) per minute. Every 15 seconds, there should be about four complete breaths. Increased respiration rate may be due to respiratory distress. However, the sympathetic nervous system does increase respiration, so fear and anxiety result in more rapid breaths.
- *What areas of the client's body move during respiration? Does the client do diaphragmatic* (abdominal) or costal breathing? Are there any postural deviations that affect breathing (e.g., barrel chest, kyphosis, forward head posture) (Figure 8-4)? Unless massage is contraindicated, these movements or postures help the massage therapist decide on which muscles to focus treatment.
- *During respiration, are there any respiratory-related sounds?* The massage therapist should listen for high-pitched sounds, wheezing, rattling, crackling, and deep or harsh sounds. Wheezing indicates a narrowing of respiratory passageways, perhaps as a result of illness such as asthma, hay fever, common cold or flu, or more serious illness such as tuberculosis. Crackling or rattling may indicate that the respiratory passageways contain mucus. These sounds can be heard with a stethoscope and with the human ear.
- *What are the client's breathing patterns? Are there signs of shortness of breath? Is the client a nose breather? A mouth breather?* Shortness of breath can indicate anything from rushing to make the massage appointment, to anxiety, to a respiratory disorder. Mouth breathing can indicate constrictions or blockages in the air passageways.

GENERAL MANIFESTATIONS OF RESPIRATORY DISEASE

If a client has any of the following, the massage therapist needs to refer the client to the client's health care provider for diagnosis and treatment.

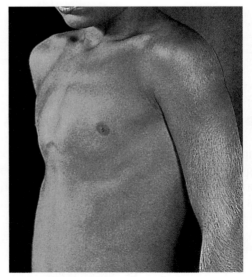

Figure 8-4. Barrel chest.

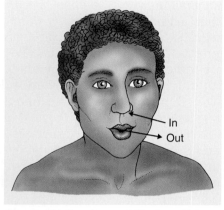

Figure 8-5.   Pursed lip breathing.

- Altered breathing patterns (e.g., rapid, difficult, prolonged, or labored breathing)
- Change in breathing sounds (may be high-pitched, a rattle, or a deep, harsh sound, or an absence of breathing sounds)
- Wheezing
- Nasal flaring during inhalation
- Pursed lips during exhalation (Figure 8-5)
- Chest or facial pain
- Pale skin
- Cyanosis of lips or fingertips
- Clubbed finger and toes (nails may curve downward)
- Sore throat
- Swollen lymph nodes
- Any signs of respiratory infection such as sneezing, coughing, watery eyes, running nose, hoarseness, chills, or fever
- Sputum (color may vary from yellowish-greenish, to rusty; may be thick or thin; may have a foul odor; may be tinged with blood)

RESPIRATORY PATHOLOGIES

Apnea (ap´·nee·uh)

Gr. Without; Breathing

Description—Apnea is a temporary cessation (usually lasting 15 seconds) or absence of spontaneous breathing. Sleep apnea occurs during sleep. It can be due to abnormalities in the respiratory center in the brain or to obstruction of airflow in the mouth or pharynx while sleeping. Individuals with sleep apnea may have loud snoring, insomnia, sleepiness during the day, early morning headaches, and possibly depression.

Massage Consideration/s—The massage therapist needs to ask the client with sleep apnea about the cause of the apnea and adjust the massage accordingly. The massage therapist also needs to ask if the client is comfortable prone or supine. If prone and/or supine positions are not possible, side or semi-reclining positions can be used. A general, relaxing massage can help give the client with sleep apnea a chance to rejuvenate and perhaps alleviate some symptoms of depression, if the client has any.

Asthma

Gr. Panting

Description—Asthma is a chronic, inflammatory disorder caused by airway sensitivity to various stimuli; this can lead to airway obstruction. Triggers of asthmatic attacks include allergens (substances that produce allergic reactions) such as pollen, dust mites, molds, certain foods, emotional upset, aspirin, exercise, cold air, and cigarette smoke. An early phase or acute attack of asthma results in smooth muscle spasm in the smaller bronchi and bronchioles accompanied by excessive mucus secretion that further clogs airways and worsens the attack. The person having an acute asthmatic attack needs to be medically treated immediately by being given an inhaled medication to help relax the smooth muscle in the bronchioles and reopen the airways. The late phase or chronic asthmatic response is characterized by airway inflammation, edema, and death of cells lining the airways. Long-term treatment of asthma includes antiinflammatory medications. In the United States 3% to 5% of the population have asthma; it is more common in children than in adults. Asthma is partially reversible, either with treatment or spontaneously. See Figure 8-6 for signs and symptoms of an asthma attack.

Massage Consideration/s—The therapist needs to make sure from the client's intake form and pre-massage interview that there are no allergens in the massage office that would trigger an attack. If the client uses a bronchodilator, the massage therapist should make sure it is handy for the client to reach. Side-lying or semi-reclining positions to help with breathing may be the most comfortable for the client. A full-body, relaxing massage is helpful. The massage treatment should focus on the primary and secondary muscles of respiration (Table 8-2). Techniques such as deep friction, kneading, ischemic compression, and deep gliding strokes can help loosen these tight muscles. The postural muscles also need to be addressed because many clients with chronic asthma develop kyphosis. Vibration and percussion over the rib cage may help loosen mucus. The massage therapist needs to communi-

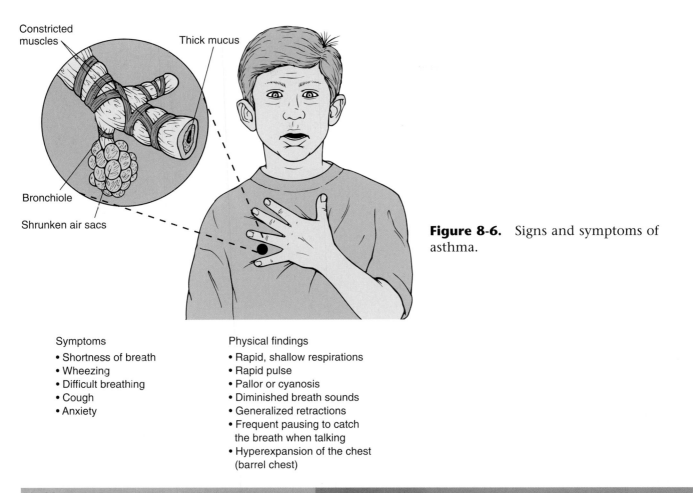

Figure 8-6. Signs and symptoms of asthma.

Symptoms
- Shortness of breath
- Wheezing
- Difficult breathing
- Cough
- Anxiety

Physical findings
- Rapid, shallow respirations
- Rapid pulse
- Pallor or cyanosis
- Diminished breath sounds
- Generalized retractions
- Frequent pausing to catch the breath when talking
- Hyperexpansion of the chest (barrel chest)

Table **8-2** **MUSCLES OF RESPIRATION**

	PRIMARY NORMAL, QUIET BREATHING	SECONDARY DEEP, FORCEFUL BREATHING
Muscles of exhalation	None (passive process)	Abdominals, internal intercostals, serratus posterior inferior
Muscles of inhalation	Diaphragm, external intercostals	Scalenes, sternocleidomastoid, pectoralis minor, serratus posterior superior

cate with the client about the pressure and effectiveness of techniques.

Bronchitis (brahng·kai´·tis)

Gr. Windpipe; Inflammation

Description—Bronchitis is inflammation of the bronchial mucosa that causes swelling of bronchial tubes and production of extra mucus. The two types of bronchitis are acute and chronic. Acute bronchitis is caused by an upper respiratory tract infection; it results in a productive cough and high fever. Chronic bronchitis involves copious secretions of mucus with a productive cough that typically lasts 3 full months of the year for 2 successive years (Figure 8-7). Cigarette smoking is the most common cause of chronic

bronchitis. The inhaled irritants lead to chronic inflammation and excessive mucus production. The thick mucus narrows airways and impairs ciliary action, thus making it difficult for the person to expel debris-laden mucus. Inhaled pathogens easily embed in the airways and multiply rapidly.

Massage Consideration/s—Massage is contraindicated if the client has acute bronchitis and a fever. Massage would only exacerbate the symptoms and make the client feel worse. If the client has chronic bronchitis, the massage therapist needs to ask the client what positions on the massage table are comfortable. A full-body relaxing massage is helpful. Postural drainage is very useful in clearing the respiratory tract of mucus. The massage therapist should position the client so that the head is lower

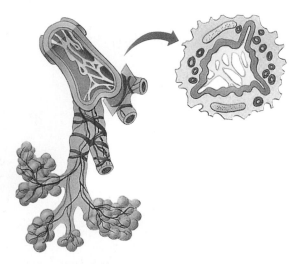

Figure 8-7. Thick mucus of chronic bronchitis.

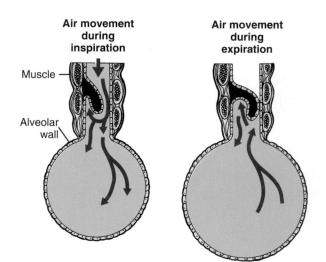

Figure 8-8. Mechanisms of restricted air flow in chronic obstructive pulmonary disease (COPD).

than the rest of the body. This can be done by putting pillows under the client's abdomen or by making the head of the massage table lower than the foot of the table. Percussion and vibration are then performed on the ribcage for up to 5 minutes. A menthol-based cream can be applied to help clear air passageways; ask the client if he or she can tolerate menthol before applying it. The massage therapist also needs to focus on the muscles of respiration (see Table 8-2). Techniques such as deep friction, kneading, ischemic compression, and deep gliding strokes can help loosen these tight muscles. The massage therapist needs to communicate with the client about the pressure and effectiveness of techniques.

Chronic Obstructive Pulmonary Disease (COPD)

Description—COPD is a group of pulmonary disorders characterized by persistent or recurring obstruction of airflow, such as asthma, emphysema, cystic fibrosis, pneumoconiosis, or chronic bronchitis (Figure 8-8). The individual is unable to breathe freely and can be classified medically as "pink puffers" (predominately emphysema) or "blue bloaters" (predominately bronchitis) (Figure 8-9).

Massage Consideration/s—See entries for asthma, emphysema, cystic fibrosis, pneumoconiosis, and chronic bronchitis.

Common Cold (Head Cold, Infectious Rhinitis, Upper Respiratory Infection, URI) (in·fek´·shuhs rai·nai´·tis)

M.E. Infect; Gr. Nose; Inflammation

Description—A cold is an acute inflammation of the mucosa of the upper respiratory tract, usually confined to the nose and throat, but

the larynx can be involved as well. Symptoms include coughing, sneezing, watery eyes, nasal congestion and discharge, sore throat, and hoarseness. Fever and chills may accompany a cold.

Massage Consideration/s—A person is infectious for 2 to 3 days after the cold symptoms start, so massage is contraindicated during this time. After the infectious stage, massage can be performed as long as the symptoms are not severe. Once symptoms are no longer acute, massage may be done, only if the client understands that the treatment may exacerbate symptoms for a short time, but decreases the overall recovery time.

Cystic Fibrosis (sis´·tik fai·broh´·sis)

Gr. Bladder; Fiber; Condition

Description—Cystic fibrosis is a genetic disorder involving the overproduction of secretions of all exocrine glands, especially the pancreas, and the lining of the respiratory system (Figure 8-10). The bronchi secrete thick mucus, which obstructs and narrows the airway. Individuals with cystic fibrosis often have poor nutrition and a small stature (Figure 8-11). The prognosis is poor and there is no known cure.

Massage Consideration/s—Clearance for massage from the client's health care provider is recommended. Once clearance is obtained, inquire about what positions on the massage table are comfortable for the client. A full-body relaxing massage is helpful. Postural drainage is useful in clearing the respiratory tract of mucus. The massage therapist would position the client so that the head is lower than the rest of the body. This can be done by

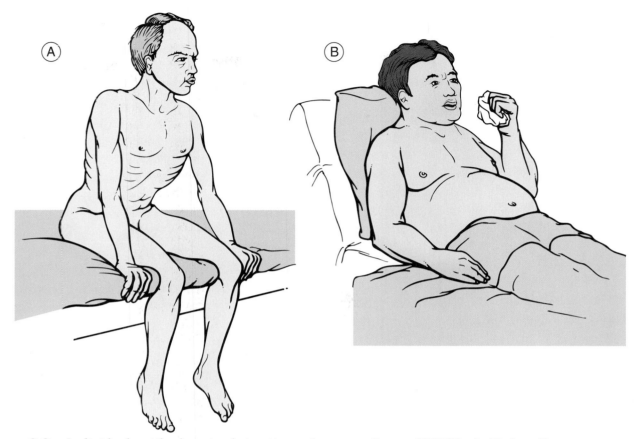

Figure 8-9. Individuals with chronic obstructive pulmonary disease (COPD). **A,** Pink puffers, or **B,** blue bloaters.

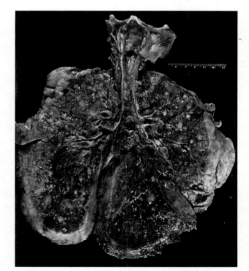

Figure 8-10. Lungs of a dying patient with cystic fibrosis.

putting pillows under the client's abdomen or by making the head of the massage table lower than the foot of the table. Percussion and vibration are then performed on the ribcage for up to 5 minutes. The massage therapist also needs to be sure to focus on the muscles of respiration (see Table 8-2). Techniques such as deep friction, kneading, ischemic compression, and deep gliding strokes can help loosen these tight muscles. The massage therapist needs to communicate with the client about the pressure and effectiveness of techniques.

Emphysema (em`·fuh·zee´·muh)

Gr. To Inflate

Description—Emphysema involves gradual destruction of elasticity in the walls of the alveoli. This produces abnormally large air spaces that remain filled with air during expiration (Figure 8-12). With the loss of elasticity in the alveoli, the person may inhale easily, but has to labor to exhale (Figure 8-13). The added exertion increases the size of the rib cage, resulting in a barrel

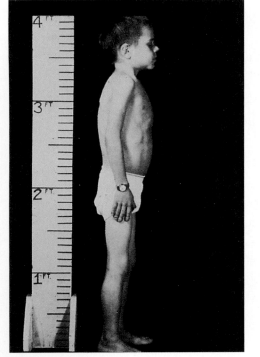

Figure 8-11. Individual with poor nutrition often seen in cystic fibrosis.

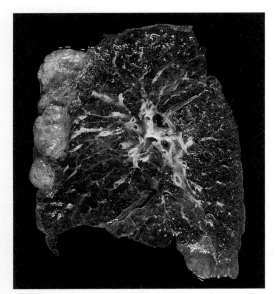

Figure 8-12. Lung of individual with emphysema due to smoking.

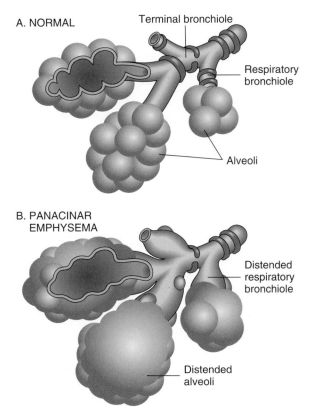

Figure 8-13. Changes in alveoli in emphysema. **A,** Close-up of normal alveoli. **B,** Close-up of alveoli in emphysema.

chest. Emphysema is caused by long-term irritation (e.g., cigarette smoke, air pollution) and exposure to industrial dust.

Massage Consideration/s—The massage therapist needs to ask the client what positions on the massage table are comfortable. The client may need to be propped in a semireclining position for ease of breathing (Figure 8-14). The muscles of respiration will be especially tight, so the massage treatment should focus on them (see Table 8-2). In particular, the sternocleidomastoid, intercostals, scalenes, and pectoralis minor need to be addressed with techniques such as deep gliding, deep friction, kneading, and ischemic compression. During the later stages, a soothing rather than vigorous massage may be indicated if the client fatigues easily. The massage therapist should ask the client how quickly he or she tires. The massage therapist should also communicate with the client about the pressure and effectiveness of techniques.

Hay Fever (Allergic Rhinitis)

Gr. Other; Work; Nose; Inflammation

Description—Hay fever is a general term used to denote any allergic reaction of the nasal mucosa and is characterized by sudden attacks of sneezing, swelling, and profuse water discharge of the nasal mucosa, with itching and watering of

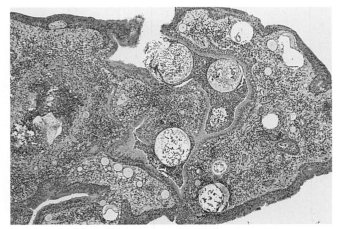

Figure 8-14. Client in semireclining position.

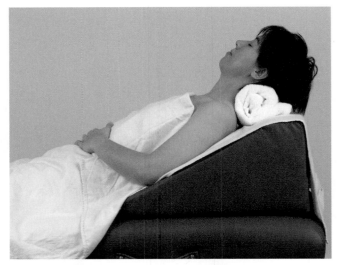

Figure 8-15. Swollen and inflamed nasal mucosa.

the eyes. Often occurring perennially, it is caused by allergens such as house dust, pet dander, and pollen (Figure 8-15).

Massage Consideration/s—Massage is contraindicated during an acute allergic attack as it may make the symptoms worse. If the client is not having an acute attack but has congestion, the massage therapist needs to ask the client if the client is comfortable lying prone and/or using the face cradle, as both can cause nasal passages to drain. The massage therapist needs to make sure the massage treatment area is free of dust and as many allergens as possible. The massage therapist should ask if the client is currently experiencing any symptoms. General massage can be performed as long as the client is not experiencing any acute allergic attack.

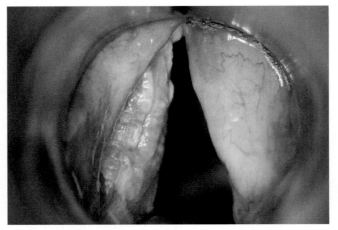

Figure 8-16. Chronic laryngitis. This lesion appears as thickened vocal cords.

Influenza (Flu) (in·floo·en´·zuh)

It. Influence; Note: from the belief that the stars influenced epidemics

Description—Influenza is an acute viral infection of the respiratory tract caused by different strains of viruses *(influenzaviruses)* designated A, B, and C. These viruses have a 3-day incubation period, with the illness lasting between 3 and 10 days. Influenza is characterized by an inflamed nasal mucosa and pharynx with fever and chills. Headaches, muscle aches, and pains may also be noted. The most serious complication is bronchopneumonia.

Massage Consideration/s—Massage is contraindicated for a client with influenza, which is a contagious disease. Also, because the client would be experiencing system-wide effects, the manipulation of tissues with massage would only make the client feel worse.

Laryngitis (lar`·uhn·jai´·tis)

Gr. Larynx; Inflammation

Description—Laryngitis is inflammation of the larynx that often results in loss of voice (Figure 8-16). Respiratory infections or irritants such as cigarette smoke cause laryngitis. Most long-term smokers acquire a permanent hoarseness from the damage created by chronic irritation and inflammation. Edema of the vocal cords, as well as coughing and a scratchy throat, often accompanies this disorder.

Massage Consideration/s—The massage therapist needs to ask the client the cause of the laryngitis. If it is due to an infectious disease, massage is contraindicated. If it is not due to an infection, general massage can be performed.

Pleurisy (Pleuritis) (plur´·uh·see) (plur´·ai·tis)

Gr. Side; Inflammation

Description—Pleurisy is inflammation of the pleural membranes characterized by burning or stabbing pain during breathing. Painful breathing is caused by friction created as the swollen pleural membranes rub against each other. Chronic pleurisy may result in permanent pleural adhesions.

Massage Consideration/s—The massage therapist needs to obtain clearance for massage from the client's health care provider. Massage is contraindicated if the pleurisy is due to bacterial infection. Otherwise, a full-body, relaxing massage is helpful. The massage treatment should focus on the primary and secondary muscles of respiration (see Table 8-2). Techniques such as deep friction, kneading, ischemic compression, and deep gliding strokes can help loosen these tight muscles. The massage therapist needs to communicate with the client about the pressure and effectiveness of techniques.

Pneumoconiosis (noo`·moh·koh`·nee·oh´·sis)

Gr. Lung; Dust; Condition

Description—Pneumoconiosis is a respiratory condition resulting from long-term exposure to irritating dust or particles. Pneumoconioses types can range from harmless forms to destructive or fatal conditions. They are named for the type of exposed substance, such as aluminosis (aluminum), asbestosis (asbestos) (Figure 8-17), coal worker's pneumoconiosis (coal dust) (Figure 8-18), siderosis (iron), silicosis (silica), and welder's lung (iron oxide).

Massage Consideration/s—Clearance for massage from the client's health care provider is recommended. If the client is severely debilitated, massage is contraindicated because the manipulation of tissues would only make the client feel worse. If permission for massage is given, a general, relaxing massage including ribcage vibration and percussion would be helpful. It helps to orient the client with the head lower than the chest by using pillow bolsters under the abdomen and chest to induce positional drainage (Figure 8-19). The client may cough as a natural reflex, so tissues should be kept handy. The massage treatment should focus on the primary and secondary muscles of respiration (see Table 8-2). Techniques such as deep friction, kneading, ischemic compression, and deep gliding strokes can help loosen these tight muscles. The massage therapist needs to communicate with the client about the pressure and effectiveness of techniques.

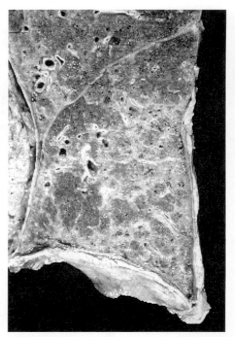

Figure 8-17.   Lung with asbestosis.

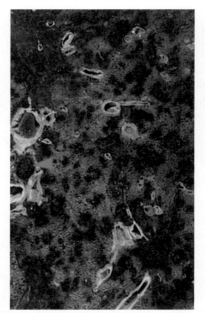

Figure 8-18.   Lung of individual with coal dust pneumoconiosis.

Pneumonia (nuh·moh´·nyuh)

Gr. Lung; Condition

Description—Pneumonia is an infection or inflammation of the alveoli caused by the bacterium *Streptococcus pneumoniae*, but other infectious agents, such as protozoans, viruses, and fungi, may also be responsible (Figure 8-20). During pneumonia, the alveoli fill with fluid and exudates such as dead white blood cells and pus. Exudates are substances that have been slowly discharged from cells or blood vessels as waste products. Pneumonia is the most common infectious cause of death in the United States, affecting, in particular, older adults, infants, immunocompromised individuals, and cigarette smokers.

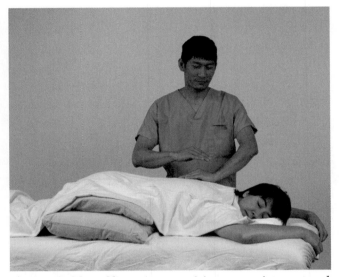

Figure 8-19. Client in a position to assist postural drainage, receiving percussion.

Massage Consideration/s—Massage is contraindicated during the acute phase because it is infectious. Also, massage would exacerbate the symptoms and make the client feel worse.

If the client is not acute, obtain physician clearance. Percussion and vibration on the ribcage can help drain secretions. The massage treatment should also focus on the primary and secondary muscles of respiration (see Table 8-2). Techniques such as deep friction, kneading, ischemic compression, and deep gliding strokes can help loosen these tight muscles. The massage therapist needs to communicate with the client about pressure and effectiveness of techniques.

Stretching, joint mobilizations, and massage on the extremities can help prevent muscle atrophy from prolonged bed rest.

Pulmonary Edema

L. Lung; Gr. Swelling

Description—Pulmonary edema is a condition involving excessive amounts of blood in the pulmonary blood vessels, known as pulmonary hypertension, and interstitial fluid in the tissues of the lungs (Figure 8-21). Common causes of pulmonary edema are near drowning, congestive heart failure, infection (e.g., pneumonia, tuberculosis), renal failure, and cerebrovascular accidents.

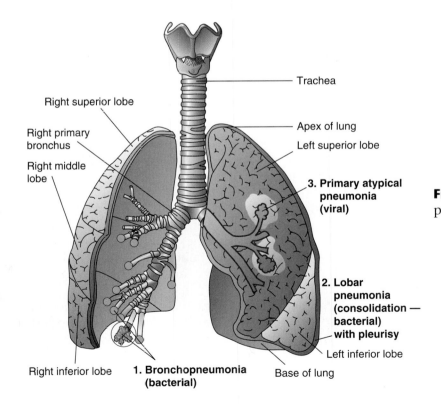

Right superior lobe

Right primary bronchus

Right middle lobe

Right inferior lobe

1. Bronchopneumonia (bacterial)

Trachea

Apex of lung

Left superior lobe

3. Primary atypical pneumonia (viral)

2. Lobar pneumonia (consolidation — bacterial) with pleurisy

Left inferior lobe

Base of lung

Figure 8-20. Three main types of pneumonia.

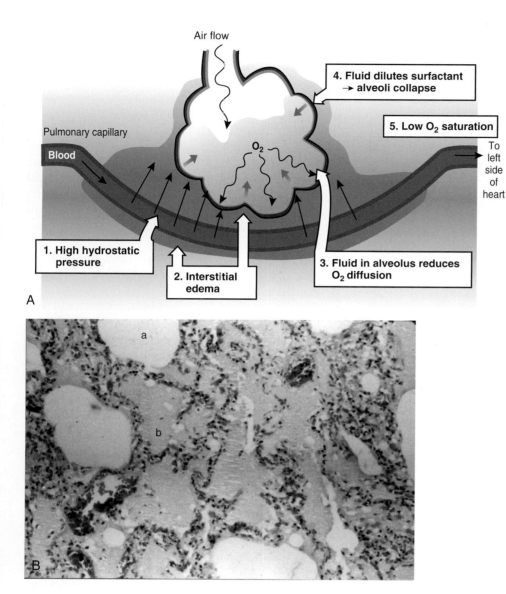

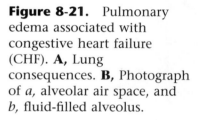

Figure 8-21. Pulmonary edema associated with congestive heart failure (CHF). **A,** Lung consequences. **B,** Photograph of *a,* alveolar air space, and *b,* fluid-filled alveolus.

Massage Consideration/s—If the symptoms are severe, massage is contraindicated because, as massage helps move tissue fluids back into the blood, the increased blood volume can make the edema in the lungs worse. Also, if the pulmonary edema is due to congestive heart failure, the increased blood volume could overload the already debilitated heart. If the symptoms are less severe, the massage therapist needs to obtain clearance for massage from the client's health care provider. The massage therapist needs to ask the client what positions on the massage table are comfortable. If the client tires easily, a lighter massage of shorter duration may be indicated.

Pulmonary Embolism

Lung; Gr. Plug; Condition

Description—Pulmonary embolism is the partial or complete closure of the pulmonary artery or one of its branches by an embolus (a blood clot, bubble of air, or any piece of debris transported by the bloodstream) (Figure 8-22).

Massage Consideration/s—Because immediate medical attention is needed for someone experiencing a pulmonary embolism, massage is contraindicated.

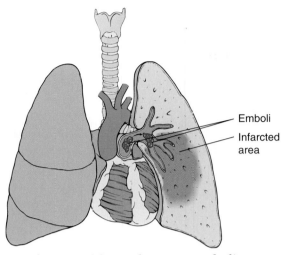

Figure 8-22. Pulmonary embolism.

Emboli

Infarcted area

Box **8–1**

Common Causes of Adult Respiratory Distress Syndrome (ARDS)
Shock
Trauma
Burns
Acute cardiac failure
Pneumonia
Bacterial
Viral
Toxic lung injury
Toxic fumes
Cytotoxic drugs
Bacterial toxins
Aspiration of fluids
Near-drowning

*From Damjanov I: Pathology for the health-related professions,
ed 2, Philadelphia, 2000, WB Saunders.*

Respiratory Distress Syndrome (RDS, Infant and Adult [ARDS], Hyaline Membrane Disease)

L. Breathing; To Draw Apart; Together; Course

Description—Respiratory distress syndrome is a type of respiratory failure in which the respiratory membranes are severely leaky. Hypoxia, or inadequate oxygen at the tissue level, results. RDS is accompanied by a respiration rate of more than 60 breaths per minute and nasal flaring (Box 8-1). RDS can result from near drowning, aspiration of the acidic gastric juice, reactions from medications, inhaling an irritating gas such as ammonia, lung infections such as pneumonia or tuberculosis, and pulmonary hypertension. In premature infants, RDS is also known as hyaline membrane disease. Infants born before their lungs have had time to fully develop will not have enough surfactant to be able to breathe easily. The walls of the alveoli collapse in on each other and tend to stick together when air is exhaled. Surfactant is a substance in the lungs that keeps the walls of the alveoli from adhering to each other, thus making them easier to fill up with air again. Without surfactant, infants with RDS have a difficult time getting air into their alveoli. These infants are given a synthetic surfactant.

Massage Consideration/s—Massage is contraindicated. Adults and infants with RDS will be under medical treatment because they will be very debilitated. RDS is a life-threatening disorder.

Severe Acute Respiratory Syndrome (SARS)

Nonapplicable

Description—SARS is a severe respiratory illness reported in parts of Asia, Europe, and North America. Symptoms begin with a mild fever, head and body aches, and an overall feeling of discomfort. Some individuals experience mild respiratory complaints. Within 2 to 7 days after

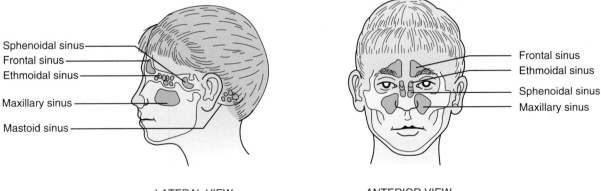

Sphenoidal sinus
Frontal sinus
Ethmoidal sinus
Maxillary sinus
Mastoid sinus

Frontal sinus
Ethmoidal sinus
Sphenoidal sinus
Maxillary sinus

LATERAL VIEW   ANTERIOR VIEW

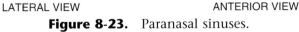

Figure 8-23. Paranasal sinuses.

symptoms begin, individuals may develop a dry cough and have difficulty breathing.

Massage Consideration/s—SARS is a life-threatening disorder. Massage is contraindicated. Individuals with SARS will be under medical treatment because they will be very debilitated.

Sinusitis

L. A Curve; Hollow; Gr. Inflammation

🚦 **Description**—Sinusitis is an inflammation of the paranasal sinuses (Figure 8-23). Causes range from dental infection, a complication of an upper respiratory tract infection, a change in atmosphere (as in air travel or underwater diving), or a structural defect in the nose. Swelling of nasal

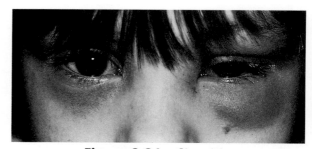

Figure 8-24. Sinusitis.

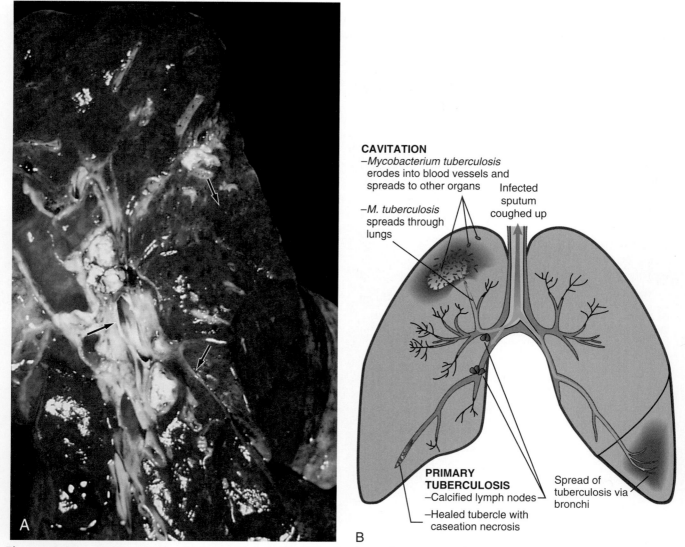

Figure 8-25. Tuberculosis. **A,** Upper lobe of tubercular lung (top arrow shows ischemia and lower arrows show lymph nodes with caseation). **B,** Types and events of tuberculosis.

mucosa may obstruct the openings from sinuses, resulting in an accumulation of sinus secretions and causing local tenderness, pain, headache, and fever (Figure 8-24).

Massage Consideration/s—If the client has a fever, massage is contraindicated because massage would only exacerbate the symptoms and make the client feel worse. If the client does not have fever, general massage can be performed. The massage therapist needs to ask if the client is comfortable lying prone and/or using the face cradle, as both of these situations can cause an increase in sinus congestion. Local moist heat applications and deep ischemic pressure applied over the frontal and sphenoidal sinuses may help to relieve pain. Steam inhalation may help to relieve congestion.

Tuberculosis (Consumption, White Plague)
(tu`·buhr·kyuh·loh´·suhs)

L. Little Swelling; Gr. Condition

Description—Tuberculosis is a chronic lung infection caused by the bacterium *Mycobacterium tuberculosis*. It is typically transmitted by the inhalation and exhalation (or consumption) of infected droplets (Figure 8-25). Even though the lungs are the disease's primary target, the liver, bone marrow, and spleen may be involved as well. During tuberculosis, lung tissue is destroyed by bacteria and is replaced by fibrous connective tissue, limiting gas exchange. The primary lesions are called *tubercles*. These break down into cheeselike masses of tissue in a process known as caseation. Cavities form within the lungs as a result of the destructive events that occur as tuberculosis progresses. Primary tuberculosis is the type of tuberculosis that occurs during childhood. Tuberculosis is still one of the most widespread diseases in the world.

Massage Consideration/s—Massage is contraindicated unless the client is no longer infective. Generally, tuberculosis is not infectious from 2 to 4 weeks after the start of treatment with medications. Check with the client's health care provider to make this determination. The massage therapist needs to ask the client about his or her vitality. A client who still feels weak may require a lighter massage of shorter duration. A client who is feeling more robust may want a more vigorous massage.

SUMMARY

Respiration is achieved by a combination of the respiratory and circulatory systems. The respiratory system is the primary provider of gas exchange that keeps the human body alive. The respiratory system takes in air, extracts oxygen from it, and expels heat, moisture, carbon dioxide, and other waste gases back out of the body. Pulmonary ventilation is made up of two processes: inhalation and exhalation.

During inhalation air is drawn in through the airway, which is made up of the nasal cavities, mouth, pharynx, larynx, and trachea. This air then enters the lungs through the bronchi. In the lungs the alveoli allow for gas exchange with the bloodstream. Oxygen is taken into the blood from the air, and carbon dioxide moves from the blood into the air. The oxygenated blood is carried to all cells so that the cells can use it for energy production. During exhalation air is forced from the lungs back through the airways. Other functions of the respiratory system include olfaction, sound production, and regulation of pH.

Respiratory pathologies include apnea, asthma, bronchitis, chronic obstructive pulmonary disease, common cold, cystic fibrosis, emphysema, hay fever, influenza, laryngitis, pleurisy, pneumoconiosis, pneumonia, pulmonary edema, pulmonary embolism, respiratory distress syndrome, SARS, sinusitis, and tuberculosis.

Respiratory pathologies may be suspected when symptoms include altered breathing patterns, change in breathing sounds, wheezing, nasal flaring during inhalation, pursed lips during exhalation, chest pain, facial pain, pale skin, cyanosis of lips or fingertips, clubbed fingers and toes, sore throat, swollen lymph nodes, sputum, and any signs of respiratory infection such as sneezing, coughing, watery eyes, or runny nose. The massage therapist needs to refer the client to a physician immediately when these symptoms are present. Other signs to look for during assessment include lymphedema, breathing rate, breathing patterns, and the use of inhalers or medication for respiratory illness.

Resources

American Academy of Allergies, Asthma, and Immunology
611 East Wells Street
Milwaukee, WI 53202
800-822-ASMA
www.aaaai.org

American Lung Association
1740 Broadway
New York, NY 10019
800-LUNG-USA (800-586-4872)
www.lungusa.org

Asthma and Allergy Foundation of America
1125 15th Street NW
Washington, DC 20005
800-7-ASTHMA
www.aafa.com

Asthma Information Line
800-822-ASMA

Cystic Fibrosis Foundation
6931 Arlington Road
Bethesda, MD 20814-5200
800-FIGHT-CF

National Jewish Center for Immunology and Respiratory Medicine
1400 Jackson Street
Denver, CO 80206
800-222-LUNG
303-355-LUNG (in Denver)

National Institute of Allergies and Infectious Diseases
www.niaid.nih.gov

List the letter of the answer to the term or phrase that best describes it.

A. Apnea
B. Asthma
C. Bronchitis
D. Chronic obstructive pulmonary disease
E. Cystic fibrosis
F. Emphysema
G. Hay fever
H. Laryngitis
I. Pleurisy
J. Pneumoconiosis
K. Pneumonia
L. Pulmonary edema
M. Sinusitis
N. Tuberculosis

_____ 1. A respiratory condition resulting from long-term exposure to irritating dust or particles.

_____ 2. A genetic disorder involving the overproduction of secretions of all exocrine glands, especially the pancreas, and the lining of the respiratory system. The bronchi secrete thick mucus, which obstructs and narrows the airway.

_____ 3. Inflammation of the larynx that often results in loss of voice.

_____ 4. A chronic lung infection caused by the bacterium *Mycobacterium tuberculosis* that is typically transmitted by the inhalation and exhalation of infected droplets.

_____ 5. A group of pulmonary disorders characterized by persistent or recurring obstruction of air flow, such as asthma, emphysema, cystic fibrosis, pneumoconiosis, or chronic bronchitis.

_____ 6. Inflammation of the pleural membranes characterized by burning or stabbing pain during breathing.

_____ 7. An infection or inflammation of the alveoli caused by the bacterium *Streptococcus pneumoniae,* but other infectious agents such as protozoans, viruses, and fungi, may also be responsible.

_____ 8. Inflammation of the paranasal sinuses.

_____ 9. Gradual destruction of elasticity in the walls of the alveoli caused by a long-term irritation such as cigarette smoke, air pollution, and exposure to industrial dust.

_____ 10. A chronic, inflammatory disorder caused by airway sensitivity to various stimuli.

_____ 11. A general term used to denote any allergic reaction of the nasal mucosa and is characterized by sudden attacks of sneezing, swelling, and profuse water discharge of the nasal mucosa, with itching and watering of the eyes; caused by allergens such as house dust, pet dander, and pollen.

_____ 12. A temporary cessation or absence of spontaneous breathing.

_____ 13. A condition involving an excessive amount of blood in the pulmonary blood vessels; common causes are near drowning, congestive heart failure, infection (e.g., pneumonia, tuberculosis), renal failure, and cerebrovascular accidents.

_____ 14. Inflammation of the bronchial mucosa that causes the bronchial tubes to swell and extra mucus to be produced.

9

Gastrointestinal Pathologies

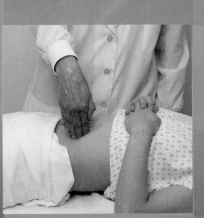

GASTROINTESTINAL SYSTEM OVERVIEW

Because the digestive system is responsible for processing the food necessary for life, it is an important system for massage therapists to understand. Massage can affect the digestive system both directly and indirectly. Abdominal massage is one way to directly affect the digestive system. It stimulates the intestines and helps substances move forward, which can be especially helpful in a client with constipation. Digestion proceeds more smoothly and efficiently in a relaxed person than in a person under stress, so massage plays a vital, although indirect, role in a client's energy level.

The nutrients the body needs for energy, synthesis of new tissues, and repairing damaged or worn-out tissues come from food taken into the body. Most food, however, needs to be broken down into molecules small enough to enter body cells. There are six classes of nutrients: *carbohydrates, proteins, lipids (fats), vitamins, minerals,* and *water*. Of these, only vitamins, minerals, and water do not need to be broken down further; they can enter body cells as they are. Carbohydrates, proteins, and lipids are very complex (and large) structures that need to be broken apart chemically into smaller molecules. This process is called digestion.

Carbohydrates are deconstructed into their building blocks called *monosaccharides*, which are single unit sugars. The most common monosaccharide is glucose. Proteins are deconstructed into their building blocks called *amino acids*. The most common lipids are *triglycerides*. A triglyceride consists of a molecule of glycerol with three molecules called fatty acid chains attached to it. The different types of fats depend on the chemical composition of the fatty acids. Lipids are hydrophobic ("water-fearing") and tend to stick together in large clumps. Before the triglycerides can be deconstructed effectively, the large clumps need to be dispersed, or emulsified, into small droplets. Then the triglycerides will be broken down into their building blocks, glycerol, and fatty acids.

Certain foods that cannot be digested also need to be taken into the body. This is called roughage (i.e., bulk or fiber). Roughage comes from the skins of fruits and vegetables. These are necessary because they help form the mass that the large intestine needs to move substances forward and out of the body.

The digestive system is responsible for breaking down the nutrients into their building blocks. The digestive system is made up of two groups of organs: the gastrointestinal (GI) tract or alimentary canal (alimentary = nourishment) (Figure 9-1) and the

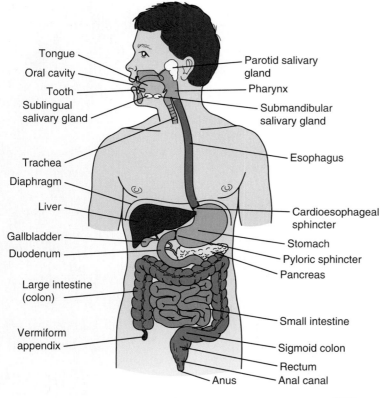

Figure 9-1. Gastrointestinal structures and accessory organs.

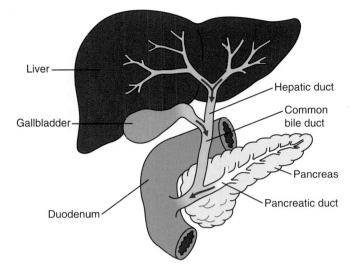

Figure 9-2. Accessory organs and their ducts; liver, pancreas, and gallbladder in relationship to duodenum.

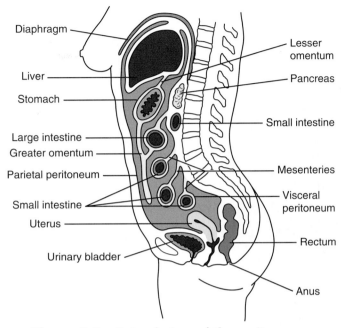

Figure 9-3. Lateral view of the peritoneum.

accessory digestive organs (Figure 9-2). The GI tract is a long tube that extends from the mouth to the anus. It is about 30 feet long in a cadaver, but is much shorter in a living person as a result of muscle tone in the wall of the GI tract. Organs and structures of the GI tract include the oral cavity (mouth), pharynx (throat), esophagus, stomach, small intestine, and large intestine (colon). Accessory digestive organs include the teeth, tongue, salivary glands, liver, gallbladder, and pancreas. Most of the organs of the digestive system are found in the abdominal pelvic cavity. They are connected to each other and to the inside of the cavity by a membrane called the peritoneum (Figure 9-3).

The digestive system performs six basic processes:
- *Ingestion* is eating and drinking.
- *Secretion* refers to the 7 liters of water, acid, buffers, and enzymes secreted by the wall of the GI tract and accessory organs of digestion in a 24-hour period.
- *Mixing and propulsion* (i.e., peristalsis) is the blending of food with digestive secretions, and the forward movement of the food through the GI tract.
- *Digestion* involves mechanical and chemical processes that break food into small molecules. In mechanical digestion, food is chewed into smaller pieces by the teeth, and is further ground into tiny bits by churning in the stomach and small intestine. In chemical digestion, enzymes break carbohydrates down into monosaccharides, break proteins down into amino acids, and

break triglycerides down into glycerol and fatty acids.
- *Absorption* involves the movement of the products of digestion into the blood and lymph.
- *Defecation* involves eliminating undigested and unabsorbed substances from the body.

Digestion begins in the mouth. The teeth mechanically break down ingested food. Salivary glands secrete saliva, which contains digestive enzymes, into ducts that empty into the mouth. The tongue helps mix food with saliva. The digestive enzymes initiate the chemical digestion of carbohydrates and lipids. After the food is formed into a soft, easily swallowed mass called a bolus, it is ingested. It moves from the oral cavity into the pharynx, then into the esophagus. The esophagus then transports the bolus to the stomach.

In between the esophagus and the stomach is the cardioesophageal sphincter. The stomach is a hollow, muscular organ (Figure 9-4). The layers of muscle in its wall contract to grind the bolus into a thin, soupy liquid called chyme. The stomach also secretes a digestive enzyme that initiates protein digestion. From the stomach, the chyme enters the small intestine. Between the stomach and the small intestine is the pyloric sphincter.

The small intestine is about 10 feet long in a living person. The first part is called the duodenum. It extends from the pyloric sphincter for about 10 to 12 inches. The second part is the jejunum. It is about 3 feet long and extends from the duodenum. The third part is the ileum, which is about 6 feet long. It extends from the ileum and connects to the large intestine at the ileocecal sphincter.

Most digestion and absorption occur in the small intestine. In addition to secretions from the wall of the small intestine itself, secretions from the liver, gallbladder, and pancreas enter the small intestine via ducts. Bile is made by the liver and is responsi-

ble for emulsifying fats. Once the fats are emulsified, enzymes from the pancreas finish their chemical digestion into glycerol and fatty acids. The gallbladder stores excess bile. When a meal high in fats is eaten, bile will be ejected from the gallbladder into the small intestine. Chemical digestion of carbohydrates into monosaccharides and proteins into amino acids is completed in the small intestine as a result of enzymes from both the small intestine and the pancreas.

Once the chemical digestion of nutrients is complete, absorption into the blood and lymph occurs. Small molecules such as water, ions, glucose, amino acids, and water-soluble vitamins are absorbed into blood capillaries. Because lymphatic vessels are larger in diameter than blood capillaries, larger molecules such as large fatty acids and fat-soluble vitamins are absorbed into them. Lymph, with its absorbed molecules, eventually drains into the bloodstream. The blood then circulates these nutrients to all the cells of the body.

By the time the chyme enters the large intestine, most of the substances and water have been absorbed. The large intestine is about 6 feet long and consists of four main parts. The first part is the cecum and it is about 2.5 inches long. The appendix is attached to the cecum. The appendix is a tube about 3 inches long with lymphatic tissue inside it.

The next part of the large intestine is the colon proper (Figure 9-5). The ascending colon rises supe-

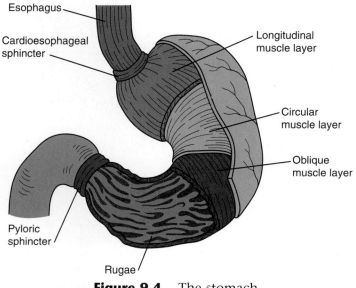

Figure 9-4. The stomach.

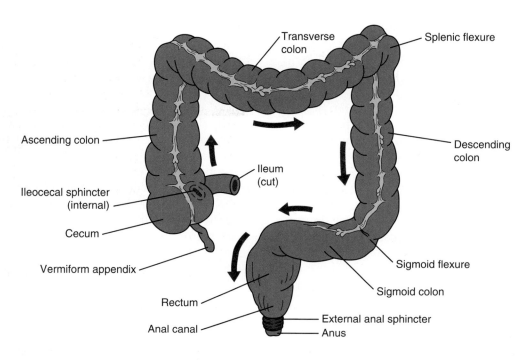

Figure 9-5. The colon.

riorly from the cecum. The colon makes a 90-degree turn under the liver, and the transverse colon continues across the abdomen where it makes another 90-degree turn under the spleen. From there, the colon continues inferiorly as the descending colon. Near the left iliac crest, the colon turns posteriorly to form an S-shape, and is called the sigmoid colon.

The sigmoid colon connects with the last part of the large intestine, the rectum. The rectum is 8 inches long and is anterior to the sacrum and coccyx. The last inch of the rectum is the anal canal, and the opening to the outside is the anus. The internal anal sphincter is made of smooth muscle and operates involuntarily. The external anal sphincter is made of skeletal muscle and operates voluntarily.

After chyme has been in the large intestine for anywhere from 3 to 10 hours, most of the water and some electrolytes have been absorbed. Bacteria, normally found in the large intestine, also make some B vitamins and vitamin K that are absorbed from the colon.

After absorption in the large intestine occurs, the chyme becomes feces. Feces consists of water, inorganic salts, cells sloughed off the wall of the GI tract, bacteria, products of bacterial decomposition, unabsorbed digested material, and indigestible parts of food (roughage). Defecation occurs when both the internal and external anal sphincters open and expel the feces.

THERAPEUTIC ASSESSMENT OF THE GASTROINTESTINAL SYSTEM

The following list of pertinent questions serves as a review of how to evaluate the digestive system. Findings need to be documented.

Questions to ask the client in the premassage interview:

- *Does the client have any gastrointestinal discomfort? If so, what body positions make it better? Which make it worse?* The massage therapist needs to be prepared to use pillows or bolsters to increase the client's comfort.
- *Does the client indicate that he or she has a colostomy or an ileostomy?* If so, Box 9-1 has guidelines for massage.

Observations and palpations to make during the premassage interview and during the massage treatment:

- *Is the client overweight for his or her frame and height?* Box 9-2 has information on massaging large clients.

- *During palpation, are any hard masses felt in the abdomen?* If so, the massage therapist needs to refer the client to the client's health care provider. However, formed or partially formed stools often feel hard. If a mass is felt in the region of the descending or sigmoid colon, it may be assumed that it is a stool. In either case, the massage may proceed, avoiding the abdominal region until the source is determined.
- *During palpation, is the client experiencing rebound tenderness?* This discomfort is felt as the fingertips are lifted off the abdomen instead of during the application of pressure (Figure 9-6). Rebound tenderness is often indicative of appendicitis or peritonitis and therefore needs immediate medical attention.

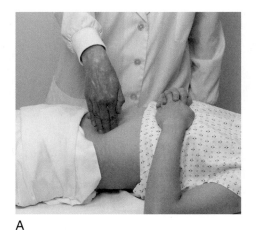

A

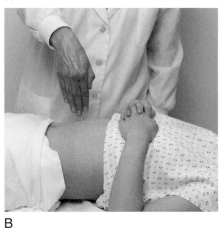

B

Figure 9-6. Testing for rebound tenderness. **A,** Pressure application. **B,** Lifting from abdomen.

Box **9-1**

Clients Who Have Had a Colostomy or Ileostomy

A colostomy is an incision in the colon to create an opening that is affixed to the exterior abdominal wall. A bag is attached outside the body to collect fecal material that passes through the opening. Colostomies are sometimes permanent; sometimes they are a temporary bypass method used in conjunction with other surgeries.

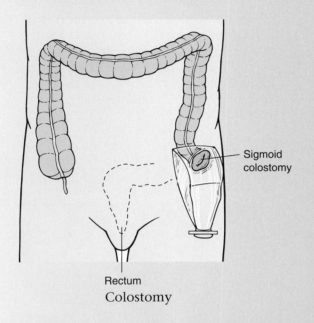

Colostomy

An ileostomy is similar to a colostomy except the *ileostomy* connects the small intestine (i.e., ileum) to the external abdominal wall. Clients who have lower colostomies can regulate their bowels. The bowel material of upper colostomies and ileostomies will be too loose to afford the client the ability to control bowel movements.

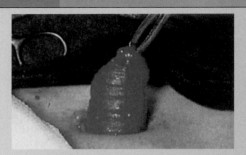

Ileostomy

When clients who have a colostomy or ileostomy make an appointment for a massage, the massage therapist should recommend that they not eat 2 hours before their scheduled appointment time. This 2-hour delay decreases bowel motility. Because of the anterior abdominal opening, these clients may not be able to receive massage in the prone position. The side-lying position can accommodate these special individuals. An extra pad may be placed under the massage linens in the event of bag spillage.

The massage therapist can suggest that a client empty his or her bag before the massage begins. A bag can burst or become unclipped during the session, spilling its contents. Should this occur, the massage therapist needs to remain calm and reassure the client that accidents like this do happen. The massage therapist should ask if the client would prefer to clean up or if the client would like assistance. A client with a spinal injury may require assistance. Disposable gloves and towels or washcloths should be kept handy.

Lubricant should not be applied on or near the bag opening. Oily substances interfere with the ability of the adhesive or cement to anchor the bag to the skin.

Adapted from Salvo S: Massage therapy: principles and practice, *ed 2, Philadelphia, 2003, WB Saunders.*

GENERAL MANIFESTATIONS OF GASTROINTESTINAL DISEASE

If a client has any of the following, the massage therapist needs to refer the client to the client's health care provider for diagnosis and treatment.

- Abdominal pain
- Blood reported in stools
- Difficulty when swallowing
- Masses palpated in the abdomen and not related to hard stool
- Nausea or vomiting
- Oral lesions
- Rebound tenderness
- Significant fatigue or lethargy

GASTROINTESTINAL PATHOLOGIES

Anorexia Nervosa (a·nuh·rek´·see·uh nuhr·voh´·suh)
Gr. Without Appetite; Nerve

Description—Classified as an eating disorder and an emotional disorder, anorexia nervosa is the prolonged avoidance of eating. Lack of

Box **9-2**

Massaging the Large Client

When massaging the client who is large (i.e., obese or the somatotype known as an endomorph) or who has generous amounts of fragile subcutaneous tissue, two areas require special consideration. The first consideration is psychological and requires the massage therapist to approach the client with an attitude that is compassionate, caring, and nonjudgmental, as large clients typically have a history of verbal abuse from society. The massage therapist should never badger a client about weight or blame excessive size or weight on lack of morality or self-control. No one has a body that is perfect in all aspects. After necessary accommodations are made for the client's comfort, the massage therapist proceeds with the session.

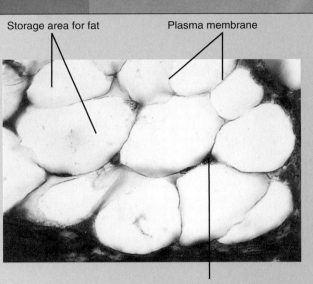

Storage area for fat   Plasma membrane

Nucleus of adipose cell

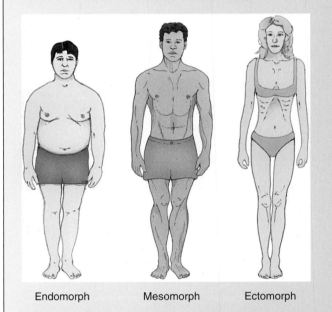

Endomorph   Mesomorph   Ectomorph

The second consideration is physiological. Pressure must be applied carefully to areas that contain large quantities of adipose tissue, thus reducing the possibility of tissue damage. Adipose tissue is extremely vascular, with each pound of tissue having copious amounts of capillaries. This makes adipose tissue extremely susceptible to bruising. The massage therapist needs to avoid deep stroking of adipose tissue because it can damage and break these vessels. The back, neck, shoulders, hips, and sometimes legs of many larger clients may require extra massage work

because these muscles have become overdeveloped to support the extra weight.

Palpation must be used to discern the difference between muscle and adipose tissue. If muscle fiber cannot be felt with gentle pressure, the massage therapist needs to avoid working deeply into the tissue. The massage therapist can ask the client to contract a specific muscle or muscle group to help distinguish the difference. If the tissue does not respond with an increase in tone, it is probably adipose tissue, and deep pressure should be avoided. Sometimes it is possible to gently retract adipose tissue to access muscle tissue underneath. Clients who have had recent weight loss may have areas that tend to hang in folds until the skin tightens. These areas should never be worked deeply or pinched; folds can be moved to the side while working on adjacent muscle and may be flattened out against the area to be worked so that the therapist can work through these areas while remaining attentive to pressure.

The massage therapist should inquire about the client's activity level. Just because someone is large does not necessarily mean that the person is sedentary. For those who are inactive, edema may occur. If the client does have edema, the legs can be elevated during the massage treatment to promote drainage, and lymphatic drainage massage techniques can be used.

Continued

Box **9-2**

Massaging the Large Client—cont'd

Another area of consideration when working with larger clients is the therapist's body mechanics and efficiency. It may help to either lower the table height before the client's visit or have a small platform to stand on to gain height and leverage. Most table manufacturers offer electric lift or hydraulic tables that can be raised or lowered to a comfortable height.

The massage therapist needs to use a sheet or an extra-large towel as a top drape to provide adequate coverage. A client who is obese or excessively large may feel awkward or unsafe getting on and off the massage table. A foot stool should be available, and the massage therapist needs to be willing to offer assistance. If there is an electric or hydraulic lift massage table, it should be set in a lower position while the client is getting on and off. A client who does not feel comfortable on the massage table may need to receive the massage on the floor. A comfortable floor mat or futon can be used in such cases. Some portable tables can be placed on the floor while the table legs are folded underneath to accommodate clients who need to be treated on the floor.

Adapted from Salvo S: Massage therapy: principles and practice, *ed 2, Philadelphia, 2003, WB Saunders.*

---

nutrients results in emaciation, amenorrhea (cessation of menstruation), decreased sleep, and psychological disturbance. When people with anorexia nervosa do eat, they often prefer foods low in calories. Although cases among young males are on the rise, most people with anorexia nervosa are young Caucasian females. Treatment consists of increasing dietary intake and psychological counseling, as many people with this condition have a negative body image (Figure 9-7).

Massage Consideration/s—Massage therapy can be a helpful adjunct to psychological counseling. The massage therapist needs to obtain clearance for massage from the client's health care provider if symptoms are severe. A gentle, nurturing massage to physically and psychologically connect areas of the client's body may help improve the client's self-image and may decrease anxiety.

Appendicitis (uh·pen`·duh·sai´·tis)

L. Hang On; Gr. Inflammation

Description—An inflammation of the vermiform appendix, appendicitis is often detected by acute pain in the right lower quadrant of the abdomen, vomiting, fever, and elevated white blood cell count. Appendix is caused by obstruction of the hollow center of the appendix by food, inflammation, a foreign body, a tumor or abnormal narrowing, or kinking of the organ (Figure 9-8).

Massage Consideration/s—Massage is contraindicated for clients with appendicitis because of the pain and need for immediate medical attention.

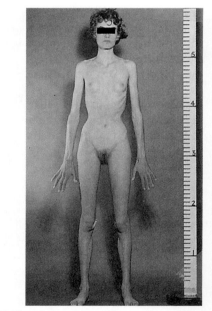

Figure 9-7. Anorexia nervosa in a 20-year-old woman.

Bulimia (Boulimia) (buh·lee´·mee·uh) (boo·lee´·mee·uh)

Gr. Hunger

Description—Bulimia is characterized by an insatiable craving for food, often resulting in episodes of continuous eating (bingeing), followed by vomiting (purging), depression, and self-deprivation. Individuals who are bulimic may also abuse laxatives and diuretics. The teeth can become eroded from stomach acid during vomiting, and the esophagus can be torn from continual vomiting, to

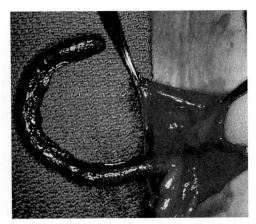

Figure 9-8.   Acute appendicitis.

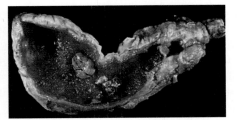

Figure 9-9.   Cross section of gallbladder with chronic cholecystitis.

the point that the person coughs up blood. If the tear is severe enough, hemorrhaging can occur. Like anorexia nervosa, bulimia is classified as an eating and an emotional disorder, treated by psychological counseling.

Massage Consideration/s—Massage therapy can be a helpful adjunct to psychological counseling. A gentle, nurturing massage to physically and psychologically connect areas of the client's body may help improve the client's self-image and may decrease anxiety.

Cholecystitis (koh`·luh·sis·tai´·tis)

Gr. Bile; Bag; Inflammation

Description—Chronic or acute inflammation of the gallbladder is called cholecystitis (Figure 9-9). Acute cholecystitis is often due to gallstones that cannot pass through the bile duct. Pain is felt in the right upper quadrant of the abdomen, accompanied by nausea and vomiting. Chronic cholecystitis is more common than acute cholecystitis. Pain is often felt at night after eating a large, fatty meal, and gradually increases in intensity.

Massage Consideration/s—Massage is contraindicated during acute stage because the pressure of massage can make the pain worse. For chronic cholecystitis, the massage therapist needs to ask the

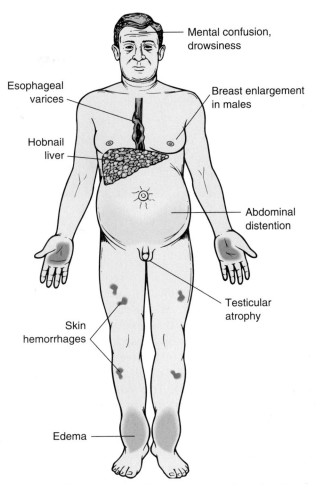

Figure 9-10.   Signs and symptoms of cirrhosis of the liver.

client how much pain the client is experiencing at the time of the massage treatment. If the pain is severe, massage is contraindicated; if it less severe, or absent, general massage may be performed, avoiding the abdominal area. The massage therapist needs to ask the client what positions are comfortable for the client on the massage table. For added comfort, the client may need propping under the low back while supine, or under the abdomen while prone, or the side-lying position may need to be used.

Cirrhosis of the Liver (suh·roh·sis uhv thuh li·vuhr)

Gr. Orange Yellow; Condition

Description—Cirrhosis of the liver is a chronic regenerative/degenerative disease in which the hepatic cells are destroyed and replaced with fibrous connective tissue, giving the liver a yellow-orange color. Liver functions deteriorate as hepatic cells are destroyed. Jaundice is a

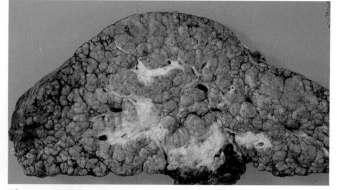

Figure 9-11. Alcoholic cirrhosis. Note the fibrosis and the orange color.

hallmark symptom of cirrhosis along with edema of the legs. As the disease progresses, gastrointestinal hemorrhage, ascites, hemorrhoids, and kidney failure may also occur. Ascites is an abnormal accumulation of fluid in the peritoneal cavity, up to several liters. Cirrhosis is usually the result of chronic alcohol abuse, infections such as hepatitis, intestinal bypass, and hepatic/biliary obstruction (Figures 9-10 and 9-11). The symptoms of cirrhosis are nausea, fatigue, and loss of appetite.

Massage Consideration/s—Massage is contraindicated. Jaundice indicates that the liver is not functioning properly, with the blood flow through it possibly impaired. Massage can indirectly increase that blood flow (when a client relaxes, more blood moves to the viscera) and exacerbate the jaundice. Also, as the liver synthesizes many clotting factors, an impaired liver greatly increases the chance of bruising. The edema in this case is also a contraindication for massage. Massage increases fluid return to the blood, which would increase the blood volume and, as the blood flows through the liver, further tax that debilitated organ.

Constipation

L. To Press Together

Description—Constipation is infrequent or difficult passing of stools. Common causes of constipation are insufficient intake of fluid or dietary fiber, lack of physical activity, emotional disturbance, diverticulitis, pregnancy, enema abuse, and painful defecation.

Massage Consideration/s—The massage therapist needs to ask the client the cause of the constipation. If it is due to diverticulitis, more information can be found under that entry in this chapter. Otherwise, abdominal massage can help relieve constipation by stimulating the forward movement of intestinal contents. Gliding strokes,

kneading and vibration, within the client's tolerance, can be helpful (gliding clockwise). The massage therapist should ask the client what positions on the massage table are comfortable and may need to prop the client with a pillow under the abdomen while prone. Or, if the client cannot lie prone comfortably, the side-lying position may need to be used.

Crohn's Disease (Regional Ileitis, Regional Enteritis) (ree´·juh·nuhl i`·lee·ai´·tis) (ree´·juh·nuhl en·tuh·rai´·tis)

Burrill B. Crohn; American Gastroenterologist; 1884-1983.

Description—A type of chronic inflammatory bowel disease, Crohn's disease affects the colon and/or ileum. Early symptoms are severe abdominal pain, diarrhea, fever, nausea, blood in the stools, and loss of appetite (Figure 9-12). Inflammation helps to thicken the intestinal walls, giving it a cobblestone appearance. Typically, normal colon segments separate diseased colon segments. The cause of Crohn's disease is unknown.

Massage Consideration/s—Because the symptoms of Crohn's disease can vary from day to day, the massage therapist needs to ask the client about the severity of pain and other symptoms before each massage treatment. The massage therapist also needs to ask the client what positions on the massage table are comfortable. Propping with a pillow under the client's abdomen while the client is prone may be necessary, or, if the client cannot lie prone comfortably, the side-lying position may need to be used. Generally, the abdomen should be avoided because the pressure of massage could cause undue pain.

Diarrhea

Gr. Through; To Flow

Description—The frequent passing of unformed, loose, watery stools is called diarrhea. Factors that cause diarrhea include stress, diet, infection, medication side effects, or inflammation. The stool may also contain blood, pus, or mucus. Other symptoms are abdominal pain and cramping. Diarrhea may also lead to dehydration.

Massage Consideration/s—The massage therapist needs to ask the client the cause of the diarrhea. Because acute onset of diarrhea is often due to infection, clients with this type of diarrhea should not be massaged until all symptoms are gone. Furthermore, it is unlikely that a client with acute diarrhea will tolerate a massage. If a client has chronic diarrhea (lasting more than 3 weeks), it is usually due to

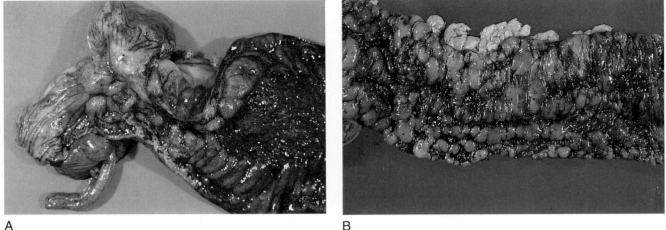

A   B

Figure 9-12. Crohn's disease. **A,** Thickened intestinal wall. **B,** Cobblestone-like appearance of intestinal mucosa.

conditions such as inflammatory bowel disease. The massage therapist needs to refer the client to the client's health care provider for diagnosis and treatment. After obtaining clearance for massage from the client's health care provider, general massage may be performed, within the client's tolerance, but the abdomen may need to be avoided. The massage therapist would need to communicate with the client about abdominal sensitivity.

Diverticulitis (dai`·vuhr·ti`·kyuh·lai´·tis)

L. To Turn Aside; Gr. Inflammation

Description—Diverticula are pouchlike herniations of the colon wall where the muscle has become weak (Figure 9-13). Diverticulitis is an inflammation of one or more diverticula. This condition can lead to obstruction, perforations, and abscess formation. People with diverticulitis often have pain and/or a mass in the left lower quadrant and a change in bowel habits such as an increase or decrease in constipation or diarrhea, or alteration between the two.

Massage Consideration/s—Because the symptoms of diverticulitis can vary from day to day, the massage therapist needs to ask the client about the severity of pain and other symptoms before each massage treatment. The massage therapist also needs to ask the client what positions on the massage table are comfortable. Propping with a pillow under the client's abdomen while the client is prone may be necessary, or, if the client cannot lie prone comfortably, the side-lying position may need to be used. Generally, the abdomen should be avoided because the pressure of massage could cause undue pain.

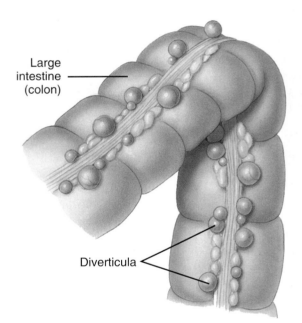

Large intestine (colon)

Diverticula

Figure 9-13. Inflamed diverticula as seen in diverticulitis.

Diverticulosis (dai`·vuhr·ti`·kyuh·loh´·sis)

L. To Turn Aside; Gr. Condition

Description—Diverticula are pouchlike herniations of the colon wall where the muscle has become weak (Figure 9-14). Diverticulosis involves small mucosal herniations through the muscular wall anywhere in the colon, but most typically in the sigmoid colon. Other colon changes include bleeding, abscesses, stenosis, and the presence of pericolonic fat. Fistulas may form between the colon and the small intestines. This condition is most likely to be found in individuals more than

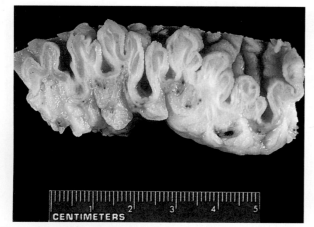

Figure 9-14. Cross section of colon in person with diverticulosis. Note the pericolonic fat.

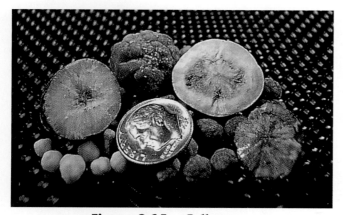

Figure 9-15. Gallstones.

50 years old who have a low-fiber diet. Even though people who have diverticulosis have no symptoms, 15% will develop diverticulitis (inflammation of the diverticula; see prior entry) and associated abdominal pain.

Massage Consideration/s—Massage considerations are the same as for diverticulitis.

Gallstones (Choledocholithiasis, Biliary Calculi) (koh·luh·doh·kuh·luh·thai´·uh·sis) (bi´·lee·er`·ee kal´·ku-li)

Gr. Bile; Stone; Condition

Description—Gallstones are crystals of cholesterol that form in the gallbladder or bile duct. They grow gradually in size and number and may cause minimal to complete obstruction of bile flow into the duodenum (Figure 9-15). Treatments include lithotripsy and surgery. Lithotripsy is the use of sound waves to break the stones apart so they can be eliminated through the large intestine. Surgery can be used to remove either the stones or the entire gallbladder.

Massage Consideration/s—Same as for cholecystitis.

Gastritis

Gr. Stomach; Inflammation

Description—Inflammation of the stomach's lining is called gastritis. It occurs in two forms: acute and chronic. Acute gastritis may be caused by food poisoning, a virus, bacteria, or chemical toxin (Table 9-1). Chronic gastritis is often the sign of an underlying illness, such as an ulcer (Figures 9-16 and 9-17). One of the main symptoms of gastritis is pain in the abdominal area. Alcohol or medication use is a common cause of both types of gastritis.

Massage Consideration/s—Massage is contraindicated for acute gastritis. Because gastritis is caused by a pathogen or toxin and has systemic effects, massage would only make the client feel worse. For chronic gastritis, massage may be performed. The massage therapist needs to ask the client if the client is comfortable lying flat in the prone position. If not, propping under the abdomen may be necessary, or the side-lying position could be used. The head of the massage table could be elevated slightly above the foot of the table so that gravity could aid in digestion. If the client indicates that the abdomen is sensitive, massage in that area should be avoided.

Gastroenteritis (Enterogastritis) (gas`·troh·en`·tuh·rai´·tis) (en`·tuh·roh·gas`·trai´·tis)

Gr. Stomach; Intestine; Inflammation

Description—Gastroenteritis is an inflammation of the lining of the stomach and intestines, characterized by nausea, vomiting, diarrhea, abdominal pain, lack of appetite, and weakness. Causes of gastroenteritis include food poisoning caused by infection with such organisms as *Escherichia coli* or *Salmonella*, consumption of irritating food or drink, or psychological factors such as anger, stress, and fear (see Table 9-1).

Massage Consideration/s—The massage therapist needs to ask the client the cause of the gastroenteritis. If the gastritis is due to an infectious agent, massage is contraindicated until the client has completely healed. Also, massage would only make the client feel worse. If the gastroenteritis is due to other factors, massage may be performed. The massage therapist needs to ask the client if the client is comfortable lying flat in the prone position. If not, propping under the abdomen may be necessary, or the side-lying position could be used.

Table 9-1 COMMON INFECTIONS TRANSMITTED BY FOOD AND WATER

PATHOGEN	SOURCE	INCUBATION	MANIFESTATIONS
Staphylococcus aureus	Food handlers; inadequate cooking or refrigeration of custards, salad dressing, cold meats	1-7 hours (2-4 average)	Sudden severe nausea, vomiting, and cramps, sometimes diarrhea; subnormal body temperature and low blood pressure
Escherichia coli	Fecal contamination of food and water	10-12 hours	Profuse watery diarrhea, sometimes with blood or mucus; vomiting and abdominal cramps often present
Salmonella	Fecal contamination of food or undercooked or raw eggs, poultry, shellfish; contaminated work surfaces	6-72 hours	Sudden diarrhea, abdominal pain, and fever; sometimes vomiting
Viral: rotavirus	Oral-fecal contamination of shellfish	24-72 hours	Vomiting and diarrhea, fever
Entamoeba histolytica (amebic dysentery)	Fecal contamination of water and vegetables	2-4 weeks	Diarrhea with blood and mucus, may alternate with constipation; fever and chills
Clostridium botulinum	Spores in poorly canned food or prepared meat	12-36 hours	Visual problems, dysphagia, then flaccid paralysis and respiratory failure; possibly early vomiting or diarrhea

Modified from Gould BE: Pathophysiology for the health professions, *ed 2, Philadelphia, 2002, WB Saunders.*

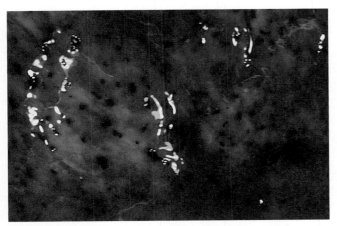

Figure 9-16. Acute gastritis caused by aspirin use. Note the inflamed mucous membrane.

The head of the massage table could be elevated slightly above the foot of the table so that gravity could aid in digestion. If the client indicates that his abdomen is sensitive, massage in that area should be avoided.

Gastroesophageal Reflux Disease (GERD)
(gas`·troh·uh·sah`·fuh·jee´·uhl ree´·fluhks duh·zeez´)

Gr. Stomach, Gullet; L. Back; Flow

Description—If the lower gastroesophageal sphincter fails to close normally after food has reached the stomach, hydrochloric acid from the stomach can enter the inferior portion of the esophagus. This condition is referred to as gastroesophageal reflux disease (GERD). The hydrochloric acid irritates the esophageal wall and causes a burning sensation. It is often called heartburn because the sensation is near the heart, not because of cardiac problems. Antacids neutralize the hydrochloric acid and decrease the burning sensation. If food is eaten in smaller amounts and the person does not lie down right after a meal, symptoms are less likely to occur. Irritation of the esophageal wall by chronic GERD can cause ulcer-like lesions that are called Barrett's syndrome or Barrett's esophagus (Figure 9-18). This could possibly cause a premalignant change in the esophageal lining.

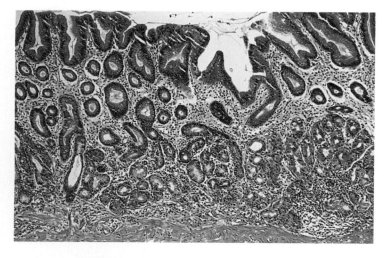

Figure 9-17. Chronic gastritis associated with pernicious anemia.

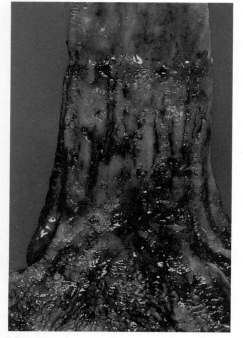

Figure 9-18. Barrett esophagus with early carcinoma.

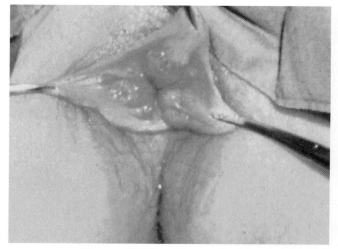

Figure 9-19. Hemorrhoids.

Massage Consideration/s—If a client is prone to GERD, the massage therapist should urge the client not to eat a large meal at least one hour before the scheduled appointment. The massage therapist needs to ask the client about the severity of the symptoms before each massage treatment. If the client indicates that the abdomen is sensitive, massage in that area should be avoided. The massage therapist needs to ask the client if the client is comfortable lying flat in the prone position. If not, propping under the abdomen may be necessary, or the side-lying position could be used. The head of the massage table could be elevated slightly so that gravity could aid in digestion.

Hemorrhoids (Piles)

Gr. Vein Unable To Bleed

Description—Hemorrhoids are varicosities of the rectal veins (Figure 9-19). The veins in the rectal area lack internal valves, which make them particularly susceptible to vascular congestion (Figure 9-20). Prolonged sitting, pregnancy, obesity, constipation, and straining to defecate can contribute to hemorrhoid development.

Massage Consideration/s—General massage may be performed on a client with hemorrhoids.

Hepatitis

Gr. Liver; Inflammation

Description—Hepatitis is an inflammation of the liver that can be caused by alcohol, drugs, toxins, and infection by the hepatitis virus, of which there are several types. Symptoms include muscle and joint pain, fatigue, loss of appetite, nausea, vomiting, diarrhea or constipation, abdom-

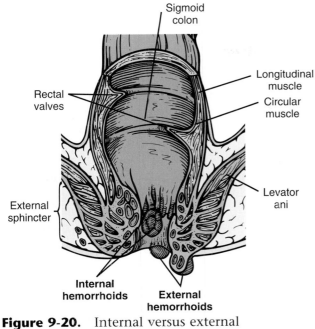

Figure 9-20. Internal versus external hemorrhoids.

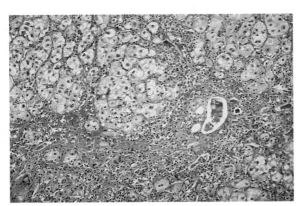

Figure 9-21. Hepatitis B infection.

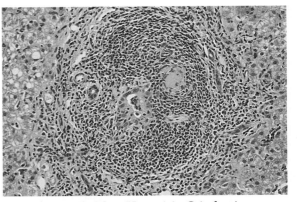

Figure 9-22. Hepatitis C infection.

inal discomfort, tea-colored urine, white stools, and jaundice (Figures 9-21 and 9-22). Severity ranges from mild and brief to chronic and life threatening (Table 9-2). Chronic hepatitis can lead to cirrhoses. (See prior entry.)

Massage Consideration/s—Massage is contraindicated during the acute phases because it is often infectious. Jaundice indicates that the liver is not functioning properly and that blood flow through it may possibly be impaired. Massage can indirectly increase that blood flow (when a client relaxes, more blood moves to the viscera) and exacerbate the jaundice. Also, as the liver synthesizes many clotting factors, an impaired liver greatly increases the chance of bruising. If a client has chronic hepatitis (lasting more than 6 months), massage

should be performed only after receiving a health care provider's clearance to make sure the client is not infectious and that the debilitated liver will not be stressed by massage. If clearance is given, abdominal massage is contraindicated because the pressure of massage can put undue pressure on the liver.

Hernia

L. An Opening; Rupture

Description—A hernia is a protrusion of an organ or part of an organ through its surrounding connective tissue membranes or cavity wall. This condition may be congenital, resulting from failure of structures to completely close after birth, or it may develop as a result of obesity, injury, chronic illness, or surgery. The four most common types of hernia are *hiatal, inguinal, femoral,* and *umbilical.* The esophagus pierces the diaphragm though a hole called the esophageal hiatus. A hiatal hernia occurs when part of the stomach protrudes through the esophageal hiatus (Figure 9-23). The main complaint is gastroesophageal reflux. Surgery is usually not necessary; instead, management of the gastroesophageal reflux is needed (see previous entry on GERD). The inguinal canal is a narrow passage through the muscle of the lower abdominal wall. In males, it contains the spermatic cord, a supporting structure of the male reproductive system that ascends from the scrotum. In females, it contains the round ligament, a supporting structure of the uterus. An inguinal hernia occurs when a loop of intestine enters the inguinal canal (Figures 9-24 and 9-25). In males, it sometimes fills the entire scrotal sac. They are usually repaired surgically to prevent the herniated segment of the intestine from becoming obstructive or gangrenous and blocking waste passage through the bowel. A femoral hernia occurs when a loop of intestine descends through the femoral canal into the groin (Figure 9-26). The usual

Table **9-2**   **TYPES OF HEPATITIS**

DISEASE	TRANSMISSION	INCUBATION PERIOD	COMMENTARY
Type A (HAV)	Fecal contamination	2-6 weeks, followed by complete recovery	Infection provides lifelong immunity.
Type B (HBV)	Blood contact, shared needles or other instruments, sexual contact	1-6 months (average of 60-90 days)	Can cause rapid death or develop into chronic disease. Risk of progressing into liver cancer.
Type C (HCV)	Blood contact, shared needles or other instruments	2 weeks to 6 months (average 6-9 weeks)	Can lead to cirrhosis, liver failure, or cancer.
Type D (HDV)	Blood contact, shared needles or other instruments, sexual contact	2-10 weeks	Occurs as a coinfection with HBV. Responsible for half of all total liver failure cases.
Type E (HEV)	Usually occurs from fecal contaminated food or water from natural disasters	2-9 weeks	Usually occurs in epidemics in the Middle East and Asia. Resembles Hepatitis A and can be fatal in pregnant women.

Modified from Gould BE: Pathophysiology for the health professions, *ed 2, Philadelphia, 2002, WB Saunders.*

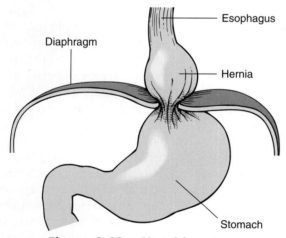

Figure 9-23.   Hiatal hernia.

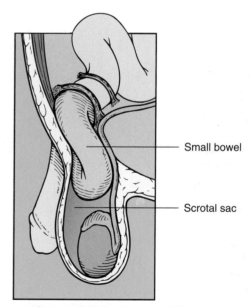

Figure 9-24.   Inguinal hernia.

treatment is surgical repair. An umbilical hernia is usually found in newborns. It is a skin-covered protrusion of intestine through a weakness in the abdominal wall around the umbilicus (navel) (Figures 9-27 and 9-28). It usually closes spontaneously in 1 to 2 years. Large hernias, however, may require surgery.

Massage Consideration/s—The massage therapist needs to ask if the client is in pain from the hernia. If so, massage should not be performed and the client needs to see the health care provider immediately. If the client is not experiencing pain from the hernia, general massage may be performed, but local massage is contraindicated because the pressure of massage could cause pain and damage to the tissues in the area. The massage

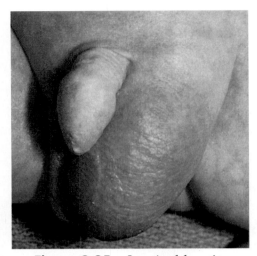

Figure 9-25.   Inguinal hernia.

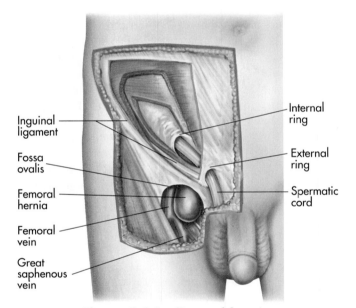

Inguinal
ligament

Fossa
ovalis

Femoral
hernia

Femoral
vein

Great
saphenous
vein

Internal
ring

External
ring

Spermatic
cord

Figure 9-26.   Femoral hernia.

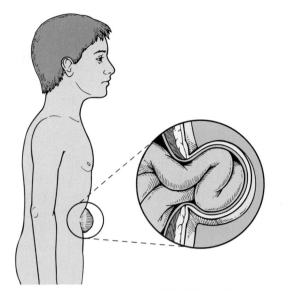

Figure 9-27.   Umbilical hernia.

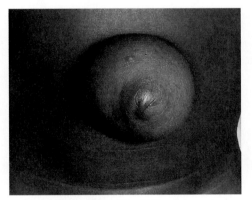

Figure 9-28.   Umbilical hernia.

therapist needs to ask if the client is comfortable lying flat in the prone position. If not, propping under the abdomen may be necessary, or the side-lying position could be used.

If the client has a surgical mesh as a result of surgery, use only gentle pressure over the mesh site, especially during the first 3 months after surgery. Moderate or deep pressure may disrupt the tissue-mesh relationship and cause damage. These devices must adhere to the surrounding tissues, so techniques such as deep friction and myofascial release that are used to release adhesions are contraindicated. Additionally, most surgical meshes are placed in the anterior abdominopelvic wall, so the thera-

pist will not be able to perform abdominal massage to increase intestinal peristalsis or go through the abdominal wall to massage the iliopsoas.

Intestinal Obstruction

Description—An intestinal obstruction is any blockage to the passage of intestinal contents. Common causes are blockages resulting from adhesions from past abdominal surgeries and, in rare cases, impacted feces (Figure 9-29) or tumors of the bowel. Small intestinal obstruction causes severe pain, vomiting, dehydration, and eventually a drop in blood pressure. Most small intestinal obstructions are due to mechanical reasons (Figure 9-30). Large intestinal obstruction causes less severe pain, marked abdominal distention, and constipation.

Massage Consideration/s—Massage is contraindicated because this is a very serious condition that requires medical attention.

Irritable Bowel Syndrome (Spastic Colon)

L. To Tease; O. Fr. Intestines; Gr. Together; Course

Description—Irritable bowel syndrome is a condition of the large intestine characterized by abnormal muscular contraction (peristalsis isn't working properly) and excessive mucus in stools. It is generally associated with young adults under extreme emotional stress. Early symptoms are diarrhea, nausea, and cramping in the lower abdomen. Many individuals benefit from adding roughage to their diets. Other positive steps to take in reducing irritable bowel syndrome are counseling, stress reduction, change in dietary habits, and antispasmodic medications.

Massage Consideration/s—Because the symptoms of irritable bowel syndrome can vary from day to day, the massage therapist needs to ask the client about the severity of pain and other symptoms before each massage treatment. The massage therapist also needs to ask the client what positions on the massage table are comfortable. Propping with a pillow under the client's abdomen while the client is prone may be necessary, or, if the client cannot lie prone comfortably, the side-lying position may need to be used. Generally, the abdomen should be avoided because the pressure of massage could cause undue pain.

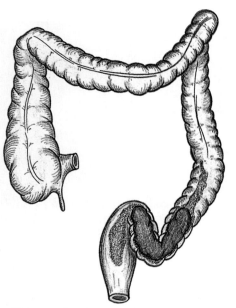

Figure 9-29. Fecal impactions.

Jaundice (Icterus) (jahn´·dis)

Fr. Yellow

Description—Characterized by a yellow discoloration of the skin, mucous membranes, and sclerae of the eyes, jaundice is caused by greater than normal amounts of bilirubin in the blood (Figure 9-31). Jaundice is often a symptom of other disorders, such as liver diseases (cirrhosis of the liver, hepatitis), as well as GI obstruction and anemia. Individuals with jaundice may also experience nausea, vomiting, and abdominal pain (Figure 9-32).

Massage Consideration/s—Massage is contraindicated. Jaundice indicates that the liver is not functioning properly; blood flow through the liver is possibly impaired. Massage can indirectly increase that blood flow (when a client relaxes, more blood moves to the viscera) and exacerbate jaundice. Also, as many of the clotting factors are synthesized by the liver, an impaired liver greatly increases the chance of bruising.

Mumps (Parotitis) (par`·uh·tai´·tis)

D. Sulken

Description—Mumps is an acute infectious viral disease caused by a paramyxovirus (an airborne member of the herpes family). Symptoms are enlargement of the parotid salivary glands, fever, and extreme pain during swallowing (Figure

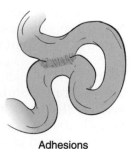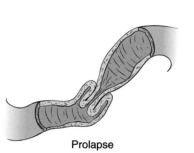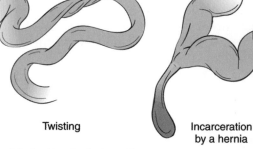

Adhesions   Prolapse   Twisting   Incarceration by a hernia

Figure 9-30. Mechanical causes of intestinal obstruction.

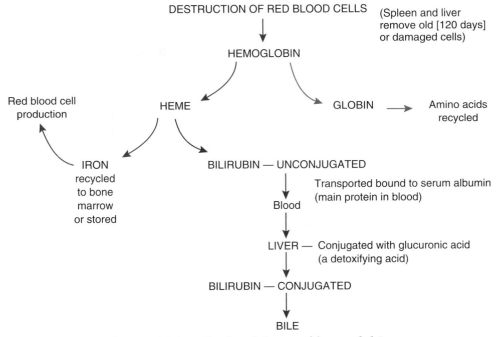

DESTRUCTION OF RED BLOOD CELLS   (Spleen and liver
                                      remove old [120 days]
                                      or damaged cells)

HEMOGLOBIN

Red blood cell   HEME   GLOBIN → Amino acids
production   recycled

IRON   BILIRUBIN — UNCONJUGATED
recycled
to bone   Transported bound to serum albumin
marrow   Blood   (main protein in blood)
or stored
                       LIVER — Conjugated with glucuronic acid
                               (a detoxifying acid)

                       BILIRUBIN — CONJUGATED

                       BILE

Figure 9-31. The breakdown of hemoglobin.

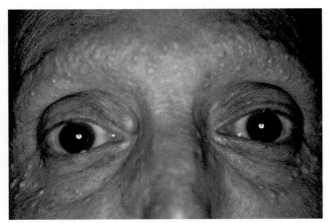

Figure 9-32. Severe jaundice.

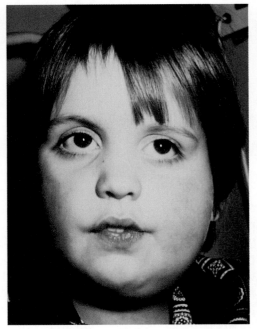

Figure 9-33. Child with mumps.

9-33). Transmitted by contact with infectious droplets, mumps is most likely to be contracted by children between 5 and 15 years old, but the disease may occur in adults.

Massage Consideration/s—Massage is contraindicated because mumps is a contagious disease.

Obesity

L. Corpulence

Description—Obesity is characterized by an abnormal increase in subcutaneous fat, primarily in visceral regions of the body (Figure 9-34).

Generally, an individual is regarded as obese if the body weight is 30% above desired body weight for age, height, frame size, and sex. Normal (nonathlete) body fat is 18% in men and 25% in women.

Massage Consideration/s—Box 9-2 has information on massaging the large client.

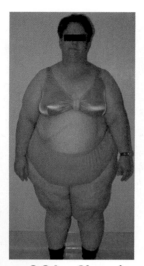

Figure 9-34.   Obese female.

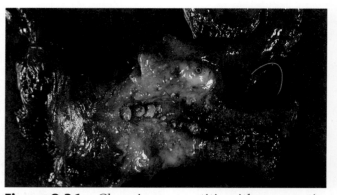

Figure 9-36.   Chronic pancreatitis with pancreatic atrophy.

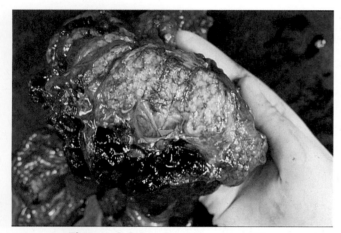

Figure 9-35.   Acute pancreatitis.

Pancreatitis

Gr. All Flesh; Inflammation

Description—An acute or chronic inflammation of the pancreas, pancreatitis is usually the result of alcohol abuse. Other causes are trauma, infection, or certain medications that damage the pancreas (Figures 9-35 and 9-36). Symptoms may be severe abdominal pain that is referred to the back, fever, lack of appetite, nausea, vomiting, and a decreased production of pancreatic enzymes.

Massage Consideration/s—Clients with acute pancreatitis should not be massaged and require medical attention. With chronic pancreatitis, the massage therapist needs to obtain clearance for massage from the client's health care provider. If given, the massage therapist needs to ask the client

about his or her symptoms before each massage treatment. A gentle, nurturing massage is indicated when symptoms are more severe; a more vigorous massage may be performed when symptoms are less severe.

The massage therapist should ask the client what positions on the massage table are comfortable. Propping with a pillow under the client's abdomen while the client is prone may be necessary, or, if the client cannot lie prone comfortably, the side-lying position may need to be used. Generally, the abdomen should be avoided because the pressure of massage could cause undue pain.

Peritonitis (pe`·ruh·tuh·nai´·tis)

Gr. Around; To Stretch; Inflammation

Description—An acute inflammation of the peritoneum, peritonitis is produced by bacteria or irritating substances that gain access into the abdominal cavity (Figure 9-37). These substances are introduced into the cavity by a ruptured organ, penetrating wound, perforation of the gastrointestinal or urogenital tract (e.g., ectopic pregnancy), or a ruptured appendix.

Massage Consideration/s—Because the peritoneum covers almost all the abdominal organs, the inflammation could be widespread. Usually, the person is debilitated and should not be massaged. However, massage may be administered in the hospital to reduce stress and pain, but only after obtaining the health care provider's clearance. The massage therapist needs to communicate with the client and the client's health care provider about areas of the client's body that can be massaged, what techniques can be used, and appropriate pressure. Generally, the abdomen should be avoided.

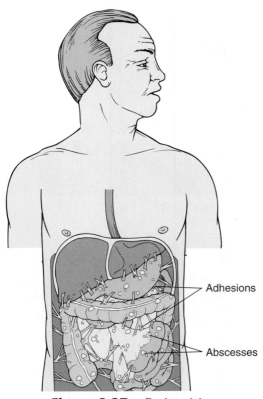

Figure 9-37. Peritonitis.

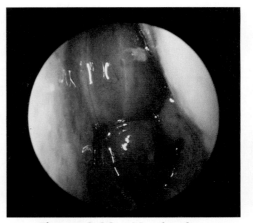

Figure 9-38. Nasal polyp.

Pharyngitis (Sore Throat) (far`·uhn·jai´·tis)

Gr. Throat; Inflammation

Description—Inflammation or infection of the pharynx is called pharyngitis. Causes range from viral and bacterial to irritation from nasal secretions. Strep throat, a type of pharyngitis, is caused by *Streptococcus* infection, and is accompanied by fever, chills, and enlarged cervical lymph nodes.

Massage Consideration/s—The massage therapist needs to ask the client the cause of the pharyngitis. If the pharyngitis is due to infection, massage is contraindicated until the client has completely recovered. For noninfective causes of pharyngitis, massage can be performed.

Polyps

Gr. Foot

Description—Polyps can be single or multiple growths on mucous membranes, but they most commonly occur in the nose, uterus, or the colon (Figure 9-38). Most polyps are benign, but their presence is a risk factor for the future development of cancer. There may be no symptoms, or there could be rectal bleeding and abdominal pain.

Massage Consideration/s—In the case of cancerous polyps, the massage therapist needs to obtain clearance for massage from the client's health care provider and follow the guidelines outlined in Chapter 12. If the polyps are noncancerous, massage can be performed. The massage therapist also needs to ask the client what positions on the massage table are comfortable. If the client cannot lie prone comfortably, the side-lying position may need to be used. Generally, the affected area (e.g., face, abdomen) should be avoided because the pressure of massage could cause undue pain.

Tonsillitis (tahn`·suh·lai´·tis)

L. Almond; Inflammation

Description—Tonsillitis is inflammation of the tonsils, especially the palatine tonsils. Acute tonsillitis, frequently caused by streptococcal infection, is characterized by severe sore throat, high fever, dull headache, difficulty in swallowing, earache, and enlarged lymph nodes in the neck (Figure 9-39).

Massage Consideration/s—Because tonsillitis is due to an infection, massage is contraindicated until the client has completely recovered.

Ulcerative Colitis (Colitis)

Gr. Colon; Inflammation

Description—A type of chronic inflammatory bowel disease, colitis is an inflammation of the mucosa of the large intestine and rectum. It is characterized by weight loss, intestinal ulcerations, diarrhea, and bleeding of the colon wall (Figure 9-40). The origins of colitis are not known, although it is thought to be an autoimmune disease. Some treatment recommendations are increased fluid intake, dietary alterations, antibiotics, and immune response modifiers (e.g., steroids).

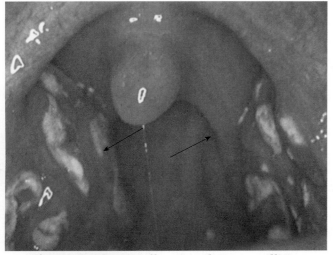

Figure 9-39. Swollen tonsils in tonsillitis.

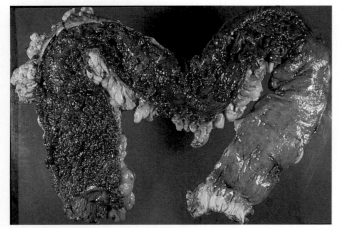

Figure 9-40. Cross section of intestinal segment affected by ulcerative colitis.

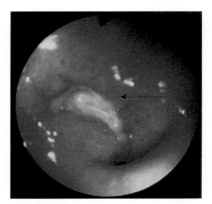

Figure 9-41. Duodenal ulcer.

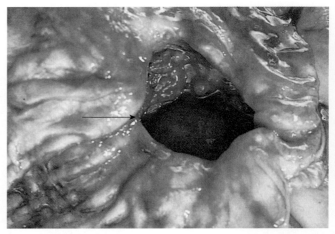

Figure 9-42. Perforating gastric ulcer.

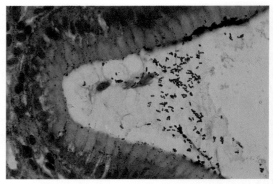

Figure 9-43. *Helicobacter pylori.*

Massage Consideration/s—Because the symptoms of ulcerative colitis can vary from day to day, the massage therapist needs to ask the client about the severity of pain and other symptoms before each massage treatment. The massage therapist should ask the client what positions on the massage table are comfortable. Propping with a pillow under the client's abdomen while the client is prone may be necessary, or, if the client cannot lie prone comfortably, the side-lying position may need to be used. Generally, the abdomen should be avoided because the pressure of massage could cause undue pain.

Ulcers

L. A Sore

Description—An ulcer is a craterlike lesion of the skin or mucous membranes. It results from tissue death that accompanies an inflamma-

tory, infectious, or malignant process. A peptic ulcer can develop in parts of the digestive tract exposed to acidic gastric juice. Those that occur in the first part of the duodenum are called duodenal ulcers (Figure 9-41). Some occur in the body of the stomach and are called gastric ulcers (Figure 9-42). Symptoms of ulcers include nonradiating pain in the upper abdominal region and bleeding that could lead to anemia. There are three main causes of ulcers: (1) use of nonsteroidal antiinflammatory drugs (NSAIDs) such as aspirin, (2) hypersecretion of hydrochloric acid caused by a tumor of the pancreas, and (3) the bacterium *Heliobacter pylori* (the most common cause) (Figure 9-43). Cigarette smoking, alcohol, caffeine, aspirin, and stress can exacerbate ulcers.

Massage Consideration/s—Massage is beneficial for clients with ulcers because it is an effective stress management tool. The massage therapist needs to ask the client the severity of the symptoms before each massage treatment. Abdominal massage is contraindicated if the client's abdomen is sensitive. The massage therapist also needs to ask the client what positions on the massage table are comfortable. Propping with a pillow under the client's abdomen while the client is prone may be necessary, or, if the client cannot lie prone comfortably, the side-lying position may need to be used.

SUMMARY

The digestive system is responsible for converting food into molecules small enough to be absorbed into the blood and lymph, and small enough to enter cells where they can be used for energy, building new tissues, and repairing worn-out ones. The six classes of nutrients are carbohydrates, proteins, lipids, vitamins, minerals, and water. Vitamins, minerals, and water do not need to be broken down before being absorbed. However, carbohydrates are broken down into monosaccharides, proteins are broken down into amino acids, and lipids are broken down into glycerol and fatty acids before they are absorbed. This conversion occurs through the processes of ingestion, secretion, mixing and propulsion, digestion, absorption, and defecation. The conversion process takes place in the GI tract, which is composed of the oral cavity, pharynx, esophagus, stomach, small intestine, and large intestine. The liver, gallbladder, and pancreas are accessory organs that produce substances that aid in digestion.

Digestive pathologies are numerous and wide in variety. They include eating disorders such as anorexia nervosa and bulimia; various infections such as appendicitis, tonsillitis, cholecystitis, diverticulitis, gastritis, gastroenteritis, pharyngitis, and peritonitis; bowel disorders such as constipation, diarrhea, Crohn's disease, irritable bowel syndrome, hemorrhoids, polyps, obstructions, and ulcerative colitis; diseases of the accessory organs such as gallstones, pancreatitis, hepatitis, and cirrhosis of the liver; and miscellaneous disorders such as gastroesophageal reflux, hernia, jaundice, mumps, obesity, and ulcers.

Digestive pathologies may be suspected when symptoms include abdominal pain, blood in the stools, difficulty swallowing, nausea, vomiting, oral lesions, rebound tenderness, significant fatigue or lethargy, and palpable masses in the abdomen but not in the region of the descending or sigmoid colon. If the client has not been diagnosed, refer the client to a physician immediately when these symptoms are present.

Resources

American Anorexia/Bulimia Association, Inc.
165 W 46th Street, Suite 1108
New York , NY 10036
212-575-6200
www.4woman.gov

American Liver Foundation
75 Maiden L, Suite 603
New York, NY 10038
800-GO-LIVER (800-465-4837)
www.gi.ucsf.edu/alf

National Eating Disorders Association
603 Stewart Street, Suite 803
Seattle, WA 98101
206-382-3587
www.nationaleatingdisorders.org

List the letter of the answer to the term or phrase that best describes it.

A. Anorexia nervosa
B. Appendicitis
C. Bulimia
D. Cholecystitis
E. Cirrhosis of the liver
F. Constipation
G. Crohn's disease
H. Diarrhea
I. Diverticulitis
J. Diverticulosis
K. Gastritis
L. Gastroenteritis
M. Gastroesophageal reflux disease
N. Hemorrhoids
O. Hepatitis
P. Hernia
Q. Irritable bowel syndrome
R. Mumps
S. Pancreatitis
T. Peritonitis
U. Pharyngitis
V. Tonsillitis
W. Ulcerative colitis
X. Ulcers

_____ 1. Inflammation of the pancreas.
_____ 2. An insatiable craving for food, often resulting in episodes of continuous eating (bingeing) followed by vomiting (purging), depression, and self-deprivation.
_____ 3. Inflammation of the liver.
_____ 4. Inflammation of the tonsils, especially the palatine tonsils.
_____ 5. Infrequent or difficult passing of stools.
_____ 6. A condition of the large intestine characterized by abnormal muscular contraction and excessive mucus in stools.
_____ 7. A chronic regenerative/degenerative disease in which the hepatic cells are destroyed and replaced with fibrous con-

nective tissue, giving the liver a yellow-orange color.
_____ 8. Inflammation of one or more diverticula.
_____ 9. Inflammation of the mucosa of the large intestine and rectum.
_____ 10. Frequent passing of unformed, loose, watery stools.
_____ 11. Inflammation of the vermiform appendix.
_____ 12. Varicosities of the rectal veins.
_____ 13. Craterlike lesion of the skin or mucous membranes resulting from tissue death that accompanies an inflammatory, infectious, or malignant process.
_____ 14. Herniations of the colon wall where the muscle has become weak, most typically in the sigmoid colon.
_____ 15. Failure of the lower gastroesophageal sphincter to close normally after food has entered the stomach, causing a burning sensation.
_____ 16. Acute inflammation of the peritoneum produced by bacteria or irritating substances that gain access into the abdominal cavity.
_____ 17. Inflammation of the lining of the stomach and intestines.
_____ 18. An eating disorder and an emotional disorder characterized by prolonged avoidance of eating.
_____ 19. Acute infectious viral disease caused by a paramyxovirus; symptoms are enlargement of the parotid salivary glands, fever, and extreme pain during swallowing.
_____ 20. A type of chronic inflammatory bowel disease affecting the colon and/or ileum.
_____ 21. A protrusion of an organ or part of an organ through its surrounding connective tissue membranes or cavity wall.
_____ 22. Inflammation or infection of the pharynx; a sore throat.
_____ 23. Inflammation of the stomach's lining.
_____ 24. Inflammation of the gallbladder.

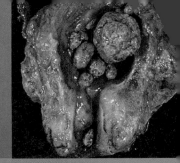

10   **Urinary Pathologies**

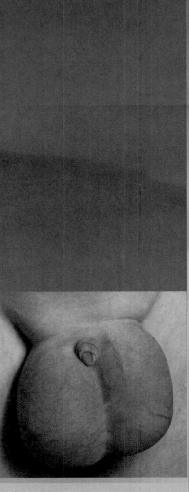

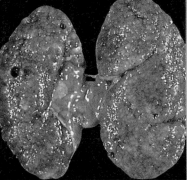

URINARY SYSTEM OVERVIEW

Although massage does not directly affect the urinary system, it is still an important system for massage therapists to be acquainted with. The kidneys perform an important function—filtering wastes out of the blood. They also play a significant role in maintaining homeostatic blood pressure. Because massage therapy techniques can affect blood flow, pathologies of the urinary system need careful consideration before massage can be performed.

The cells and tissues of the body are constantly making wastes as by-products of cellular metabolism. These wastes need to be removed quickly because, if they were to build up, cell, tissue, and even organ death could occur. In fact, high enough levels of wastes could kill the individual.

Cells export their wastes into the surrounding interstitial fluid. From there, the wastes diffuse into the blood, which transports them away from the cells to one of the body's most important waste management systems, the urinary system.

The urinary system consists of two kidneys, two ureters, one urinary bladder, and one urethra. The kidneys are the primary organs of the urinary system. The other parts are mostly passageways and storage areas (Figure 10-1).

Six main functions of the kidneys help maintain the body's homeostasis:

- Helping with the regulation of the blood levels of several ions, most importantly sodium ions, potassium ions, calcium ions, and phosphate ions
- Helping with the regulation of blood pH by eliminating acids and conserving buffers
- Adjusting blood volume by conserving or eliminating water in the urine
- Regulating blood pressure by adjusting blood volume and by initiating a mechanism to increase blood pressure when it drops below homeostatic levels
- Producing two hormones—calcitriol (the active form of vitamin D), which helps regulate blood calcium levels, and erythropoietin, which stimulates red blood cell production
- Excreting wastes and foreign substances as urine. Metabolic wastes include ammonia and urea from protein in metabolism, creatinine from muscle metabolism, and uric acid from metabolism of genetic material. Foreign substances include drugs and environmental toxins.

The kidneys are reddish, kidney bean-shaped organs located in the posterior abdominal wall, just

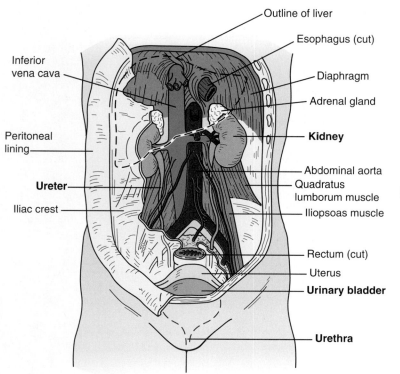

Figure 10-1. General urinary structures.

about waist level. They are about the size of a bar of bath soap. Each kidney is a separate, functioning organ. If one kidney is removed, the other will increase its filtering capacity so that it will filter at 80% of two normal kidneys.

The functional unit of the kidney is the nephron (Figure 10-2). There are about a million nephrons in each kidney. Nephrons are responsible for filtering substances out of the blood, returning useful substances to the blood (depending on the needs of the body), and forming urine.

The first portion of the nephron consists of a loop of blood capillaries called a glomerulus (plural is glomeruli) surrounded by a hollow capsule called a glomerular (Bowman's) capsule. Between the wall of the glomerular capillaries and the capsule is a filtration membrane. This membrane has pores that allow only certain substances, such as water, wastes, ions, amino acids, and glucose, to be filtered out of the blood. Blood cells and large proteins are too large to fit through the filtration membrane, so blood and protein in the urine indicate kidney dys-

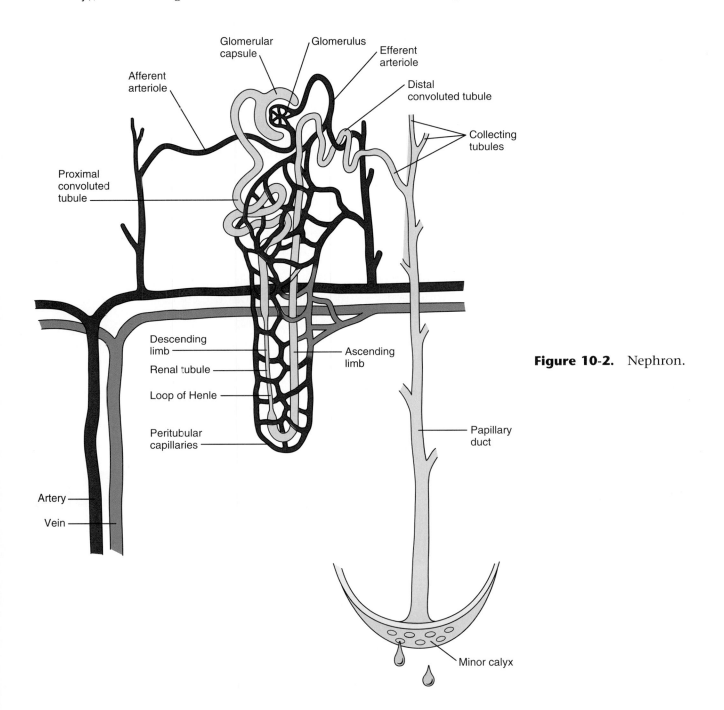

Figure 10-2. Nephron.

function. Blood pressure is the force responsible for filtration.

The second part of the nephron is the renal tubule, which is a small, hollow tube that connects to the glomerular capsule. As the fluid filtered out of the blood passes through the renal tubule, useful substances (some water, glucose, ions, amino acids) are returned to the blood. Ultimately, as this fluid is processed, it becomes urine.

Because blood pressure is the force behind filtration, the kidneys are equipped with an area that measures blood pressure called the juxtaglomerular apparatus. If blood pressure drops too low, the filtration rate can decrease. The juxtaglomerular apparatus secretes renin, which converts angiotensinogen from the liver into angiotensin I. Angiotensin I goes through the lungs and becomes angiotensin II. Angiotensin II causes the secretion of aldosterone, which increases sodium and water reabsorption from the fluid in the renal tubule back into the blood. This increases blood volume, which increases blood pressure back to normal. This pathway is called the renin-angiotensin-aldosterone system.

Because the kidneys remove wastes from the blood and regulate its volume and ionic composition, they have an abundant blood supply. At rest, a fifth to a fourth of the body's blood can be found in the kidneys being filtered. In fact, the body's entire blood volume is filtered 65 times in a 24-hour period. Renal arteries bring blood to the kidneys. Inside each kidney, the arteries divide into smaller and smaller blood vessels, until they become glomerular capillaries. After exiting the nephron, the blood vessels drain into larger and larger veins, and the renal vein carries blood away from the kidneys.

After urine is formed in the nephrons, it travels to the hollow center of each kidney, then travels down the ureters to the urinary bladder. The bladder can hold 700 to 800 ml. At 300 ml, the bladder is distended enough that the conscious sensation of needing to urinate arises. The urethra, which is 1.5 inches long in women and 6 to 8 inches long in men, then carries urine to outside the body.

THERAPEUTIC ASSESSMENT OF THE URINARY SYSTEM

The following list of pertinent questions serves as a review of how to evaluate the urinary system. Findings need to be documented.

Questions to ask the client in the premassage interview:

- *Is the client currently experiencing any lower abdominal, groin, or low back pain?* These, along with other symptoms, may be linked to kidney or bladder infections.
- *Does the client complain of frequent or painful urination, urine discoloration, or blood in the urine?* Any of these symptoms may be linked to a urinary infection. A kidney stone or bladder infection may produce blood in the urine (called hematuria). Kidney stones, bladder infections, or bladder cancer may produce hematuria.
- *Is the client taking medication for blood pressure or diuretics?* Table 7-1 has a discussion of these medications.

Observations and palpations to make during the premassage interview and during the massage treatment:

- *What is the condition of the client's skin?* The massage therapist needs to assess it for color (bruising, pallor, flushed, jaundiced, cyanotic, varicosities) and temperature (client may be cold or hot or may feel cold/hot to the touch).
- *Are there any signs of edema (i.e., pitting edema or molted skin)?* If so, caution is advised. The massage therapist needs to ascertain the cause of the edema from the client and clearance may need to be obtained from the client's health care provider before massage therapy can be performed. If the edema is not due to a serious condition such as congestive heart failure or renal failure, massage can be performed. The massage therapist should elevate the affected area during treatment to promote drainage and use lymphatic drainage techniques.

GENERAL MANIFESTATIONS OF URINARY DISEASE

If a client has any of the following, the massage therapist needs to refer the client to the client's health care provider for diagnosis and treatment.

- Discoloration or blood in the urine
- Fever accompanied by abdominal, groin, flank, or low back pain (over the kidneys)
- Painful, difficult, or frequent urination
- Nausea and vomiting
- Unusual swelling or edema
- Decreased urinary output

URINARY PATHOLOGIES

Cystitis (Bladder Infection) (sis·tai´·tis)

Gr. Bag; Inflammation

Description—Cystitis is an inflammation of the urinary bladder (Figures 10-3 and 10-4). Cystitis is often characterized by pain, blood in the urine, and by urgency and frequency of urination. This condition may either be chronic or acute. Risk factors for cystitis are diabetes mellitus, pregnancy, obstruction of the urinary tract, and improper toilet habits. Cystitis occurs more often in women than men. This may be because the urethra in women is located near the anus. Bacteria from feces can be transported to the urethra as a result of improper toilet habits (i.e., wiping from back to front rather than from front to back). Also, the urethra in women is shorter than the urethra in men. There is less opportunity to flush microbes out with the flow of urine.

Massage Consideration/s—The massage therapist needs to suggest to the client that she seek medical attention if she has not already done so. If the client has received medical attention, the massage therapist needs to encourage her to take the full course of antibiotics and to increase fluid intake. A full body massage may be beneficial to the client to help her relax and manage stress from the disease. Massage over the abdominal area is contraindicated because the pressure of massage may cause discomfort or pain. The massage therapist needs to ask the client if she is comfortable lying prone and may need to prop her with a pillow under her abdomen. A side-lying position may also be used.

Glomerulonephritis (gluh·mer`·yuh·loh`·ni·frai´·tis)

L. Little Ball; Gr. Kidney; Inflammation

Description—Glomerulonephritis is an inflammation of the glomeruli within the kidney (Figure 10-5). One of the most common causes is an allergic reaction to the toxins produced by streptococcal bacteria that have infected another part of the body such as the throat (i.e., strep throat). The glomeruli become inflamed and swollen, and the filtration membranes allow blood cells and blood proteins to pass through and end up in the urine. Signs and symptoms include blood and protein in the urine, edema, and hypertension. This condition may be either chronic or

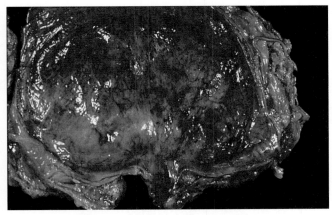

Figure 10-3. Acute cystitis.

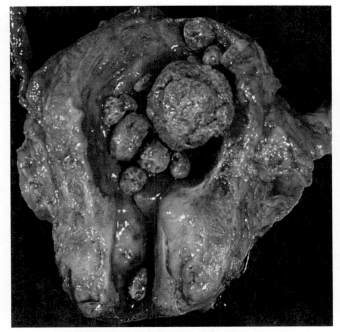

Figure 10-4. Chronic cystitis.

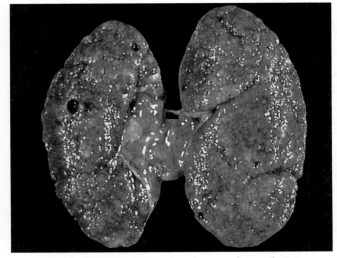

Figure 10-5. Chronic glomerulonephritis.

acute. The glomeruli may become permanently damaged, which could lead to chronic renal failure (see entry below).

Massage Consideration/s—Clearance for massage from the client's health care provider is essential. Massage strokes should be very light and soothing, and of shorter duration. The massage therapist should not try to reduce edema with lymphatic massage. Moving the fluid back into the blood may overload the heart, or the already debilitated kidneys.

Gout

L. Drop

Description—Gout is a condition characterized by high levels of uric acid (a metabolic waste) in the blood. It can occur either because an overproduction of uric acid by cells of the body, or because the kidneys are not able to excrete as much as normal. The uric acid is converted to sodium urate crystals, which are frequently deposited in joints, the kidneys, and other tissues. Gout is more common in men than in women. The great toe is a common site for the accumulation of sodium urate crystals, causing painful swelling (see Figure 4-36). When gout settles in the joints, it is called gouty arthritis (see Gouty Arthritis, Chapter 4).

Massage Consideration/s—Massage and joint mobilizations to the affected area are both contraindicated during an acute phase of gout because of the inflammation and pain. However, application of cold packs could be beneficial. If the client is not having a flare-up, light massage can be done on the surrounding areas.

Kidney Failure (Renal Failure)

Description—Kidney failure occurs when the glomeruli in the nephrons greatly decrease or stop filtering blood. In acute renal failure, the kidneys abruptly stop working. Causes include a low blood volume (such as from hemorrhage), decreased output of blood from the heart (such as from a heart attack or congestive heart failure), damaged nephrons (such as from glomerulonephritis), kidney stones, and reactions from certain medications. Chronic renal failure is a progressive and usually irreversible decline in the filtration of blood. Causes include kidney infections, polycystic kidney disease (see entry in this chapter), or trauma and/or damage to the kidneys. Kidney failure causes a host of problems. Edema results from salt and water retention. Acidosis can occur because the kidneys are unable to excrete acidic substances. Wastes build up in the blood. The blood level of potassium rises, which could lead to cardiac arrest. Anemia can occur because the kidneys no longer produce enough erythropoietin for healthy red blood cell production. If both kidneys are in kidney failure, the person needs to undergo renal dialysis, and may be a candidate for a kidney transplant. See Box 10-1 for more information on renal dialysis.

Massage Consideration/s—Massage is contraindicated for a client with kidney failure because the client is in a severely debilitated state. A more vigorous massage can indirectly increase blood flow (when a client relaxes, more blood moves to the viscera) and tax the kidneys further.

Kidney Stones (Urolithiasis, Renal Stones, Renal Calculi) (yur`·uh·li·thai´·uh·sis) (ree´·nuhl kal´·kyuh·lee)

Gr. Urine; Stone; Condition

Description—Kidney stones are crystals of salts in the urine, such as uric acid or calcium salts. Causes of kidney stones include excessive calcium intake, low water intake, or abnormally alkaline or acidic urine (Figure 10-6). When the stones lodge in the urinary tract, such as the ureter, they commonly produce intense pain in the midback region, which may radiate to the lower abdomen or genitals. If the stone is large enough to block the flow of urine from the kidney, it must be removed by either surgery or other medical procedures (Figure 10-7).

Massage Consideration/s—If a client has a history of kidney stones but none currently, massage may be performed. Massage is contraindicated if pain is severe. If a client is taking medication for treatment of kidney stones, clearance from the client's health care provider is needed for massage. Massage may help reduce pain, stress, and muscle spasms in the back. The massage therapist needs to ask the client about any referred pain, areas of the body to avoid massaging, and positions on the massage table the client finds comfortable. Propping under the abdomen while prone and under the low back while supine may be necessary, or a side-lying position may be used. The massage therapist needs to encourage the client to increase fluid intake.

Nephrotic Syndrome (nuh·frah´·tik sin´·drohm)

Gr. Kidney; Condition

Description—Nephrotic syndrome is a constellation of symptoms characterized by proteins in the urine and high blood levels of lipids and cholesterol in the blood. Protein in

Box **10-1**

Renal Dialysis

Renal Dialysis (Hemodialysis)

Gr. Through; Dissolve; Procedure

Description—If the kidneys are impaired by disease or injury to the point that they can no longer function, then the blood needs to be cleaned artificially by dialysis in an artificial kidney machine. Blood is removed from the person's body and flows through tubing made of a semipermeable dialysis (filtration) membrane. Waste products diffuse from the blood into the dialysis solution. After filtering, the cleansed blood flows back into the body. The process takes 2 to 3 hours, and must be done about two to three times a week.

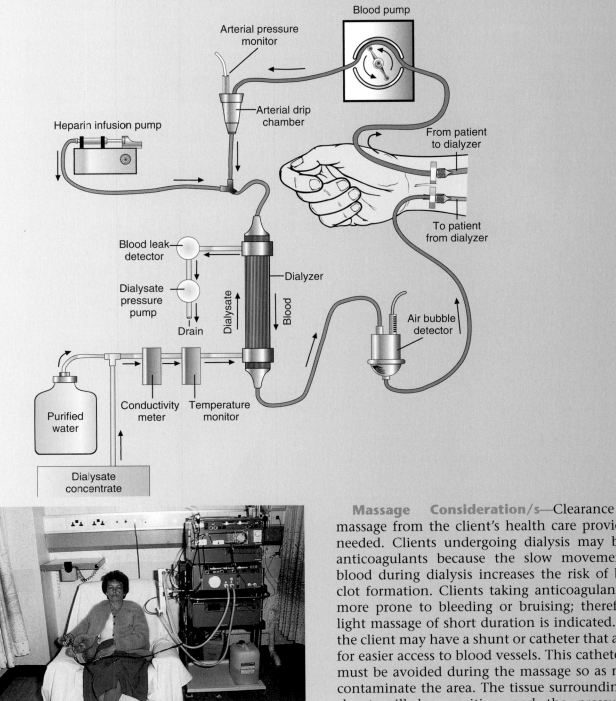

Massage Consideration/s—Clearance for massage from the client's health care provider is needed. Clients undergoing dialysis may be on anticoagulants because the slow movement of blood during dialysis increases the risk of blood clot formation. Clients taking anticoagulants are more prone to bleeding or bruising; therefore a light massage of short duration is indicated. Also, the client may have a shunt or catheter that allows for easier access to blood vessels. This catheter site must be avoided during the massage so as not to contaminate the area. The tissue surrounding the shunt will be sensitive, and the pressure of

Continued

Renal Dialysis—cont'd

massage may cause pain or damage to the tissues. Because the client may feel progressively worse as wastes build up between dialysis treatments, or the client may feel very tired immediately after a dialysis treatment, it is important for the massage therapist to ascertain from the client the best time to schedule massage treatments. The client's health and vitality will change from massage to massage, so it is important for the massage therapist to ask the client how he or she is feeling and about any symptoms the client is experiencing at each massage appointment.

Adapted from Salvo S: Massage therapy: principles and practice, ed 2, Philadelphia, 2003, WB Saunders.

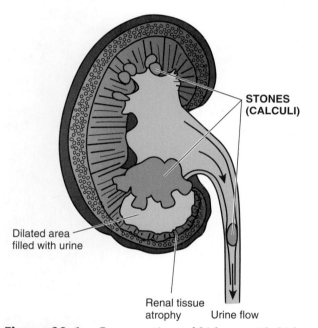

STONES (CALCULI)

Dilated area filled with urine

Renal tissue atrophy   Urine flow

Figure 10-6.   Cross section of kidney with kidney stones.

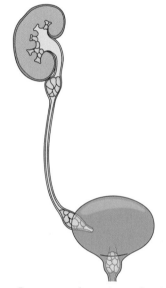

Figure 10-7.   Common locations for kidney stone formation.

the urine is due to an increase in the permeability of the filtration membrane in the nephron. Causes may be primary, such as glomerulonephritis, or secondary, such as those associated with other diseases such as cancer, lupus, and diabetes mellitus. In males, the scrotum often swells (Figure 10-8).

Massage Consideration/s—Clearance for massage from the client's health care provider is essential. The massage therapist needs to ask the client about his or her vitality, and if there is referred pain and/or other areas of the body to avoid. A light, soothing massage of short duration is best. The massage therapist should not try to reduce the edema with lymphatic massage. Moving the fluid back into the blood may overload the heart and the already debilitated kidneys.

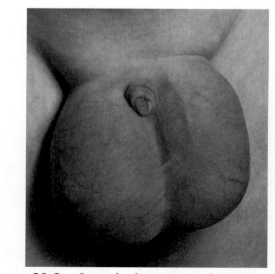

Figure 10-8.   Scrotal edema in nephrotic syndrome.

Polycystic Kidney Disease (PKD, Polycystic Kidneys)

Gr. Many; Cyst

Description—PKD is one of the most common genetic disorders. The nephrons become riddled with thousands of fluid-filled cavities (cysts) (Figure 10-9). The cells of the nephrons die, which may cause a progression to renal failure. People with PKD may also have cysts and cell death in the liver, pancreas, spleen, and gonads. They may also be at greater risk for cerebral aneurysms and heart valve defects. Medications restoring normal blood pressure, restricting protein and salt in the diet, and controlling urinary tract infections may slow the progression to renal failure. Symptoms often appear in adulthood and include abdominal masses, back pain, blood in the urine, and hypertension.

Massage Consideration/s—Clearance for massage from the client's health care provider is essential. Gentle, relaxation massage that avoids the abdomen may be helpful in relaxing the client and reducing stress from the disease.

Pyelonephritis (pai`·uh·loh`·ni·frai´·tis)

Gr. Pelvis; Kidney; Inflammation

Description—Pyelonephritis is an infection of the kidney (Figure 10-10). Acute pyelonephritis usually results from a lower urinary tract infection that has traveled up to the kidney. Onset is rapid and is characterized by fever, chills, hip pain, nausea, and frequent urination. Chronic pyelonephritis develops slowly, often after a urinary bacterial infection. It may progress to renal failure. Some form of obstruction, such as a kidney stone or constricted ureter, also characterizes most cases.

Massage Consideration/s—Massage is contraindicated. The kidney is debilitated and the blood flow through it possibly impaired. A more vigorous massage can indirectly increase blood flow (when a client relaxes, more blood moves to the viscera) and exacerbate the infection.

Uremia

Gr. Urine; Blood

Description—Often seen in renal failure and glomerulonephritis, uremia is a toxic level of urea and other waste products in the blood because of an inability of the kidneys to filter normally.

Massage Consideration/s—Clearance for massage from the client's health care provider is essential. The massage therapist needs to ask the client about his or her vitality and whether the client bruises easily. If so, a light, soothing massage of short duration is indicated. A more vigorous massage can indirectly increase blood flow (when a client relaxes, more blood moves to the viscera) and tax the kidneys further.

Urethritis (yuh·ri·thrai´·tis)

Gr. Urethra

Description—Urethritis, or inflammation of the urethra, is characterized by painful urination, discharge, urethral itching, and tenderness. If left untreated, it can escalate into a bladder or kidney infection. A total of 50% of urethritis cases are caused by gonorrhea; the other 50% are nongonococcal.

Massage Consideration/s—Massage is contraindicated during the acute stage. Urethritis is an infection, which massage would only exacerbate. Once healing is complete, massage can

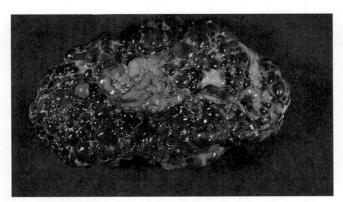

Figure 10-9. Polycystic kidney disease. Note the fluid-filled cavities.

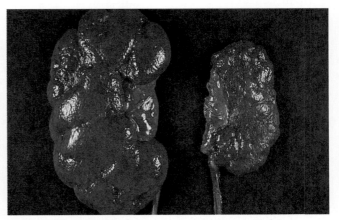

Figure 10-10. *Left,* A normal kidney. *Right,* Shrunken, irregular, scarred kidney of individual with pyelonephritis.

be performed. The massage therapist needs to ask the client if there is abdominal discomfort. If so, the abdomen should be avoided until the client is comfortable having the abdomen massaged.

Urinary Incontinence

Gr. Urine; L. Not; To Stop

Description—The involuntary loss or leakage of urine is referred to as urinary incontinence. This condition may be the result of an infection or damage to the central or peripheral nervous system, or of injury to the urinary sphincter or perineal structures, which can occur during childbirth. Of the various types of incontinence, the most common is incontinence caused by laughing, coughing, and sneezing; late stages of pregnancy; or straining while lifting heavy objects.

Massage Consideration/s—General massage can be performed. However, the massage therapist needs to ask the client if he or she is comfortable with pressure over the lower abdomen. If not, the massage therapist should not apply any pressure over the area.

Urinary Tract Infection (UTI)

Gr. Urine; L. Extend; To Taint

Description—Urinary tract infection, or UTI, is a general term for infection of one or more structures of the urinary system. For example, cystitis and urethritis (see previous entry) are infections of the bladder and ureters, respectively. Most UTIs are caused by bacteria and are more common in women. The most common symptoms of UTIs are increased need or sensation to urinate, burning and pain during urination, and, if the infection is severe, blood and pus in the urine.

Massage Consideration/s—If the client has not already done so, the massage therapist needs to encourage the client to seek medical attention, to take the full treatment of the health care provider-prescribed antibiotics, and to drink plenty of fluids (0.5 oz of fluids per body weight per day). The massage therapist needs to ask the client about the severity of symptoms. Massage is contraindicated if symptoms are severe. A general massage can be performed only if the client feels up to it. Abdominal massage is contraindicated because the pressure of massage may cause discomfort. The massage therapist needs to keep in mind that the client may need to take frequent trips to the bathroom and reassure the client that that is normal.

SUMMARY

Homeostasis is maintained in the body in part by the urinary system, which is composed of a pair of kidneys, a pair of ureters, a urinary bladder, and a urethra.

The nephrons, which are the functional unit of the kidneys, filter the metabolic waste products from the bloodstream while regulating blood volume, fluid volume, blood pressure, blood pH, and chemical composition of the blood. Kidney pathologies include kidney failure, pyelonephritis, glomerulonephritis, nephrosis, kidney stones, and gout.

The ureters transport urine to the bladder where it is stored until it is excreted from the body by the urethra. Common pathologies of these organs include incontinence and infections such as urethritis, bladder infections, and urinary tract infections.

Urinary pathologies may be suspected when symptoms include discolored urine, blood or protein in the urine, painful urination, frequent urination, or a combination of fever and low back or kidney pain. The massage therapist needs to refer the client to a physician immediately when these symptoms are present. Other signs to look for during assessment include skin condition, edema, and the use of diuretic or blood pressure medications.

Resources

American Association of Kidney Patients
100 South Ashley Drive, Suite 280
Tampa, FL 33102
800-749-2257
www.aakp.org

American Foundation for Urologic Disorders
1126 North Charles Street
Baltimore, MD 21201
800-242-2387
www.afun.org

Help for Incontinent People
PO Box 8310
Spartanburg, SC 29305-8310
800-BLADDER

Incontinence Organization
PO Box 8547
Silver Springs, MD 20907
800-358-9295

Interstitial Cystitis Association of America
51 Monroe Street, Suite 1402
Washington, DC 20850
800-435-7422
ICAmail@ichelp.org

National Kidney Foundation
30 East 33rd Street, Suite 1100
New York, NY 10016
800-622-9010
**National Kidney and Urologic Diseases
Information Clearinghouse**
3 Information Way
Bethesda, MD 20892-3580
301-468-6345

**National Organ Procurement and
Transplantation Network**
1100 Boulders Parkway, Suite 500
PO Box 13770
Richmond, VA 23225
804-330-8500
Polycystic Kidney Research Foundation
4901 Main Street, Suite 200
Kansas City, MO 64112-2634
800-PKD-CURE
pkdcure@pkrfoundation.org

List the letter of the answer to the term or phrase that best describes it.

A. Cystitis
B. Glomerulonephritis
C. Gout
D. Kidney or renal failure
E. Kidney stones
F. Nephrotic syndrome
G. Polycystic kidney disease
H. Pyelonephritis
I. Uremia
J. Urethritis
K. Urinary incontinence
L. Urinary tract infection

_____ 1. Condition that occurs when the glomeruli in the nephrons greatly decrease or stop filtering blood.

_____ 2. Involuntary loss or leakage of urine.

_____ 3. Inflammation of the glomeruli within the kidney.

_____ 4. Condition in which the nephrons become riddled with thousands of fluid-filled cavities (cysts), destroying nephronic cells.

_____ 5. Stones that are composed of substances such as uric acid and calcium salts.

_____ 6. Inflammation of the urinary bladder; also known as a bladder infection.

_____ 7. Inflammation of the urethra characterized by painful urination, discharge, urethral itching, and tenderness.

_____ 8. A kidney infection. Most cases are also characterized by some form of obstruction, such as a kidney stone or constricted ureter.

_____ 9. A general term for infection of one or more structures of the urinary system.

_____ 10. A condition characterized by high levels of uric acid in the blood.

_____ 11. This condition is characterized by a toxic level of waste products in the blood resulting from an inability of the kidneys to filter these wastes.

_____ 12. A constellation of symptoms characterized by proteins in the urine and high blood levels of lipids and cholesterol in the blood.

11

Reproductive Conditions, Reproductive Pathologies, and Sexually Transmitted Diseases

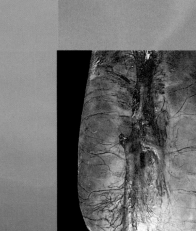

Although massage does not directly affect the reproductive system, it is an important system for massage therapists to know. Massage can be useful in decreasing anxiety and muscle tension that may accompany premenstrual syndrome and menstruation. It can help alleviate some of the physical discomforts associated with pregnancy. It may also be helpful in reducing anxiety associated with infertility issues.

Like most higher forms of life, human beings reproduce sexually. Sexual reproduction is the process by which male and female sex cells unite to produce offspring. Male sex cells are called spermatozoa (i.e., sperm cells) and carry genetic information from the male that produced them. Female sex cells are called oocytes (i.e., eggs) and carry genetic information from the female that produced them. When a sperm unites with an egg, the process is called fertilization. The resulting cell, called an ovum, contains genetic information from each parent.

Reproductive organs are divided into two groups, primary and secondary. The primary reproductive organs are called gonads. They produce hormones and the cells necessary for reproduction. In the male they are the testes; in the female they are the ovaries. The secondary set of organs is a combination of ducts used to transport the reproductive cells for possible fertilization, and then transport the fertilized ovum to a place of incubation. This secondary set of organs in the male includes the epididymis, ductus deferens, ejaculatory ducts, seminal vesicles, prostate gland, bulbourethral glands, and penis (Figure 11-1).

The scrotum is the supporting structure for the testes. It is a sac made of loose skin that hangs down from the penis and is attached to the body. As stated previously, sperm production, or spermatogenesis, occurs in the testes. The testes also produce the hormones testosterone, dihydrotestosterone (DHT), and inhibin. Luteinizing hormone from the anterior pituitary gland stimulates the production of testosterone. Follicle-stimulating hormone from the anterior pituitary gland, testosterone, and inhibin control the process of spermatogenesis. Testosterone and DHT are responsible for the development of the male sex organs and masculine secondary sexual characteristics that occur at puberty. These include the muscular and skeletal system growth that results in wide shoulders and narrow hips; facial, axillary, pubic, and chest hair; and deepening of the voice.

The epididymis is a comma-shaped organ next to the testes. It is a site for the maturation of sperm. The ductus (vas) deferens is also called the seminal duct. It carries sperm from the epididymis to the ejaculatory duct. The ejaculatory duct is a tube that transports sperm from the ductus deferens to the urethra. Other testicular structures are listed in Figure 11-2.

Semen is a milky fluid that is a mixture of sperm and seminal fluid. Seminal fluid is a transport medium and source of nutrients for sperm. Seminal vesicles, the prostate gland, and bulbourethral

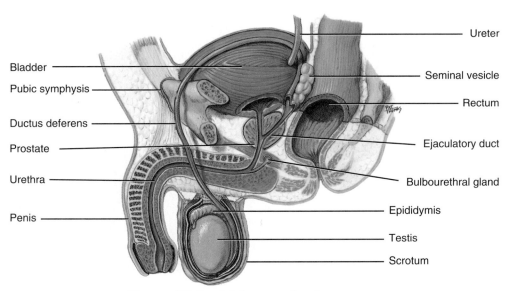

Bladder

Pubic symphysis

Ductus deferens

Prostate

Urethra

Penis

Ureter

Seminal vesicle

Rectum

Ejaculatory duct

Bulbourethral gland

Epididymis

Testis

Scrotum

Figure 11-1. Male reproductive organs.

glands all secrete fluids that together make up the seminal fluid. Seminal vesicles are located posterior to the base of the urinary bladder and anterior to the rectum. The prostate gland, or prostate, is inferior to the bladder and surrounds the urethra. The bulbourethral glands are located inferior to the prostate gland. The seminal vesicles, prostate gland, and bulbourethral glands all have ducts that conduct the fluids they secrete into the urethra.

In males, the urethra is the tube that caries urine from the urinary bladder and semen from the male reproductive system to outside the body. The penis contains the urethra and is a passageway for the ejaculation of semen and the excretion of urine.

In females the secondary organs include the fallopian tubes, uterus, cervix, vagina, clitoris, and labia (Figure 11-3). The breasts are also considered accessory organs of reproduction, as they produce the milk that will feed the young. Within the breasts are mammary glands.

In the female reproductive system, the uterus is located in the pelvic cavity between the urinary bladder and the rectum. The ovaries are located in the superior part of the pelvic cavity, lateral to the uterus. As stated previously, the ovaries produce oocytes, and they produce the hormones progesterone, estrogens, relaxin, and inhibin. These hormones, along with luteinizing hormone and follicle-stimulating hormone from the anterior pituitary gland, regulate the female reproductive cycle (discussed shortly). Estrogens and progesterone are responsible for the development of the female sex organs and feminine secondary sexual characteristics that occur at puberty. These include distribution of adipose tissue in the breasts, hips, and abdomen; a wide pelvis; and pubic and axillary hair.

Two fallopian (uterine) tubes or oviducts extend laterally from the uterus to the ovaries (Figure 11-4). The vagina is a 4-inch long muscular canal that extends from the cervix to outside the body. The vulva comprises the external genitals of the female. It is made up of the mons pubis, labia, and clitoris. The mons pubis is a mound of adipose tissue covered by skin and pubic hair, cushioning the pubic symphysis. The labia major and minor are

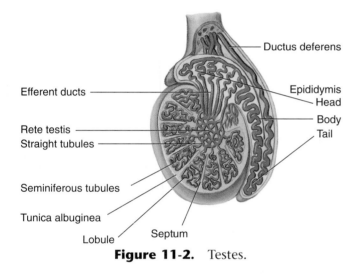

Figure 11-2.   Testes.

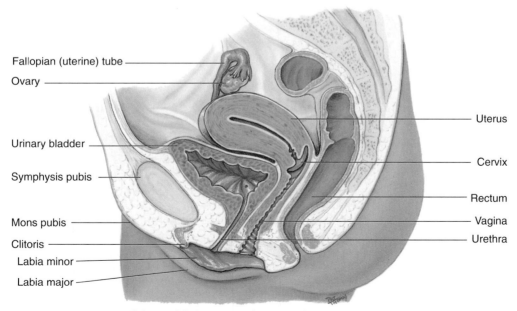

Figure 11-3.   Female reproductive system.

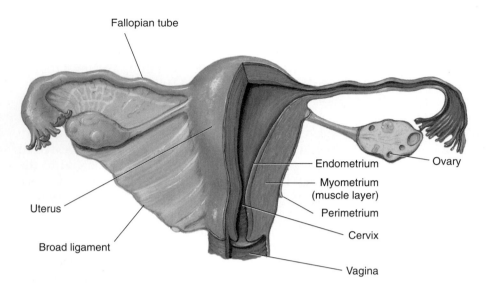

Figure 11-4. Uterus and fallopian tubes.

longitudinal folds of skin that extend inferiorly and posteriorly from the mons pubis. The clitoris is a small mass of erectile tissue and nerves located at the anterior of the labia. It plays a role in sexual excitement in the female.

At puberty, the female begins a fertility cycle about every 28 days. The monthly cycle usually continues until menopause, unless interrupted by pregnancy, disease, stress, or other factors. The cycle is divided into four phases and is dependent on hormones.

The menstrual phase (menstruation) is the first phase. Day 1 of menstruation is day 1 of the fertility cycle. Menstruation is the shedding of built-up uterine lining from the previous fertility cycle. Menstruation lasts about 5 days.

After menstruation occurs, the next phase is the preovulatory phase. It lasts from 6 to 13 days in a 28-day cycle. The production of estrogens is stimulated by follicle-stimulating hormone. These estrogens, along with luteinizing hormone, promote the development and release of the oocyte from the ovary in a process called ovulation. Estrogens also stimulate the uterine lining to proliferate and thicken with tissue and blood vessels in anticipation of a fertilized ovum.

Ovulation is the third phase. It usually occurs on day 14 in a 28-day cycle. The oocyte is released from its follicle and travels down the fallopian tube toward the uterus (Figure 11-5). If fertilization occurs, it normally happens in the fallopian tube. The levels of estrogens continue to rise. The portion of the follicle that remains after the oocyte departs becomes the corpus luteum. This glandular structure secretes progesterone and some estrogens. If the oocyte fertilizes, hormone secretion will cease

only after the placenta develops. If the oocyte does not fertilize, the corpus luteum remains functional for about 10 days, then develops into a corpus albicans, which is primarily scar tissue. At this time, hormone production ceases.

The fourth stage is the postovulatory phase. It lasts from day 15 to day 28. Luteinizing hormone stimulates the ovaries to secrete progesterone, a small amount of relaxin, and inhibin, and to continue secreting estrogens. Progesterone and estrogens continue to stimulate the buildup of the uterine lining. Progesterone also slightly elevates body temperature, creating an incubating effect. Relaxin relaxes the uterus to facilitate implantation of a fertilized ovum. Inhibin inhibits the secretion of follicle-stimulating hormone and luteinizing hormone.

If the oocyte is not fertilized, the level of progesterone decreases over 2 weeks, causing menstruation; the unfertilized egg is flushed out of the body. If, however, the oocyte is fertilized, it continues to develop (i.e., zygote, morula, blastocyst) and travels through the fallopian tube to implant in the uterus (Figure 11-6). The developing embryo secretes human chorionic gonadotropin (hCG), which stimulates the continual production of estrogens and progesterone so that the uterus can maintain the pregnancy (Figure 11-7). Pregnancy tests detect the presence of hCG in the mother's blood or urine. During pregnancy, the ovaries and placenta produce large amounts of relaxin. It increases the flexibility of the pubic symphysis and helps the cervix dilate to ease delivery of the baby.

After a gestation period of about 40 weeks, the uterus begins a complex process called labor (Figure 11-8). The hormone oxytocin from the posterior

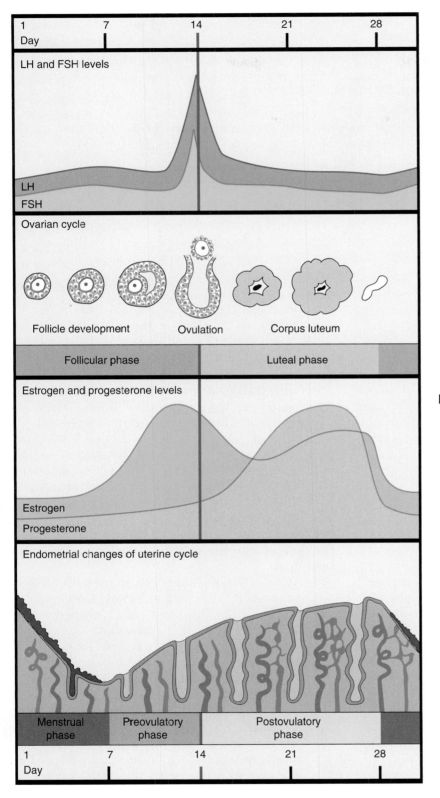

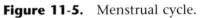

Figure 11-5. Menstrual cycle.

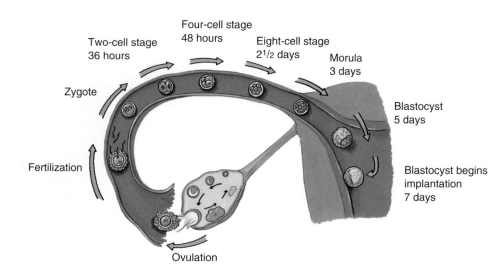

Figure 11-6. First week of prenatal development.

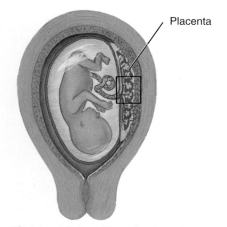

Figure 11-7. Developing fetus.

pituitary gland initiates and strengthens uterine contractions that continue until the baby is expelled through the vaginal opening. Oxytocin is also responsible for milk ejection from the mammary glands.

THERAPEUTIC ASSESSMENT OF THE REPRODUCTIVE SYSTEM

The following list of pertinent questions serves as a review of how to evaluate the reproductive system. Findings need to be documented.

Questions to ask the client in the premassage interview:

- *Is the client currently experiencing any abdominopelvic or groin pain?* These symptoms, if accompanied by others, may indicate a urogenital infection, and the client may not be a good candidate for

massage. The massage therapist needs to ask the client the cause of the inflammation, and if it is unknown, refer the client to the client's health care provider for diagnosis and treatment.

- *Does the client report any vaginal or penile discharge? Any genital inflammation?* These symptoms indicate a urogenital infection, and the client may not be a good candidate for massage. The massage therapist needs to ask the client the cause of the inflammation, and if it is unknown, refer the client to the client's health care provider for diagnosis and treatment.

Observations and palpations to make during the premassage interview and during the massage treatment:

- *What is the condition of the client's skin?* The massage therapist should assess the client's skin for color (bruising, pallor, flushed, jaundiced, cyanotic, varicosities), temperature (client may be cold or hot or may feel cold/hot to the touch), or rashes. Also, look for lesions. If found, query the client as to their cause. If unknown, refer the client to his or her health care provider.
- *Are there any signs of edema (i.e., pitting edema or molted skin)?* If so, caution is advised. The massage therapist needs to ascertain the cause of the edema from the client, and clearance needs to be obtained from the client's health care provider before massage therapy can be performed. If the edema is not due to a serious condition such as congestive heart failure, renal failure, or

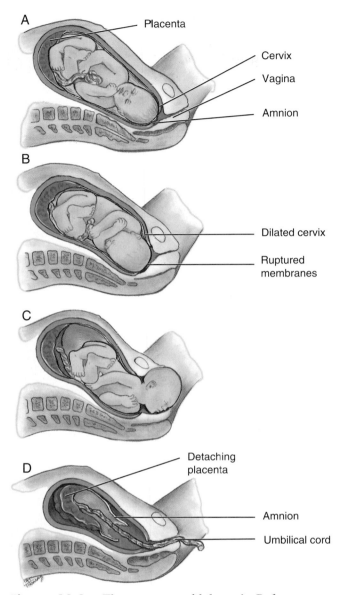

Figure 11-8. Three stages of labor. **A,** Before labor. **B,** Dilation stage. **C,** Expulsion. **D,** Placental stage.

toxemia, massage can be performed. In this case, the massage therapist should elevate the affected area during treatment to promote drainage and perform lymphatic drainage techniques.

GENERAL MANIFESTATIONS OF REPRODUCTIVE DISEASE

If a client reports any of the following, the massage therapist needs to refer the client to the client's health care provider for diagnosis and treatment.

- Genital discharge
- Breast discharge (unless the client is a lactating woman)
- Fever accompanied by groin pain
- Palpable masses in the female breast
- Palpable masses in the abdominopelvic region
- Unexplained skin lesions

REPRODUCTIVE PATHOLOGIES AND CONDITIONS

Abortion (Spontaneous and Elective, Miscarriage)

L. Away From; To Be Born

Description—The spontaneous or induced termination of pregnancy before the fetus has developed to the stage of viability (24 weeks) is abortion. The symptoms of spontaneous abortion are uterine contractions, uterine hemorrhage, dilation of the cervix, and expulsion of all or part of the fetus.

Massage Consideration/s—A gentle, nurturing massage can be soothing and help the client relax. Deep abdominal massage is contraindicated until the client has completely healed because of any possible pain in the area that deep pressure may cause. The massage therapist needs to ask the client if she is experiencing abdominal sensitivity, and may need to prop the client with a pillow under her abdomen while she is prone or, if the client cannot lie prone comfortably, the side-lying position may be used.

Amenorrhea (Amenia) (ah`·me`·nuh·ree´·uh)

Gr. Without; Month; To Flow

Description—The abnormal absence of menses, or amenorrhea, may be caused by dysfunction of the hypothalamus, pituitary gland, ovaries, uterus, or certain medications. This condition is normal before puberty, during pregnancy, after menopause, or after surgical removal of both ovaries, or of the uterus (hysterectomy).

Massage Consideration/s—General massage can be performed on women with amenorrhea. If the client has had surgery to remove her uterus, deep abdominal massage is contraindicated until the client has completely healed. Deep pressure can cause pain in the area, and possibly damage the healing tissues. The client may need to be propped with a pillow under her abdomen while she is prone or, if the client cannot lie prone comfortably, the side-lying position may be used.

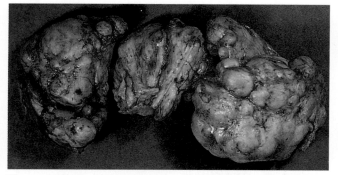

Figure 11-9. Benign prostatic hypertrophy. The prostate may contain numerous nodules.

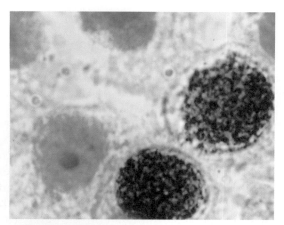

Figure 11-10. *Chlamydia trachomatis.*

Benign Prostatic Hypertrophy (Benign Prostatic Hyperplasia, BPH)
(buh·nain´ pruh·sta´·tik hai`·puhr·troh´·fee)
(buh·nain´ pruh·sta´·tik hai`·puhr·play´·zhee·uh)

L. Kind; Gr. Prostate; Gr. Nourishment

Description—BPH is an enlargement of the prostate gland, which is common among men after age 50 years (Figure 11-9). This is not a malignant or inflammatory condition, but is usually progressive and can obstruct the urethra and interfere with the flow of urine. Possible accompanying symptoms include frequency of urination, need to urinate at night, pain, and urinary tract infections. Treatments include heat packs, medication, balloon dilation, and sometimes surgery.

Massage Consideration(s)—A gentle, nurturing massage can help the client relax. The massage therapist needs to ask the client if his abdomen is tender. If so, abdominal massage is contraindicated. The client may also need to be propped with a pillow under the abdomen while he is prone or, if the client cannot lie prone comfortably, the side-lying position may need to be used.

Chlamydia (kluh·mi´·dee·uh)

Gr. Cloak

Description—Caused by the microorganism *Chlamydia* (Figure 11-10), chlamydia is one of the most common sexually transmitted diseases (STDs) in North America and is a frequent cause of sterility. In women, early symptoms are thick vaginal discharge with localized burning and itching. Men infected with chlamydia experience a penile discharge with painful urination (caused by urethritis), as well as localized burning and itching. The scrotum may be enlarged. Both infected men and women may have swollen lymph nodes. Infants born to an infected mother may acquire this disease during the birth process. It is often called the silent STD because symptoms of chlamydia may be absent and sexual transmission can occur unknowingly (Box 11-1). Chlamydia is the leading cause of pelvic inflammatory disease in women.

Massage Consideration/s—Because chlamydia is an infection, massage is contraindicated until the client has completely healed. If the client is dealing with issues of infertility, the massage therapist can ask her if she would like a referral to a mental health counselor.

Dysmenorrhea (dis`·me`·nuh·ree´·uh)

Gr. Difficult, Painful; Month; To Flow

Description—Painful menstruation, or dysmenorrhea, is extremely common, occurring at least occasionally in almost all menstruating women. Pain occurs in the abdominopelvic or low back region of the body. The sensations are felt as cramps, occurring in successive waves or as a constant cramp. The discomfort usually begins just before, or at the start of, menstrual flow and may last from 1 day to the entire period. In approximately 10% of women, dysmenorrhea is severe enough to cause episodes of partial or total disability.

Massage Consideration/s—Massage can be performed on clients with dysmenorrhea. The massage therapist needs to ask the client about location and severity of the pain. If the client's abdomen is tender, massage over the area may be contraindicated because the pressure of massage may cause more pain. The client may need to be propped with a pillow under her abdomen while she is prone or, if the client cannot lie prone comfortably, the side-lying position may be used. If pain and muscle tension in the low back are occurring, muscles such as quadratus lumborum, latissimus dorsi, the paraspinals, and possibly the gluteals, can be addressed specifically with techniques such as deep gliding, deep friction, kneading, and stretches. A moist hot pack placed on the abdomen when the client is supine or placed on the low back while the client is prone can help soothe the achy feeling associated with menses. The massage therapist needs to communicate with the client about the pressure and effectiveness of techniques. The massage therapist also needs to keep in mind that if the client has severe cramps before or during the massage treatment, the client may not feel up to receiving massage.

Endometriosis (en`·doh·mee`·tree·oh´·sis)

Description—Endometriosis is a gynecological condition characterized by painful cramping before and during menstruation. It is caused by the growth of the lining of the uterus (endometrial tissue) that grows outside the uterus. Endometriosis is a frequent cause of infertility (Figure 11-11).

Massage Consideration/s—Massage can be performed on clients with endometriosis, and may help relax them. The massage therapist needs to ask the client if she is experiencing abdominal

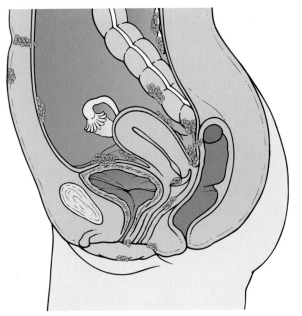

Figure 11-11. Common sites of endometriosis.

discomfort. If so, the client may need to be propped with a pillow under her abdomen while prone or, if the client cannot lie prone comfortably, the side-lying position may need to be used. Abdominal massage is contraindicated if the pressure of massage causes pain. If the client is dealing with issues of infertility, the massage therapist can ask her if she would like a referral to a mental health counselor.

Fibrocystic Breast Disease

L. Fiber; Gr. Cyst

Description—Fibrocystic breast disease consists of the presence of single or multiple cysts that are palpable in the breasts (Figure 11-12). Cysts can increase or decrease in size with the woman's menstrual cycle. The benign cysts are fairly common, yet must be observed carefully for any change in growth, which could be related to a malignancy. Women with fibrocystic breast disease are at greater risk of developing breast cancer later in life. (See Chapter 12.)

Massage Consideration/s—Massage can be performed on clients with fibrocystic breast disease. The massage therapist needs to ask the client if she is comfortable lying prone and may need to prop her with a pillow under her breasts. (See Box 11-2 for more positional suggestions.) If the client cannot lie prone comfortably, the side-lying position may need to be used. Breast massage (see

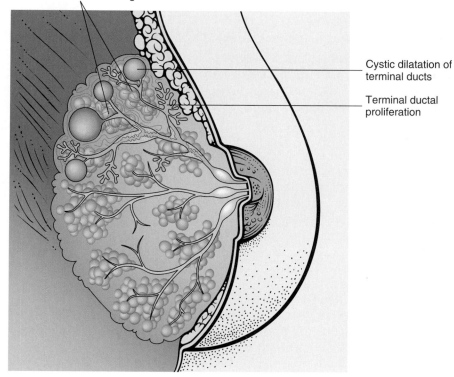

Fibrous tissue "strangles" the ducts

Cystic dilatation of terminal ducts

Terminal ductal proliferation

Figure 11-12.   Fibrocystic breast disease.

Chapter 12) can be helpful in addressing fibrocystic breast disease.

Fibroids (Fibroma, Fibroid Tumors, Leiomyoma) (lay`·oh·mai´·oh·muh)

L. Fiber

Description—A fibroid is a benign tumor composed largely of smooth muscle and fibrous tissue (Figure 11-13). Uterine fibroids can be a cause of dysmenorrhea (see page 295) and infertility (Figure 11-14).

Massage Consideration/s—Massage can be performed on clients with uterine fibroids. The massage therapist needs to ask the client if she is experiencing abdominal discomfort. If so, the client may need to be propped with a pillow under his abdomen while prone or, if the client cannot lie prone comfortably, the side-lying position may need to be used. Abdominal massage is contraindicated if the pressure of massage causes pain. If the client is dealing with issues of infertility, the massage therapist can ask her if she would like a referral to a mental health counselor.

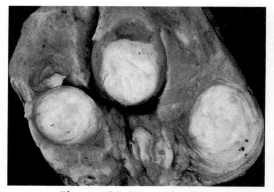

Figure 11-13.   Fibroids.

Genital Herpes (Herpes Genitalis, Herpes Progenitalis, Condylomata Acuminata)

(her´·pees proh`·je`·nuh·ta´·lis)
(kahn`·duh·loh·mah´·tuh a`·kyoo·muh·nah´·tuh)

L. Belonging to Birth; Gr. Creeping Skin Disease

Description—Genital herpes is a chronic infection caused by type 2 herpes simplex virus (Figure 11-15). It is primarily transmitted by sexual contact (via genital secretions). Infection

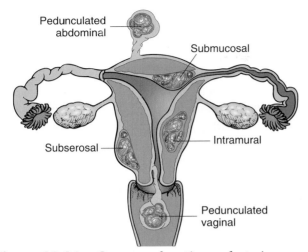

Figure 11-14. Common locations of uterine fibroids.

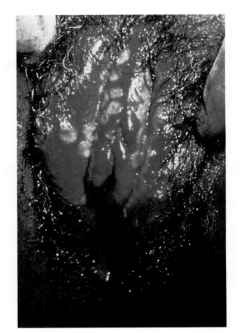

Figure 11-16. Genital herpes in the female.

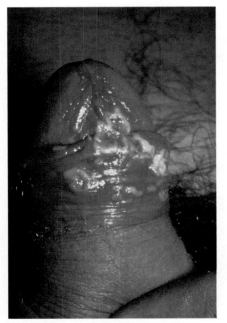

Figure 11-15. Genital herpes in the male.

causes painful vesicular eruptions on the skin and mucous membranes of the genitalia of males and females (Figure 11-16) that are similar to cold sores; symptoms are more severe in females than in males (see Box 11-1). An infected pregnant woman can pass the virus onto the infant either through the placenta or by direct contact of the fetus during birth with infected tissues.

Massage Consideration/s—As massage therapists do not massage the genitals, general massage can be performed on clients with genital herpes. The massage therapist needs to ask the client if his abdomen is tender. If so, abdominal massage is contraindicated. The client may need to be propped with a pillow under the abdomen while the client is prone or, if the client cannot lie prone comfortably, the side-lying position may need to be used. If the client is having symptoms such as general body aches or fever, massage is contraindicated because these are systemic symptoms indicating infection.

Genital Warts (Condyloma Acuminatum, Acuminate Warts, Venereal Warts)

(kahn`·duh·loh´·muh uh·kyoo`·muh·nay´·tuhm)

L. Belonging to birth; L. Wart

Description—Genital warts are a soft, wart-like or papillomatous growth common on warm and moist skin and the mucous membranes of the genitalia and perianal region of men and women (Figure 11-17). It is caused by the human papillomavirus (HPV). This virus is the cause of common warts of the hands and feet, as well as lesions of the mucous membranes of the oral, anal, and genital regions (Figure 11-18). More than 50 types of HPV have been identified, some of which are associated with cancerous and precancerous conditions. The virus can be transmitted through sexual contact and is a precursor to cancer of the cervix. Transmission has occurred without the presence of warts, indicating that transmission may occur through body fluids, such as semen or vaginal secretions. There is no specific cure for an

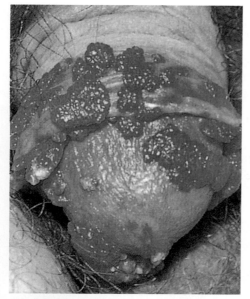

Figure 11-17. Genital warts on male penis.

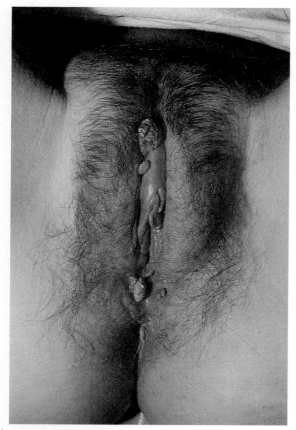

Figure 11-18. Genital warts on female genitalia.

HPV infection, but the virus often can be controlled by medications, and the warts can be removed by cryosurgery, laser treatment, or conventional surgery.

Massage Consideration(s)—As massage therapists do not massage the genitals, general massage can be performed on clients with genital warts. The massage therapist needs to ask the client if the abdominal area is tender. If so, abdominal massage is contraindicated. The client may need to be propped with a pillow under the abdomen while the client is prone or, if the client cannot lie prone comfortably, the side-lying position may need to be used.

Gonorrhea (gah`·nuh·ree´·uh)

Gr. Genitals; Flow

Description—A common sexually transmitted disease, gonorrhea is an infection of the mucous membranes of the urogenital tract and occasionally the pharynx, eyes, and rectum (see Box 11-1). Infection results from contact with an infected person, specifically contact with secretions containing the causative organism *Neisseria gonorrhoeae*. Systemic infection may cause gonococcal arthritis, endocarditis, and septicemia. It can also be passed from the infected pregnant woman to her newborn at birth. In males, infection is characterized by urethritis (inflammation of the urethra), penile discharge, and pain on urination (Figure 11-19). Females often have a vaginal discharge and

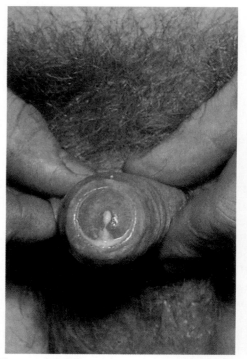

Figure 11-19. Gonorrhea in the male.

painful urination (Figure 11-20). In the United States, gonorrheal infections must be reported to local health departments.

Massage Consideration/s—Massage is contraindicated until the client has fully recovered. Gonorrhea is a systemic infection.

Mastitis

Gr. Breast; Inflammation

Description—Mastitis, or inflammation of the mammary gland (breast), is usually caused by a streptococcal or staphylococcal infection. Acute mastitis is most common in the first 2 months of lactation. It is marked by local redness, pain, swelling, and fever (Figure 11-21). Rest, antibiotics, and warm compresses are usually recommended.

Massage Consideration/s—Massage can be performed on clients with mastitis. The upper chest area should be avoided, as massage could possibly make the infection worse. The massage therapist needs to ask the client if she is comfortable lying prone and may need to prop her with a pillow under her breasts. If the client cannot lie prone comfortably, the side-lying position may need to be used. See Box 11-2 for more positional suggestions.

Menopause

Gr. Month; Cessation

Description—Regarded as a life stage and not a disease, menopause is the cessation of ovarian hormone function and menstruation in the human female. Most commonly, menopause refers to the period leading up to the end of menstruation as well as its cessation. Menses naturally becomes more irregular and eventually stops between 35 and 60 years of age but sometimes earlier as a result of illness or surgical removal of the uterus or both ovaries. Symptoms include dry skin, vaginal irritation, and hot flashes. Symptoms can be severe and debilitating enough to require hormone replacement treatment.

Massage Consideration/s—Massage can be performed on clients with menopause. Because of the prevalence of hot flashes, the massage therapist may

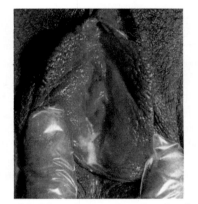

Figure 11-20. Gonorrhea in the female.

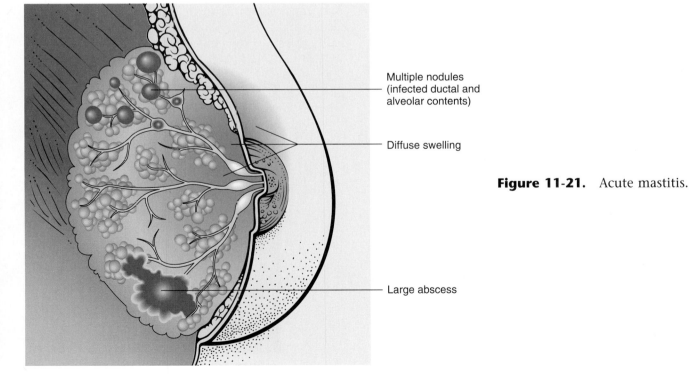

Multiple nodules (infected ductal and alveolar contents)

Diffuse swelling

Large abscess

Figure 11-21. Acute mastitis.

need to adjust the room temperature for the client's comfort, perhaps have a fan blowing, and/or remove the drape from the legs and arms. Massage should be tailored to how the client is feeling at the time of the treatment because symptoms vary from day to day. The massage therapist needs to ask the client to assess her own symptoms each time she comes in for a massage therapy treatment.

Menstruation

L. To Discharge the Menses

Description—Regarded as a normal physiological process and life stage, menstruation is the cyclic discharge of the mucosal lining of the nonpregnant uterus through the vagina. This cycle is under hormonal control and normally occurs about every 28 days during the reproductive period (puberty through menopause) of the human female. It lasts approximately 5 days.

Massage Consideration/s—When a female client is menstruating, she may feel physically and emotionally uncomfortable. Because she will be wearing some kind of feminine protection (e.g., pads or tampons), it is not uncommon for undergarments to be left on. Should any breakthrough bleeding occur while she is on the massage table, the massage therapist needs to wash the linens separately in hot water with detergent and a quarter cup of chlorine bleach after the massage, and dry them using hot air. Massage tables and related equipment should then be wiped down with a solution of 1 part chlorine bleach to 10 parts water.

Abdominal work is contraindicated, particularly if the client is having cramps. A moist hot pack placed on the abdomen when the client is supine or placed on the low back while she is prone can help soothe the achy feeling associated with menses. She may need relief from low back pain. Deep gliding, kneading, deep friction, and ischemic compression on trigger points on the quadratus lumborum, the paraspinals, latissimus dorsi, and possibly the gluteals may be helpful. The massage therapist needs to communicate with the client about the pressure of massage and effectiveness of techniques.

Ovarian Cysts

Gr. Bladder, Sac

Description—Ovarian cysts are saclike structures filled with fluid or semisolid material. Most cysts are benign, but they can be painful (Figure 11-22).

Massage Consideration/s—Massage can be performed on clients with ovarian cysts. The massage therapist needs to ask the client if she is feeling pain from the cysts. If so, abdominal massage should be avoided, as the pressure of massage could make the pain worse. If the client is experiencing abdominal pain, she may need to be propped with a pillow under her abdomen while she is prone or, if the client cannot lie prone comfortably, the side-lying position may need to be used.

Pelvic Inflammatory Disease (PID)

L. Basin; L. To Flame Within; Fr. From; Ease

Description—Caused primarily by a bacterial infection, PID is an inflammatory condition of the female pelvic organs. It is characterized by fever, foul-smelling vaginal discharge, irregular vaginal bleeding, pain in the lower abdomen, and painful intercourse (Figure 11-23). A mass may be palpated in the lower abdomen if there are abscesses. Severe or recurrent PID may result in infertility. PID can also be a secondary complication to a sexually transmitted disease.

Massage Consideration/s—Because PID involves infection and fever, massage is contraindicated until the client is fully recovered. If the client is dealing with issues of infertility, the massage therapist can ask her if she would like a referral to a mental health counselor.

Preeclampsia (Toxemia, Pregnancy-Induced Hypertension, PIH)

L. Before; Gr. Out; To Flash

Description—Preeclampsia is a serious complication of pregnancy characterized by hypertension, protein in the urine, and edema. Occurring in about 5% to 7% of pregnancies, it typically does not develop until after 24 weeks of ges-

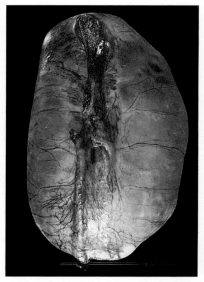

Figure 11-22. Ovarian cyst.

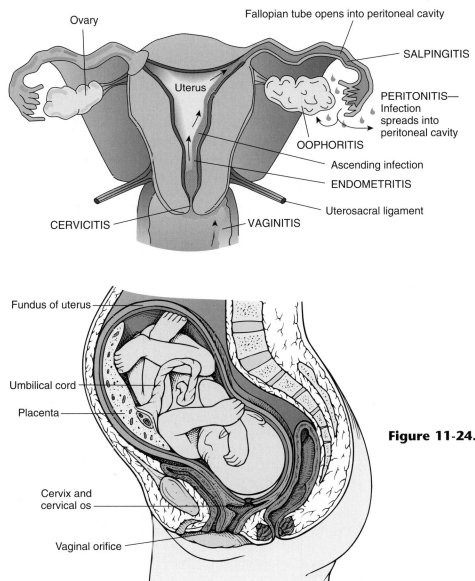

Ovary
Fallopian tube opens into peritoneal cavity
Uterus
SALPINGITIS
PERITONITIS—
Infection
spreads into
peritoneal cavity
OOPHORITIS
Ascending infection
ENDOMETRITIS
Uterosacral ligament
CERVICITIS
VAGINITIS

Figure 11-23. Pelvic inflammatory disease, causing inflammation of the fallopian tubes, the peritoneum, the ovaries, the endometrium, the cervix, and the vagina.

Fundus of uterus
Umbilical cord
Placenta
Cervix and cervical os
Vaginal orifice

Figure 11-24. Normal uterine pregnancy.

tation. The occurrence of this condition increases with advanced maternal age and when the mother carries multiple babies. Complications include premature separation of the placenta, pulmonary edema, fetal malnutrition, and low fetal birth weight. The most serious complication is maternal and fetal death. If it cannot be controlled with medication and rest, delivery by induction of labor or cesarean section may be required.

Massage Consideration/s—The accompanying hypertension, as it is difficult to control, makes preeclampsia contraindicated for massage unless it is performed under strict supervision of the client's health care provider. Avoid massage strokes that target the flow of lymphatic fluids, as they also encourage fluid to move into the blood, increase

blood volume, and tax an already stressed heart and kidneys.

Pregnancy

L. Pregnant

Description—Regarded as a life stage and not pathology, the gestational process, or pregnancy, is the growth of a developing embryo or fetus after union of an ovum and spermatozoon. Pregnancy is marked by cessation of the menses. Other symptoms are nausea (morning sickness), enlarging and tender breasts, hyperpigmentation of the nipples, and progressive enlargement of the abdomen (Figure 11-24). Other symptoms may include increased heart rate, increased blood volume, a decrease in the number of red blood cells and subsequent anemia (caused by dilution from the increased blood volume), increased respiration, increased urination, heartburn, constipation, increased perspiration, and telangiectasia.

An abnormal condition, ectopic, or extrauterine pregnancy, is the implantation of a fertilized ovum outside the uterine cavity. These pregnancies either end with spontaneous abortion or need to be surgically removed. Types of ectopic pregnancies are tubal (Figure 11-25), ovarian, and abdominal.

Massage Consideration/s—During the premassage interview, the massage therapist needs to inquire about the female client's current, as well as past pregnancies, breast soreness, and nausea. If there is a history of spontaneous abortion (miscarriage), massage is contraindicated in the first trimester because everything, including massage, is suspect should she miscarry. If the pregnant client reports that she is healthy with no past complications, then massage can be performed. In the first trimester, the client's position on the table is not a concern unless she is uncomfortable lying in a specific position. Deep abdominal massage should be avoided during the entire pregnancy and for 3 months after childbirth because the pressure of massage may damage the uterus. If the client has breast soreness or is nursing, the massage therapist needs to make modifications to her position while prone or, if the client cannot lie prone comfortably, the side-lying position may need to be used. Box 11-2 has more positional suggestions. If the pregnant client is experiencing nausea, rocking should be reduced or omitted from the massage treatment.

Because of intraabdominal pressure exerted during low back massage, and the added strain on the supporting ligaments and muscles when in a face-down position, prone positioning is contraindicated after the eighteenth week of pregnancy. This is not a client preference; it is up to the therapist to provide a safe and knowledgeable pregnancy massage.

Expectant mothers in their second and third trimesters should receive a massage in a modified supine (semi-reclining) and side-lying positions (Figure 11-26). In the modified supine position, the client's upper body is elevated about 30 degrees. Because of the pressure exerted on the abdominal blood vessels by the growing fetus, massage is contraindicated in the full supine position. The massage therapist should ask the client on which side she feels more comfortable lying and allow her to spend most of the time during the session lying on that particular side.

Because of the decreased clot-dissolving property of the blood during pregnancy, the client is at a higher risk for blood clots. Only gentle pressure in the medial thigh region should be used, with open, flat-hand techniques. Pregnant women tend to urinate frequently because of the growing fetus pressing on the urinary bladder. The massage therapist can suggest to the pregnant client that she visit the restroom before getting on the massage table. Most pregnant women are also sensitive to stuffy rooms and high temperatures. The use of heating blankets and hot packs should be avoided. The client may be more comfortable if there is a fan blowing in a corner of the room during the massage. If the client has swollen ankles, her knees and feet can be elevated using a bolster and pillows while she is in the modified supine position. The feet need to be placed higher than the knees to facilitate lymphatic flow.

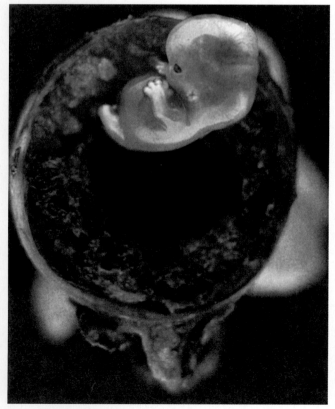
Figure 11-25. Tubal ectopic pregnancy.

Premenstrual Syndrome (PMS)

Gr. Before; Month; Together; Course

Description—PMS is a syndrome of nervous tension, irritability, weight gain, edema, headache, and lack of coordination that

Box **11-2**

Working with Clients Who Have Large or Tender Breasts

When massaging a woman with large or tender breasts or breast implants, there are several options available to make her more comfortable while she is lying prone. A rolled-up towel or cylindrical pillow can be placed under, above, or between her breasts, whichever is most comfortable. Many clients prefer a supportive device both above *and* below the breasts. A face rest that can be adjusted to above the level of the table can be used if the client is elevated due to propping. Several commercial bolsters provide support. Additionally, several massage table manufacturers now carry tables fitted with breast recesses that allow the client to lie prone more comfortably. This table option includes two small, round cushions that can be inserted to fill the breast recess spaces when not in use.

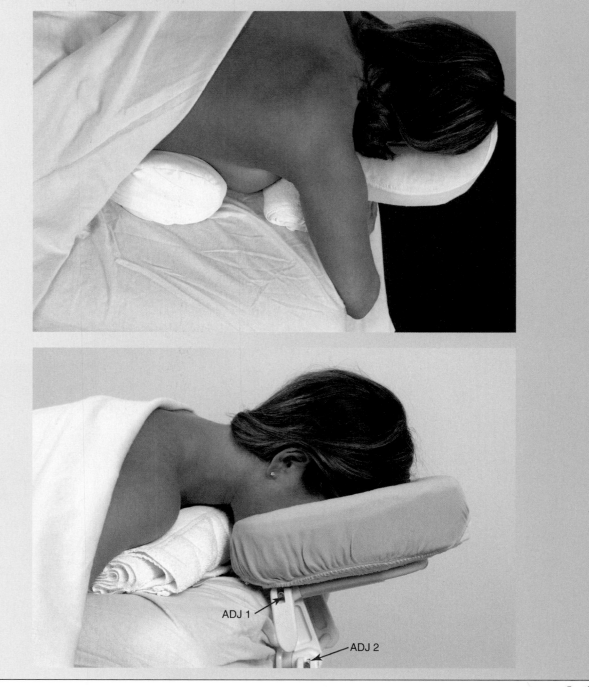

Continued

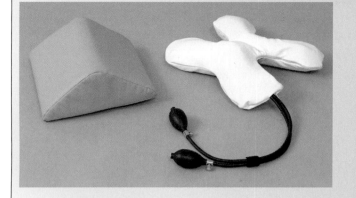

In the supine position, it is sometimes difficult to access muscles in the chest and back from the axillary region of full-figured women. If massage is needed in the pectoral region, the serratus anterior, or in the walls of the axilla, the massage therapist may ask the client to use the back side of her hand to cup the breast tissue and retract it medially. This technique establishes a safe physical boundary between client and therapist. This area may also be worked in a side-lying position with the client holding above the elbow with her bottom hand. These modifications are also useful to a postdelivery mother and a nursing mother.

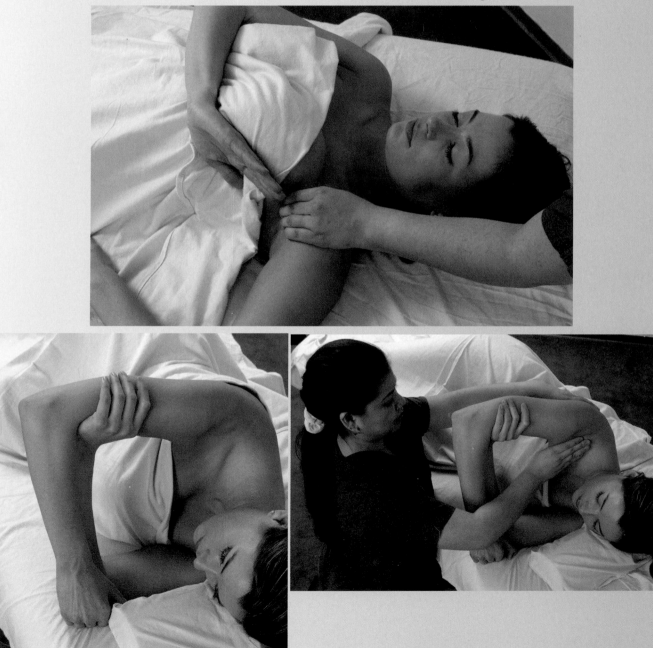

Adapted from Salvo S: Massage therapy: principles and practice, *ed 2, Philadelphia, 2003, WB Saunders.*

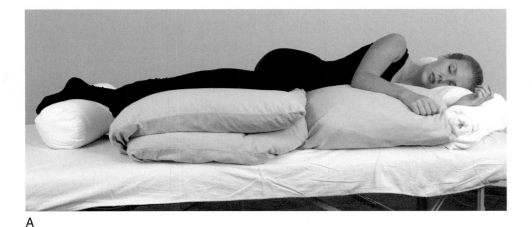

A

B

Figure 11-26. Side-lying position. **A,** Placement of supportive devices. **B,** Overhead view.

occurs a few days before the onset of menstruation. Causes range from stress and emotional disturbance to hormonal imbalance and nutritional deficiency. The following is recommended to reduce or eliminate PMS: (1) reducing caffeine and sugar intake, (2) reducing stress, and (3) receiving massage.

Massage Consideration/s—Massage can be performed on clients with premenstrual syndrome. The massage therapist needs to ask the client if she is experiencing abdominal discomfort. If so, the client may need to be propped with a pillow under her abdomen while prone or, if the client cannot lie prone comfortably, the side-lying position may need to be used. Abdominal massage is contraindicated if the pressure of massage causes pain. A gentle, relaxing massage may help the client relax.

Prostatitis (prah·stuh·tai´·tis)

Gr. Prostate; Inflammation

Description—Inflammation of the prostate, or prostatitis, is usually the result of an infection, and may be chronic or acute. The client with prostatitis usually complains of frequency and urgency of urination, and burning on urination.

Massage Consideration/s—A gentle, nurturing massage can help the client relax. The massage therapist needs to ask the client if his abdomen is tender. If so, abdominal massage is contraindicated. The client may also need to be propped with a pillow under the abdomen while he is prone or, if the client cannot lie prone comfortably, the side-lying position may need to be used.

Syphilis

L. Shepherd Having The Disease In A Latin Poem of Fracastorius (1530); Literally means "lover of swine"

Description—Syphilis is a subacute to chronic infectious disease mainly (Figure 11-27) transmitted by sexual contact but that can be contracted by direct contact with infected tissues and blood or contaminated fomites (see Box 11-1). The spirochetes are able to pass through the human placenta, producing congenital syphilis in infants. Untreated, syphilis is seen in three distinct stages of effects over a period of years (Figures 11-28 and 11-29): primary formation of primary lesions (chancre); secondary skin eruptions and infectious patches on or near mucous membranes; tertiary development of generalized lesions (gummas); and destruction of tissues resulting in aneurysm, heart disease, and degenerative changes in nervous tissue.

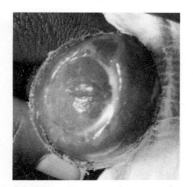

Figure 11-27. Primary lesion of syphilis.

Massage Consideration/s—Massage is contraindicated until the client has fully recovered. Syphilis is a systemic infection. Massage would exacerbate the symptoms and make the client feel worse.

Trichomoniasis (tri`·kuh·muh·nai´·uh·sis)

Gr. Hair; Unit; Condition

Description—Trichomoniasis is a sexually transmitted disease that manifests itself as a urogenital infection of the parasitic flagellated protozoa, *Trichomonas vaginalis* (Figure 11-30). In women, it is characterized by a frothy, pale yellow

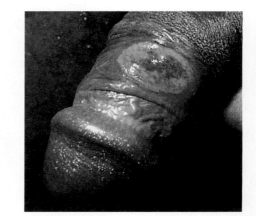

Figure 11-28. Primary skin lesions of syphilis (chancre).

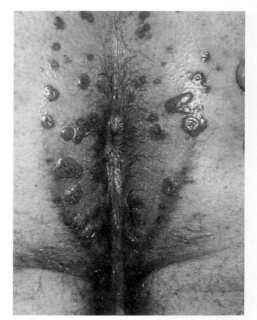

Figure 11-29. Secondary lesion of syphilis.

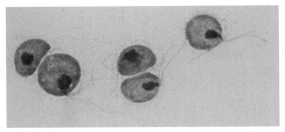

Figure 11-30. *Trichomoniasis vaginalis.*

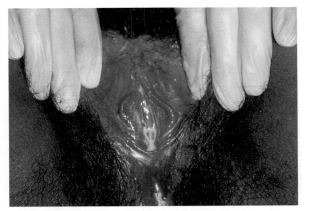

Figure 11-31. Trichomoniasis in female.

to green, odorous vaginal discharge (Figure 11-31), with local itching and redness (see Box 11-1). If the infection is chronic, symptoms may disappear even though the parasite is still present. Men infected with trichomoniasis are usually asymptomatic, but they may experience persistent or recurrent urethritis. The parasite can be transmitted to a newborn during birth. If sexual partners are not treated simultaneously, reinfection is common.

Massage Consideration/s—Massage is contraindicated until the client has fully recovered. Trichomoniasis is a systemic infection.

Vaginal Candidiasis (Candidiasis Vaginitis)

(va´·ji·nuhl kan`·duh·dai´·uh·sis)

(kan`·duh·dai´·uh·sis va`·ji·nai´·tis)

L. Sheath; White; Gr. Condition

Description—Vaginal candidiasis is a vaginal infection caused by the fungus *Candida*, usually *C. albicans*. A thick creamy vaginal discharge, local itching, and redness characterize it.

Massage Consideration/s—Massage can be performed on a client with vaginal candidiasis. If the candidiasis develops into *acute systemic candidiasis*, however, massage is contraindicated because it is a systemic infection.

SUMMARY

Because humans reproduce sexually, reproductive pathologies may be categorized as either a gender-specific disorder or a sexually transmitted disease that may be common to either sex. Some pathologies may initially infect the reproductive organs and then spread systemically throughout the entire body.

In the male, the reproductive organs include the prostate, testicles, and penis. An example of a male-specific pathology is prostatitis.

The reproductive organs of the female include the vagina, uterus, ovaries, and breasts. Female-specific disorders include amenorrhea, dysmenorrhea, ovarian cysts, endometriosis, fibrocystic breast disease, fibroid tumors, mastitis, vaginal candidiasis, premenstrual syndrome, pelvic inflammatory disease, and preeclampsia. There are other female-specific conditions that, although not considered diseases, do require special considerations for massage. These are menstruation, pregnancy, miscarriage, abortion, and menopause.

Sexually transmitted diseases that are common to either gender include chlamydia, genital herpes, genital warts, syphilis, trichomoniasis, and gonorrhea.

Reproductive pathologies may be suspected when the client reports symptoms of any of the following: fever accompanied by groin pain, palpable masses in the breast, palpable masses in the abdominopelvic region, unexplained skin lesions, genital discharge, and breast discharge (unless the client is a lactating woman). If not already diagnosed, the massage therapist needs to refer the client to the client's health care provider immediately when these symptoms are present.

Resources

American College of Obstetricians and Gynecologists

409 12th Street SW

PO Box 96920

Washington, DC 20090-6920

800-673-8444

American Society for Reproductive Medicine

1209 Montgomery Highway

Birmingham, AL 35216-2809

205-978-5000

asrm@asrm.org

American Venereal Disease Foundation
Box 385
University of Virginia
Charlottesville, VA 22908

Endometriosis Association
8585 North 76th Place
Milwaukee, WI 53223
800-992-3636

North American Menopause Society
PO Box 94527
Cleveland, OH 44101
216-844-8748
info@menopause.org

Planned Parenthood Federation of America
810 7th Avenue
New York, NY 10019
212-541-7870

Sex Information and Education Council of the US
130 West 42nd Street, Suite 2500
New York, NY 10036
212-819-9770

SELF-TEST

List the letter of the answer to the term or phrase that best describes it.

A. Amenorrhea
B. Benign prostatic hypertrophy
C. Chlamydia
D. Dysmenorrhea
E. Endometriosis
F. Fibrocystic breast disease
G. Genital herpes
H. Gonorrhea
I. Mastitis
J. Menopause
K. Menstruation
L. Pelvic inflammatory disease
M. Preeclampsia
N. Pregnancy
O. Premenstrual syndrome
P. Prostatitis
Q. Trichomoniasis
R. Vaginal candidiasis

_____ 1. An STD caused by the microorganism *Chlamydia*; a frequent cause of sterility.

_____ 2. Inflammation of the mammary gland (breast); usually caused by a streptococcal or staphylococcal infection.

_____ 3. Caused primarily by a bacterial infection, this disease is an inflammatory condition of female pelvic organs.

_____ 4. The gestational process marked by the growth of a developing embryo or fetus after union of an ovum and spermatozoon.

_____ 5. The cyclic discharge of the mucosal lining of the nonpregnant uterus through the vagina; normally occurs about every 28 days during the reproductive period (puberty through menopause) of the human female.

_____ 6. An STD that manifests itself as a urogenital infection of the parasitic flagellated protozoa, *Trichomonas vaginalis*.

_____ 7. A common STD often affecting the urogenital tract and, occasionally, the pharynx, eyes, and rectum; caused by the organism *Neisseria gonorrhoeae*.

_____ 8. A gynecological condition characterized by painful cramping before and during menstruation; it is caused by the growth of the lining of the uterus (endometrial tissue) that grows outside the uterus.

_____ 9. A chronic infection caused by type 2 herpes simplex virus.

_____ 10. Inflammation of the prostate.

_____ 11. A serious complication of pregnancy characterized by hypertension, protein in the urine, and edema.

_____ 12. The abnormal absence of menses caused by dysfunction of the hypothalamus, pituitary gland, ovaries, uterus, or certain medications.

_____ 13. A vaginal infection caused by the fungus *Candida*.

_____ 14. Painful menstruation.

_____ 15. A breast disease consisting of the presence of single or multiple cysts that are palpable; these cysts can increase or decrease in size with the woman's menstrual cycle.

_____ 16. The cessation of ovarian hormone function and menstruation in the human female; refers to the period leading up to the end of menstruation as well as the cessation of menstruation.

_____ 17. Enlargement of the prostate gland.

_____ 18. A syndrome of nervous tension, irritability, weight gain, edema, headache, and lack of coordination that occurs a few days before the onset of menstruation.

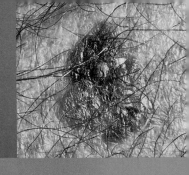

12 Cancer and Neoplasia

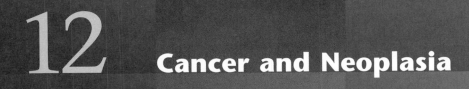

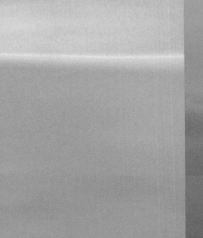

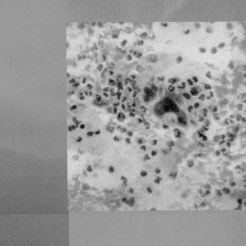

People living with cancer can benefit greatly from receiving massage. The American Cancer Society advocates massage to comfort and help improve the quality of life for cancer patients, although not to specifically treat cancer. Cancer may be a reason to begin, continue, or increase the frequency of massage treatments. Because there is an enormous amount of stress involved in dealing with a life-threatening disease, massage can play a vital role in stress reduction. This is true not only for the cancer patient but for family members and caregivers of the patient as well.

Cancer treatments, which include surgery, radiation therapy, chemotherapy, and bone marrow transplants, are enormously taxing to the body. Some of the side effects of these treatments, such as hair loss, loss of organs or limbs, or skin changes such as redness or burning from radiation, can result in anxiety, anger, depression, and negative body image for the cancer patient. A knowledgeable, skilled massage therapist can play a major role in integrating client body, mind, and spirit; reducing muscle tension; and decreasing pain by administering client-centered treatments. Besides the benefits of relaxation, improved sleep, and pain reduction, massage also bolsters immune function, reduces or prevents edema, decreases nausea and vomiting, reduces the fatigue that affects most cancer patients, and may improve the quality and survival of skin during radiation therapy. Massage can provide a relief from the pain and discomfort of medical treatments and is a human-to-human contact that is relaxing, pleasurable, and noninvasive. See Appendix B for more information about the benefits of massage with cancer patients.

In the past, cancer was automatically considered a contraindication for massage. This prevented many people living with cancer from receiving treatments that could have been beneficial for them. The prevailing thought process was that massage increased general circulation and, therefore, increased the chance of spreading the cancer throughout the client's body; however, no medical evidence supports this theory. Currently, an awareness of how to work on clients with cancer is growing within the massage community. Books and magazine articles are being published on the subject. Workshops to increase massage therapists' knowledge and skills are being offered. Because cancer and its treatments do affect the entire body and can leave the person in a fragile condition, it is important for the massage therapist to be as educated as possible. Special training in massage clients living with cancer is an avenue for massage therapists to explore.

CANCER—A PRIMER

Cancer is characterized by the uncontrollable growth of abnormal cells that form a neoplasm or tumor. The study of tumors is called oncology. The tumors can be either cancerous or harmless. A cancerous tumor is called malignant and will often metastasize or spread cancerous cells to other parts of the body (Figure 12-1). A benign tumor does not metastasize, but may become life threatening if, as it grows, it puts pressure on vital areas, such as within the brain (Figure 12-2 and Table 12-1). There are many types of cancers, and they are named for the type of tissue from which they are derived. Carcinomas arise from epithelial tissue. Melanomas grow from melanocytes—skin cells that produce the pigment melanin. Sarcomas develop from muscle cells or connective tissue. Leukemia is characterized by rapid growth of abnormal white blood cells. Lymphoma is a cancer of lymphatic tissue.

Cancerous cells can spread throughout the body via one of two routes, the bloodstream or the lymphatic system. If the cancer is metastasizing through the lymphatic system, there is a predictable pathway the cancer cells can follow based on the structure of the lymphatic vessels, and the one-way flow of lymph (see Chapter 7). Lymph nodes will often be removed and checked to see if cancerous cells have migrated to them. If the cancer is spreading through the bloodstream, however, there is no predictable pathway for them to follow, and the cancer could spread anywhere.

The most common types of cancers are lung, breast, colon, and prostate. Massage therapists and their clients need to be aware that some cancers are potentially preventable or curable if proper screening measures are followed. Such cancers include skin, oral, prostate, colon, and cervical.

The incidence of different kinds of cancer varies greatly with age, ethnicity, gender, and geographic location (Figure 12-3). For example, age-related death rate for oral cancer is almost ten times higher in Hong Kong than in Denmark. Prostate cancer is more than ten times greater in Sweden than in Japan. Additionally, prostate cancer is more common and is more aggressive in African-Americans than in Caucasians. Colon cancer is very rare in Japan, but when Japanese move to the United States, their risk of colon cancer increases. This implies that the Western diet and environment

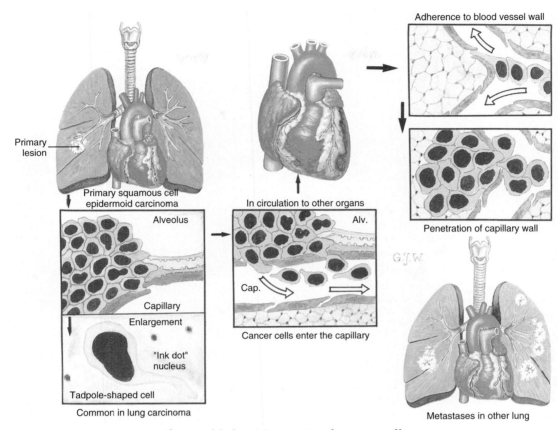

Figure 12-1.   Metastasis of cancer cells.

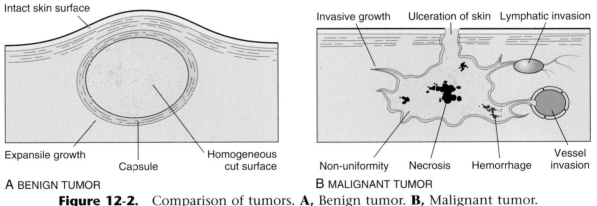

A BENIGN TUMOR

B MALIGNANT TUMOR

Figure 12-2.   Comparison of tumors. **A,** Benign tumor. **B,** Malignant tumor.

are risk factors for colon cancer. The occurrence of leukemia, however, is similar throughout the world. In the United States, cancer is second only to heart disease as a cause of mortality.

CAUSES OF CANCER

The definite cause of cancer is undetermined, but many potential causes are recognized including *carcinogens, oncogenes,* and *oncoviruses.* More than

80% of cancer cases are attributed to exposure to carcinogens, or cancer-causing agents (Figures 12-4 and 12-5). They cause permanent structural changes in the genetic material of the cell. Examples of carcinogens include cigarette tar, radon gas, and ultraviolet radiation in sunlight. Oncogenes are cancer-causing genes. When these genes are inappropriately activated, they transform a normal cell into a cancerous cell. It is unclear how oncogenes become activated. Oncoviruses cause cancer by

---

Table **12-1**   COMPARISON OF BENIGN AND MALIGNANT TUMORS

FEATURE	BENIGN	MALIGNANT
Growth	Slow and expansive	Slow and expansive or fast, invasive, and destructive
Metastases	No	Yes
Gross Appearance		
External surface	Smooth	Irregular
Capsule	Yes and no	No
Necrosis	Yes and no	Yes
Hemorrhage	Yes and no	Yes
Microscopic Appearance		
Architecture	Resembles that of tissue of origin	Does not resemble that of tissue of origin
Cells	Well differentiated	Poorly differentiated
Nuclei	Normal shape and size	Polymorphic
Cell division (mitoses)	Few	Many irregular

Modified from Damjanov I: Pathology for the health-related professions, *ed 2, Philadelphia, 2000, WB Saunders.*

stimulating cells to divide abnormally. These viruses, such as human immunodeficiency virus (HIV), the Epstein-Barr virus (EBV), human papillomavirus (HPV), and hepatitis virus B and C (HBV/HCV), have been linked to malignant cancers. There is also a high rate of malignant tumors in organ transplant recipients after receiving immunosuppressive therapy, indicating that the immune system plays a major role in controlling the proliferation of cancer (Boxes 12-1 and 12-2). Cancer is not contagious, but it can spread internally (Box 12-3). More information is found in the section Cancerous Diseases in Chapter 1.

CURRENT TREATMENTS FOR CANCER AND THEIR IMPLICATIONS FOR THE MASSAGE THERAPIST

Cancer is treated in one of three main ways: surgery, chemotherapy, or radiation therapy. Additionally, bone marrow transplants are sometimes performed. A cancer patient may receive one or a combination of these treatment methods.

Surgery

Surgical excision is commonly used to remove the tumors or cancerous organs, and often neighboring lymph nodes. The removed lymph nodes are examined to see whether cancerous cells have spread to them.

Massage therapists need to be concerned about several surgical risks. One is clot formation. Because surgery involves cutting into the body, blood clots form as part of the healing process. If the clot is dislodged, it can circulate to the brain and cause a stroke, to the heart and cause a heart attack, or to the lungs and become a pulmonary embolism, all of which are life threatening. Therefore massage around the recent incision site is contraindicated. Blood clots can also form in the lower extremities as a result of blood stasis (stagnation). Blood stasis can occur because of inactivity and bed rest, both common after a surgical procedure. Massage on the legs is contraindicated until the client is no longer at risk for blood clot formation. The massage therapist needs to consult with the client's health care provider to find out when massage can be safely administered around the incision site and on the lower extremities.

Another risk after surgery is infection. The signs and symptoms of infection are fever and redness, pain, heat, and swelling at the infection site. If it occurs, it is usually within a few days of the surgery. If there is infection, massage is contraindicated because it can exacerbate the symptoms and make the client feel worse.

Edema is another common concern after surgery, especially if lymph nodes have been removed. The edema usually occurs in limbs distal to the removed nodes. The edema is not necessarily predictable; it may come and go depending on the client's activi-

Ten Leading Cancer Sites for the Estimated New Cancer Cases and Deaths by Gender, US, 2003*

Estimated New Cases

MEN				WOMEN
Prostate	33%	32%	Breast	
Lung and Bronchus	14%	12%	Lung and Bronchus	
Colon and Rectum	11%	11%	Colon and Rectum	
Urinary Bladder	6%	6%	Uterine Corpus	
Melanoma of the Skin	4%	4%	Non-Hodgkin's Lymphoma	
Non-Hodgkin's Lymphoma	4%	3%	Melanoma of the Skin	
Kidney	3%	4%	Ovary	
Oral Cavity	3%	2%	Pancreas	
Leukemia	3%	3%	Thyroid	
Pancreas	2%	2%	Urinary Bladder	
All Other Sites	**17%**	**20%**	**All Other Sites**	

Estimated Deaths

MEN				WOMEN
Lung and Bronchus	31%	25%	Lung and Bronchus	
Prostate	10%	15%	Breast	
Colon and Rectum	10%	11%	Colon and Rectum	
Pancreas	5%	6%	Pancreas	
Non-Hodgkin's Lymphoma	4%	5%	Ovary	
Leukemia	4%	4%	Non-Hodgkin's Lymphoma	
Esophagus	4%	4%	Leukemia	
Liver	3%	3%	Uterine Corpus	
Urinary Bladder	3%	2%	Brain	
Kidney	3%	2%	Multiple Myeloma	
All Other Sites	**22%**	**23%**	**All Other Sites**	

*Excludes basal and squamous cell skin cancers and in situ carcinomas except urinary bladder.
Percentages may not total 100% due to rounding.

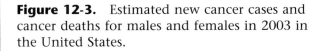

Figure 12-3. Estimated new cancer cases and cancer deaths for males and females in 2003 in the United States.

ties. For instance, if the client is sedentary, edema may increase. On the other hand, if a client starts using the limb distal to where lymph nodes have been removed, this may also increase edema. In this case, massage therapy should be performed only under supervision of the client's health care provider. Massage therapists working without this supervision may, in fact, cause an episode of edema through usual massage techniques. The massage therapist needs to work in concert with the client's physical or occupational therapist, or trained lymphatic drainage practitioner using only specific techniques. These include elevating the affected limb. The strokes should be performed lightly and toward the heart, starting proximally and working distally to clear lymph in the proximal area before moving lymph in from the distal area of the limb.

The limb should be bandaged after treatment to provide compression that would help reduce or eliminate edema.

Another risk of surgery massage therapists need to be concerned about is reduced function in the area of the incision because of pain, inflammation, scarring, and any prostheses or medical apparatus the client may be using. As a result, the client can have reduced range of motion in joints, and muscle spasms. Because of the risks of infection and damaging the healing tissues, the massage therapist needs to have proper training to work on healed scar tissue to realign collagen fibers, reduce adhesion formation, and maintain as much flexibility in the area as possible. This training should also include strokes that could help loosen adhesions and increase mobility after healing from the surgery

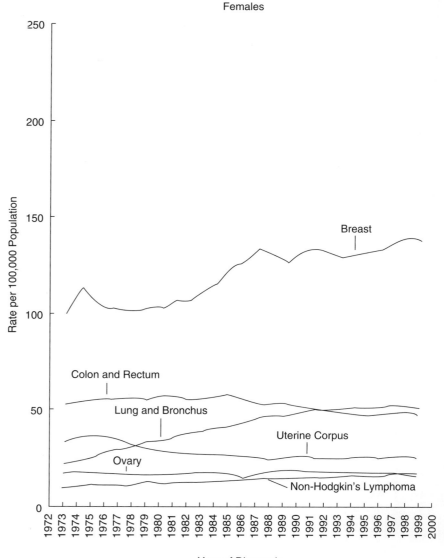

Figure 12-4. Age-adjusted cancer incidence rates for females by site, United States, 1973-1999.

is complete, such as cross-fiber friction and myofascial release techniques.

Massage therapy can be especially effective on the muscles in the area affected by the surgery. Massage can reduce or eliminate muscular spasm, decrease muscular tension, help maintain muscle strength, and increase nutrition to the muscle tissue by increasing local circulation. Helpful techniques include gliding strokes, kneading, deep friction, and ischemic compression. The massage therapist needs to communicate with the client's health care provider about specific muscles to be addressed and massage techniques to be used. Once clearance for massage has been given, the massage therapist needs to communicate with the client about the pressure and effectiveness of techniques.

Other benefits of massage therapy for clients who have had surgery include relieving anxiety the client may have before the surgery and relieving pain after surgery. When the massage therapist accepts the client's physical appearance without judgment, it may help the client who is dealing with body image issues.

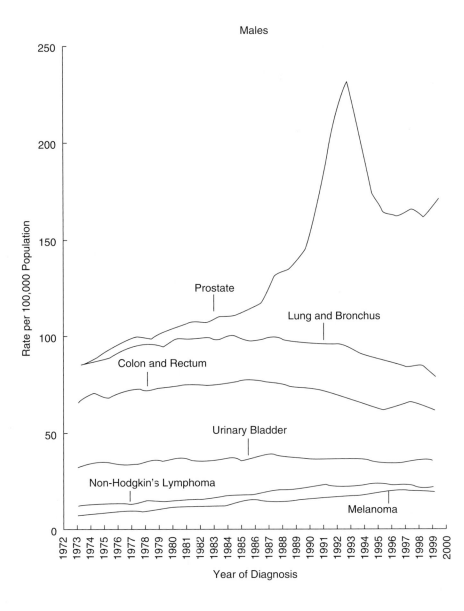

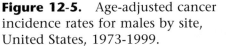

Figure 12-5. Age-adjusted cancer incidence rates for males by site, United States, 1973-1999.

Radiation Therapy

Radiation therapy uses radiation directly on tumors to decrease their size or inhibit their growth. In certain cancers, a person's entire body can be treated with radiation, or radiation can be used to prevent rejection of a transplanted tissue or organ.

The major concern for the massage therapist with a client in radiation therapy is changes that the client's skin undergoes in the radiation-treated areas. These include redness, dryness, irritation, and itching. The massage therapist needs to receive careful instruction from the client's health care provider regarding care of the client's skin, and massage must be performed within these guidelines. These areas can be thought of as being burned, as in a sunburn. A general guideline for the massage therapist is to avoid massaging the irradiated areas. Or, light pressure may be used if it is within the client's tolerance, if the health care provider approves. The health care provider must also approve the lubricant used, as certain coatings on the skin can alter the effects of the radiation beams.

Other risks of radiation therapy include fatigue, edema, nausea, and vomiting. Fatigue can espe-

Box 12-1

Seven Warning Signals of Cancer or CAUTION*

Change in bowel or bladder habits
A sore that does not heal
Unusual bleeding or discharge
Thickening of lump in breast or elsewhere
Indigestion or difficulty in swallowing
Obvious change in wart or mole
Nagging cough or hoarseness

If you have a warning signal, see your physician. These guidelines are currently under revision. Please refer to the American Cancer Society for more information.
Modified from Damjanov I: Pathology for the health-related professions, *ed 2, Philadelphia, 2000, WB Saunders.*

Box 12-2

Cancer Risk Factors

Advancing age
Lifestyle or personal behaviors
    Tobacco use
    Diet and nutrition
    Alcohol use
    Sexual and reproductive behavior
Exposure to viruses
    Epstein-Barr virus (EBV)
    Hepatitis B virus (HBV)
    Hepatitis C virus (HCV)
    Helicobacter pylori
    Herpesvirus 8
    Human immunodeficiency virus (HIV)
    Human papillomavirus (HPV)
Geographic location and environmental
    variables
Gender
Ethnicity
Socioeconomic status
Occupation
Heredity
Presence of precancerous lesions
Stress

Modified from Goodman CC, Boissonnault WG, Fuller KS: Pathology: implications for the physical therapist, *ed 2, Philadelphia, 2003, WB Saunders.*

Box 12-3

Seven Safeguards Against Cancer

Breast: Regular monthly self-examination of breast for lumps, nodules, or changes in contour; yearly check by physician
Cervix: Pap test for all adult and high-risk adolescent women
Colon-rectum: Rectal examinations and colonoscopy as routine part of annual check-ups for those over 40 years old; proctosigmoidoscopy or barium enema colon radiographs at age 50 years and every 3 to 5 years thereafter
Lung: Reduction and ultimate elimination of cigarette smoking; avoidance of smoke-filled environments
Oral: Wider practice of early detection measures; regular dental examinations
Skin: Avoidance of excessive exposure to sun or tanning lights
Basic: Routine periodic physical examination for all adults

Modified from Damjanov I: Pathology for the health-related professions, *ed 2, Philadelphia, 2000, WB Saunders.*

cially occur if a large area of the body is irradiated. The General Guidelines section in this chapter has more information on how to recognize and address fatigue in clients with cancer.

Edema is a risk that can occur if lymph nodes are damaged by radiation. As with surgery, the massage therapy needs to work with the client's health care provider on how to address the edema in the affected area. Nausea and vomiting usually occur with upper abdominal radiation, or irradiation of the entire body. If the client is nauseated or vomiting as a result of radiation therapy, massage therapy may be contraindicated. If the client does feel up to receiving massage, it can be beneficial in helping to reduce the nausea through relaxation. Gentle pressure should be used in this circumstance. Joint mobilizations, stretches, jostling, or even moving client limbs are contraindicated because all of these can increase nausea (Table 12-2).

Chemotherapy

Chemotherapy is the introduction of strong chemicals into the body. These chemicals target rapidly dividing cells, such as those found in cancers. However, the chemicals will also work against other fast-growing cells in the body, such as blood cells, cells lining the digestive tract, and hair. Therefore the side effects of chemotherapy can be systemic and debilitating.

Chemotherapy can reduce the number of functioning blood cells. If white blood cells decrease, the person will be more susceptible to infection. The

Table **12-2   SIDE EFFECTS OF THE THREE MOST COMMON CANCER TREATMENTS**

SURGERY	RADIATION THERAPY	CHEMOTHERAPY
Bleeding	Burns—skin redness	Anemia
Blood clots	Decreased platelets	Constipation
Deformity	Decreased white blood cells	Decreased bone density (with ovarian failure)
Disfigurement	Decreased red blood cells	Decreased platelets
Fatigue	Delayed wound healing	Decreased white blood cells
Fibrosis	Diarrhea	Diarrhea
Increased pain	Fatigue	Dizziness when standing
Infection	Fibrosis	Fatigue
Loss of function	Fragility of blood vessels	Fever
Lymphedema	Headaches	Fragility of blood vessels
Scar tissue	Immunosuppression	Hair loss
	Infection	Hemorrhage
	Lymphedema	Intolerance to cold
	Radiation sickness	Liver toxicity
	Skin irritation	Mouth sores
	Sterilization	Muscle weakness
	Loss of appetite and resultant weight loss	Nausea and vomiting
		Neuropathies
		Shortness of breath
		Skin rashes
		Weight loss or gain

Modified from Goodman CC, Boissonnault WG, Fuller KS: Pathology: implications for the physical therapist, ed 2, Philadelphia, 2003, WB Saunders.

massage therapist needs to communicate with the client's health care provider to find out how susceptible the client is to infection. The massage therapist should not perform massage on the client with cancer when the massage therapist is sick, or when a member of the massage therapist's household is sick, as the massage therapist could be a carrier (reservoir) of disease. If the client is receiving massage in the massage therapist's office, the treatment times need to be scheduled when few or no other clients are in the office to decrease the risk of exposure to infection.

If the client has a low platelet count, the client may bruise or bleed easily. To avoid damaging the client's tissues, do not massage using deep pressure. The massage therapist needs to communicate with the client and the client's health care provider about safe levels of pressure to be used during the massage treatment.

Anemia resulting from decreased red blood cell levels can also be a side effect of chemotherapy. Anemia can result in fatigue, dizziness when standing up, shortness of breath, and intolerance to cold. The massage therapist needs to communicate with

the client's health care provider as to the safest approaches for massaging the client. Sometimes severe anemia can cause a heart condition. The heart pumps faster to compensate for the oxygen-depleted blood. Massage may or may not be contraindicated in this case; it is up to the client's health care provider to decide. If massage is approved, the massage therapist may need to use gentler pressure so as not to overtire the client and be ready to ensure the client stays warm.

The client's skin can change during chemotherapy. It may be dry and feel "prickly"; there may be rashes. Some may look like infections but could be reactions to the medication, and/or the skin could be hypersensitive. These skin changes can change from day to day. All of these could be contraindications for local or even general massage. Any open lesions would also need to be avoided during massage. Again, the massage therapist needs to communicate with the client and the client's health care provider regarding whether massage can be performed.

Hair loss can also occur during chemotherapy. It can have a profound emotional impact on a client and affect the client's body image. It is important for the massage therapist to touch the client's body with care and accept without judgment the client's appearance, hair loss, and other physical changes as a result of the cancer and/or cancer treatments. With hair loss, the massage therapist needs to respect the client's wishes about having his or her head exposed or covered, and touched. Any lubricant used on the client's head needs to be removed so that it does not damage a hat, scarf, or hairpiece that the client may wear.

Because the digestive tract can be affected by chemotherapy, it is important to consider several factors during massage therapy. The client may have mouth sores. The massage therapist needs to ask the client if the face cradle is comfortable for the client to use. Jaw and cheek massage may be contraindicated because the pressure from massage could cause the client pain.

Nausea and vomiting are some of the most dreaded side effects of chemotherapy. Aromatherapy and scented lubricants should not be used, as they may nauseate the client. If the client is nauseated or vomiting because of chemotherapy, massage therapy may be contraindicated. If the client does feel up to receiving massage, massage can help reduce nausea by relaxing the client; however, avoid using pressure and speed that rock the client. Joint mobilizations, stretches, jostling, or even moving client limbs are contraindicated because all of these can increase nausea.

The client should be well hydrated and have enough electrolytes before receiving massage to decrease the risk of nausea and other complications. The client may also have diarrhea or constipation. In the case of diarrhea, abdominal massage is contraindicated because it could make the diarrhea worse. If a client has constipation, the abdomen may be massaged using clockwise gliding strokes to stimulate peristalsis of the large intestine. However, the massage therapist needs to obtain clearance for massage from the client's health care provider before doing this.

With certain types of chemotherapy (Cytoxan, Thioplex, Thiotepa, and Neosar), the massage therapist needs to wear gloves if the client has received the medication within 24 hours before the massage treatment. These medications can come through the client's skin and enter the massage therapist's skin if gloves are not worn. Consult with the client's health care provider if you are unsure about medications used (Table 12-3).

The client may also have extreme weight loss from chemotherapy or from the cancer itself. Weight loss can decrease the client's stamina. The massage therapist needs to adjust the massage treatment so as not to overtire the client or put undo pressure on areas of the body that do not have a lot of tissue. Adjustments include a shorter massage with gentle, but firm pressure, and propping for comfort under bony projections. The client may need to be repositioned often if he or she becomes easily sore in one position.

Another common side effect of chemotherapy is peripheral neuropathy. Symptoms include pain, tingling, or burning sensations, or numbness in the extremities. Because symptoms of neuropathy vary from day to day, the massage therapist needs to ask the client about the quality and extent of symptoms before each massage treatment. Deep pressure is contraindicated for neuropathy because the client cannot give accurate feedback about pressure. Gentle, but firm broad strokes may be performed, as long as they are done within the client's tolerance.

Fever may be present in a client undergoing chemotherapy. If the client has a fever, massage is contraindicated because it will exacerbate the symptoms and make the client feel worse.

Muscle tension is also common in clients because they may take naps in uncomfortable positions in waiting rooms or while receiving treatment. The considerations are the same as those for surgery. Massage can reduce or eliminate muscular spasm, decrease muscular tension, help maintain muscle strength, and increase nutrition to the muscle tissue by increasing local circulation. Helpful techniques include gliding strokes, kneading, deep friction, and ischemic compression. The massage therapist needs to communicate with the client's health care provider about specific muscles to be addressed and massage techniques to be used. Once clearance for massage has been given, the massage therapist needs to communicate with the client about the pressure and effectiveness of techniques.

Central venous catheters are often used to administer chemotherapy. This eliminates the need for repeated needle sticks. Avoid the area around the catheter and avoid tractioning the tissues near the catheter site. Chapter 7 has more information on central venous catheters.

Bone Marrow Transplant

A bone marrow transplant is one of the most taxing treatments a person can undergo. The cancer patient's defective bone marrow is first destroyed by chemotherapy and whole body radiation. Then red bone marrow from a healthy donor is transferred intravenously into the patient. The donor

Table **12-3 MEDICATIONS USED TO MANAGE CANCER**

MEDICATION CLASSIFICATION	MEDICATION NAME	POSSIBLE SIDE EFFECTS THAT MAY AFFECT TREATMENT
Alkylating drugs	Busulfan (Myleran), chlorambucil (Leukeran), cyclophosphamide (Cytoxan, Neosar), dacarbazine (DTIC–Dome), mechlorethamine (Mustargen, nitrogen mustard)	Convulsions, diarrhea, hair loss, nausea and vomiting, skin rashes
Antimetabolites	Cytarabine (Cytosar-U), floxuridine (FUDR), fludarabine (Fludara), fluorouracil (Adrucil), methotrexate (Folex, Mexate), Cytoxan,* Thioplex,* Thiotepa,* Neosar*	Abdominal pain, chills, convulsions, disorientation, fever, gastrointestinal irritation, hair loss, headaches, hyperpigmentation, hypertension, lethargy, nausea, skin rashes
Antinausea (antiemetic)	Chlorpromazine (Thorazine), dexamethasone (Decadron), dimenhydrinate (Dramamine), droperidol (Inapsine), granisetron (Kytril), haloperidol (Haldol), hydroxyzine (Atarax, Vistaril), meclizine (Antivert, Bonine), metoclopramide (Reglan), ondansetron (Zofran), perphenazine (Trilafon), prochlorperazine (Compazine), scopolamine (Trans-Derm Scop), thiethylperazine (Torecan)	Abdominal pain, anxiety, chills, constipation and diarrhea, disorientation, drowsiness, dry mouth, headaches, hypotension, insomnia, lethargy, skin rashes, vertigo
Antitumor antibiotics	Actinomycin D (dactinomycin), bleomycin (Blenoxane), daunorubicin (Daunomycin, Cerubidine), Doxorubicin (Adriamycin), idarubicin (Idamycin), plicamycin (Mithracin)	Abdominal pain, chills, diarrhea, fever, hair loss, hypotension, nausea and vomiting, pneumonia, shortness of breath, skin rashes, wheezing
Hormonal agents	Antiestrogenic: anastrozole (Arimidex), tamoxifen (Nolvadex), toremifene (Fareston), Antiandrogenic: bicalutamide (Casodex), flutamide (Euflex, Eulexin), nilutamide (Nilandron)	Chest pains, diarrhea, drowsiness, hair loss, headaches, hot flashes, hypotension, irregular heartbeat, lethargy, nausea and vomiting, skin rashes, vertigo
Interferons	Interferon alfa-2a (Intron A), Interferon-alpha (Veldona), Interferon beta-1b (Betaseron)	Abdominal pain, anxiety, chest pains, constipation and diarrhea, fever, hair loss, headaches, insomnia, joint pain, lethargy, nausea and vomiting, numbness, skin rashes, vertigo
Mitotic spindle drugs	Paclitaxel (Taxol), vinblastine (Velban, Velsar), vincristine (Oncovin, Vincasar), vinorelbine (Navelbine)	Abdominal pain, convulsions, diarrhea and constipation, gastrointestinal irritation, hair loss, hypotension, irregular heartbeat, joint pain, lethargy, nausea and vomiting, numbness, seizures, skin rashes

The massage therapist needs to wear gloves if the client has received the medication within 24 hours previous to the massage treatment. These medications can come through the client's skin and enter the massage therapist's skin if gloves are not worn.

marrow needs to be a close match, or tissue rejection will occur. If the bone marrow transplant is successful, stem cells from the donated marrow "reseed" and grow in the patient's red bone marrow cavities.

There are many side effects that can leave the person in a debilitated state. Immunosuppression is a major side effect. The person needs to take immunosuppressant medications to prevent rejection of the donated bone marrow, and may be required to be in protective isolation. As the person heals and recovers, he or she needs to guard diligently against infection for the rest of his or her lifetime.

Other side effects can include intensified symptoms of radiation therapy and chemotherapy such as itching, burning skin, mouth sores, severe constipation, pain, nausea, and vomiting. The massage therapist working with clients who have had bone marrow transplants needs to do in-depth research to become familiar with the challenges the client faces and then work closely with the client's health care providers to keep the client safe. Depending on the client's vitality, the massage may need to be extremely gentle and within the client's medical parameters.

If a client had a bone marrow transplant in the past and has returned to health and vigor, massage may be performed after obtaining clearance for massage from the client's health care provider. The massage therapist needs to make sure all universal precautions are in place (see Chapter 1). The massage therapist also needs to communicate with the client about the pressure and effectiveness of techniques.

THERAPEUTIC ASSESSMENT OF CLIENTS LIVING WITH CANCER

The massage therapist may find it helpful to have a premassage intake form specifically for clients living with cancer. This form will give the massage therapist information relevant to each particular client. A sample intake form is located in Box 12-4.

The following list of pertinent questions serves as a way to evaluate clients living with cancer. Findings need to be documented.

Questions to ask the client in the premassage interview:

- *What type of cancer does the client have?* The type of cancer the client has can greatly affect the choice of massage treatment. For example, avoid deep pressure over known tumor sites; avoid deep pressure or

myofascial release techniques over metastatic cancers; general massage may be too fatiguing for a client with leukemia.

- *Is the client in treatment for the cancer? If so, what type of treatment is the client undergoing?* This is important in determining massage considerations for the client. More information can be found in the section Current Treatments for Cancer in this chapter. For example, if the client is undergoing radiation treatments, lubricants should not be used on the areas to be irradiated, as substances in the lubricants can block the delivery of the radiation rays. With certain types of chemotherapy (Cytoxan, Thioplex, thiotepa, and Neosar), the massage therapist needs to wear gloves if the client has received the medication within 24 hours previous to the massage treatment. These medications can come through the client's skin and enter the massage therapist's skin if gloves are not worn.
- *Is the client receiving steroid treatment?* The client may be receiving steroids as well as chemotherapy. Long-term steroid use can lead to osteoporosis, which requires a lighter pressure during massage treatments.
- *Has the client had lymph nodes irradiated or removed? Does the client have lymphedema?* If so, more specific information regarding how to address these conditions can be found in the section Current Treatments for Cancer, Surgery, in this chapter.
- *Does the client have a history of blood clots or low platelet count?* If so, more specific information regarding how to address blood clots can be found in the section Current Treatments for Cancer, Surgery, in this chapter. If the client has a low platelet count, then he or she would be prone to bruising and bleeding. Lighter pressure for massage is indicated.
- *Does the client have a low white blood cell count or decreased immunity?* If so, the client would be much more susceptible to illness. Because the client is at high risk for becoming sick, the massage therapist should not massage the client when the massage therapist is sick. If anyone in the massage therapist's office is sick, whether it be another therapist or a client, the client living with cancer should not come to the office for massage treatment so as to reduce

Box **12-4**

Intake Form for Massaging People Living with Cancer

Client Name _____ Date _____

Address _____

Are you a cancer survivor?   Yes_____   No_____

If yes, type of cancer and location _____

Are you currently in treatment?   Yes   No   Not applicable

If yes, type of treatment currently ongoing _____

If no, when did you finish treatment? _____

What types of treatment did you receive and to what areas of your body?

_____

Please circle any of the following that may apply to you:

Fragile or sensitive skin   Scar or incision   Location _____

Low white blood cell count   Decreased immunity

Low platelet count   Easy bruising   Blood clots

Neuropathy   Decreased sensation

Lymph node treatment or removal   Lymphedema

Fatigue   Nausea   Osteoporosis

Medical device   Location _____

Arthritis   Fractures   Joint replacement

Muscle tension   Location _____

Cardiac condition   High blood pressure

Varicose veins   Diabetes   Constipation   Hearing loss

Allergy or sensitivity to oils/lotion   Yes_____   No_____

Have you ever had a therapeutic massage?   Yes_____   No_____

Do you have a preference for pressure?   Light   Moderate   Deep

(Massage therapist may advise you regarding pressure to provide safe and effective treatment in terms of current medical conditions and past medical history)

Please indicate your goals for massage therapy session today:

Relaxation   Pain Management   Stress Management   Other _____

Please provide your primary physician's name and phone number:

_____   _____
Name   Phone

Please do not hesitate to communicate your needs with your therapist at any time during treatment, and ENJOY YOUR SESSION!

_____   _____
Client signature   Phone

the possibility of the client contracting disease.

- *Does the client have any indwelling medical devices such as central venous catheters?* These devices allow chemotherapy medications to be administered to the client without repeated needle sticks. The areas of the client's body in which these devices are located are contraindicated for massage because of the risk of infection and because the pressure of massage may damage the surrounding tissues. No traction or joint mobilizations should be done to joints in the area where the devices are located so as not to damage the devices or surrounding tissues.
- *If the client is not in treatment, when did the treatment end? What types of treatment did they receive in the past?* There may be long-term effects from treatment that the massage therapist needs to consider for massage treatments. For example, chemotherapy and steroid treatment may have left the client with osteoporosis, in which case lighter pressure is indicated. There may be scar tissue and tissue sensitivity from previous surgeries that need to be avoided during massage treatments.
- *Is the client wearing a wig or other head covering because of hair loss from treatment?* If so, the massage therapist needs to ask the client if he or she wants the head covering removed for the treatment, or if the client wants the face and/or scalp massaged.

Observations to make during the premassage interview and during the massage treatment:

- *Does the client exhibit signs of fatigue?* If the client has a short attention span, labored or uneven breathing, or breathing with lots of sighs, or if the client's eyes glaze over during the premassage interview, these signs can be indicators that the client is fatigued. If so, a slow, gentle massage of shorter duration is indicated so as not to further fatigue the client. It is better to "under do" than "over do" the treatment.
- *Is the client experiencing discomfort during the treatment?* Sometimes clients living with cancer are so grateful to receive massage treatments, they may not want to "inconvenience" the therapist by telling her that certain positions and/or techniques are uncomfortable. The massage therapist needs to observe the client carefully. Is the client grimacing? Holding the breath?

Breathing rapidly? Flinching? Tightening muscles? The massage therapist needs to communicate with the client about what the client is experiencing. The massage therapist will need to adjust pressure and administration of techniques, and the client may need special propping to ensure comfort.

- *Does the client seem fatigued during the treatment? Does the client have labored or uneven breathing, or breathing with lots of sighs? Or is the client unresponsive during the treatment?* The massage treatment may be too vigorous or is lasting too long and is overtiring the client.
- *Are there signs of inflammation on the client's skin that the client has not mentioned?* If so, these areas need to be avoided and brought to the attention of the client. Inflammation in the skin over bones may be an indicator of metastasis to the bones.

GENERAL GUIDELINES FOR MASSAGE THERAPISTS WHEN WORKING WITH CANCER PATIENTS

With respect to the massage considerations delineated in the sections Surgery, Radiation Therapy, Chemotherapy, and Bone Marrow Transplant, here is a synopsis of important guidelines for massage therapists to follow:

- The massage therapist needs to obtain clearance for massage from the client's health care provider. This cannot be emphasized enough.
- The massage therapist needs to accept the client's appearance unconditionally and be respectful of what the client is going through with the cancer and medical treatments.
- The massage therapist needs to educate himself or herself thoroughly regarding the type of cancer the client has, and the treatments the client is undergoing.
- The massage therapist needs to adjust the massage to the type of cancer the client has. The massage therapist needs to know the location of the cancer. The cancer may be throughout the body as in the case of leukemia. Or, there may be primary and secondary tumor sites. Massage over the tumor sites is contraindicated because of the pain the pressure of massage may cause. Again, it is imperative for the massage therapist to communicate with the client's

health care provider to determine when administering massage would be harmful, when it would be safe, and what techniques would be helpful.

- The massage needs to be modified according to the cancer treatment the client is undergoing such as surgery, radiation therapy, chemotherapy, and/or a bone marrow transplant. More information can be obtained under these sections, which were discussed previously in this chapter.

- A major consideration is that the massage treatment needs to be adjusted to the stamina of the client. The massage therapist needs to ask the client if the medical treatments have altered the level of activity or prohibited any activities, or if the client's energy levels go through cycles based on the treatment the client is receiving, or the hours of the day. These questions can help the massage therapist and client decide on the best days and times for the massage treatment. Massage would best be performed on high-energy days and times. Massage given on low-energy days and times will deplete the client's stamina.

- The massage therapist needs to observe the client closely to determine whether the client is fatigued. If the client has a short attention span, labored or uneven breathing, or breathing with lots of sighs, or if the client's eyes glaze over during the premassage interview, the client may be fatigued. If so, a slow, gentle, but firm massage of shorter duration is indicated. A longer, deeper, more vigorous massage would overtire and further debilitate the client.

- The massage therapist needs to thoroughly document client symptoms, therapist observations, areas of the body worked, techniques used, and outcomes of techniques used. See Appendix E for abbreviations and symbols used for charting.

- The massage therapist needs to ask the client exactly what symptoms and quality of those symptoms the client is experiencing each time the client receives a massage treatment so that the massage therapist can tailor the treatment based on the client's needs.

- The massage therapist needs to be attentive about pressure, client position and comfort, and the areas to avoid. Only gentle, but firm pressure should be used, or modalities that use little or no pressure such as therapeutic

touch, polarity, Reiki, or craniosacral therapy. The massage intent is to comfort, not to stir up and release toxins.

- Side-lying position and/or special propping may need to be used to ensure client comfort, or, if the client cannot lie prone because of central venous catheters on the upper chest wall, radiation burns, or surgical wounds (Figure 12-6).

- If cancer has spread to the bones, bone integrity may be affected. Massage may be contraindicated. If clearance for massage has been obtained from the client's health care provider, deep pressure, traction, and joint mobilizations may be contraindicated or only cautiously used.

- Intravenous lines, catheters, surgical wounds over known cancer sites, radiation burns, or known tumor sites are areas to avoid during massage so as to decrease the risk of infection, pain from the pressure of massage, or damaging fragile tissues. Chapter 7 has more information on central venous catheters.

- Unless the client is debilitated or has a significant decrease in his or her stamina, the massage therapist should use moderate, firm (not deep) pressure during the massage. The pressure is critical because light stroking is generally aversive (much like a tickle stimulus) and does not produce the documented benefits of massage for cancer patients. If the client is debilitated, the massage therapist may need to use gentler pressure so as not to overtire the client, and be ready to ensure that the client stays warm.

- If the client is experiencing nausea, avoid pressure and speed that rocks the client. Joint mobilizations, stretches, jostling, or even moving client limbs are contraindicated because all of these can increase nausea.

CANCER TYPES

This section discusses the cancers themselves. Please refer to the section on General Guidelines when working on clients with cancer.

Bladder Cancer

A.S. Bladder; Gr. Crab

Description—The most common malignancy of the urinary tract, bladder cancer is characterized by blood in the urine, frequent and

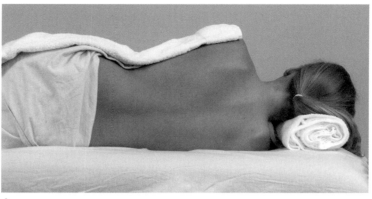

A

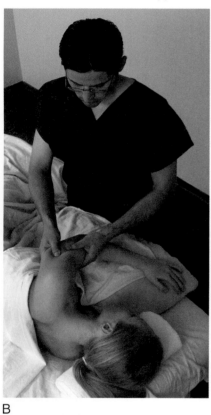

B

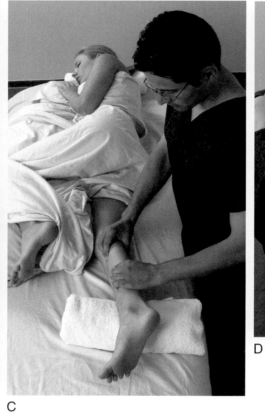

C

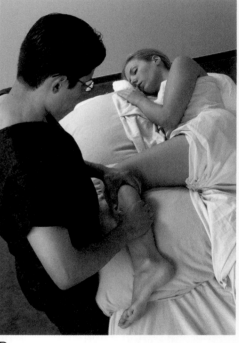

D

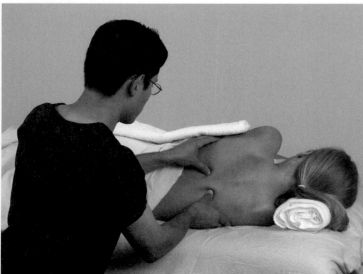

E

Figure 12-6.   Side-lying position.
A, Side-lying female client with back exposed, using a towel to anchor the drape.
B, Therapist massaging client's arm.
C, Therapist massaging inside of client's leg.
D, Therapist massaging outside of client's leg.
E, Therapist massaging client's back.

painful urination, and cystitis (Figure 12-7). Bladder cancer occurs twice as often in men than in women, is more prevalent in industrial than in rural areas. Risk factors include cigarette smoking and exposure toxic chemicals such as hydrocarbons or benzidine and its salts. These chemicals are frequently used in industries that manufacture paint, plastics, chemicals, rubber, textile, petroleum, wood products, or in medical laboratories.

Bone Cancer

A.S. Bone; Gr. Crab

Description—Bone tumors can be primary cancers. However, metastasis to the bones by cancers elsewhere in the body is more common (Figure 12-8). Even though bone cancer progress rather rapidly, it is often difficult to detect. The only symptom may be bone pain that increases at night. Radiation therapy is often used as the main form of treatment or may be given before surgery.

Brain Tumors

A.S. Brain; Gr. Crab

Description—Brain tumors can be primary cancers. However, most brain tumors are caused by cancers distant to the brain, such as breast, colon, lung, ovarian, or prostate or by skin cancers such as malignant melanoma. Symptoms of brain tumors are headaches, dizziness, nausea, vomiting, lethargy, and disorientation. Surgery is the initial treatment for most brain tumors. Radiation therapy is indicated for inoperable tumors and in removal of residual tumor tissue postsurgery (Figures 12-9 and 12-10).

Breast Cancer

A.S. Breast; Gr. Crab

Description—Breast cancer is the development of malignant tumors in the breast tissue (Figure 12-11). The tumors may occur on only one side or they may appear bilaterally. Early symptoms include the detection of a small painless lump in the breast tissue. Dimpling, skin thickness, and nipple retraction are all signs of advanced disease.

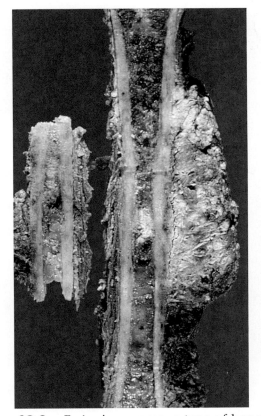

Figure 12-8. Ewing's sarcoma, a type of bone cancer.

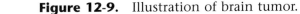

Figure 12-7. Bladder cancer.

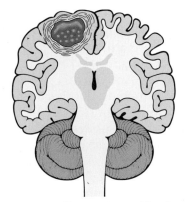

Figure 12-9. Illustration of brain tumor.

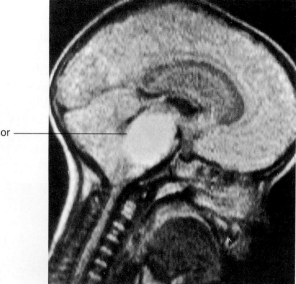

Tumor

Figure 12-10. Brain tumor.

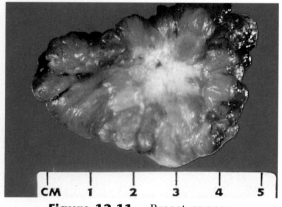

CM   1   2   3   4   5

Figure 12-11. Breast cancer.

As the malignancy advances, symptoms may include breast pain, enlargement of breast and axillary lymph nodes, discharge from the nipple, and even external ulcerations.

Suspicious lumps may be found by self-examination or by a partner (Figure 12-12). Regular breast examinations and mammograms can assist in early detection (Figure 12-13). Suspicious lumps may be biopsied for further analysis. Medical treatment may include lumpectomy, a total or simple mastectomy (removal of breast), a radical mastectomy (removal of breast, pectoral muscles, and axillary lymph nodes), or a modified radical mastectomy (removal of breast, some lymph nodes, and pectoralis minor). See Figure 12-14 and Box 12-5. Radiation and/or chemotherapy may also be used. In the case of total mastectomy, prosthetic

implants may be used, sometimes out of medical necessity, sometimes cosmetically.

Breast cancer is now the most common form of cancer in women in the United States. Breast cancer does occur in the male population, although less commonly. Besides gender, other risk factors include cystic breast disease, hypertension, diabetes, obesity, family history of breast tumors, radiation exposure to the thorax, estrogen therapy, and age.

Cervical Cancer

L. Neck; Gr. Crab

Description—Cervical cancer is curable if it is detected at an early stage by Pap (Papanicolaou) smear testing (Figures 12-15 and 12-16). There may be no symptoms in the early stages, although some women experience menstrual spotting or a watery discharge from the vagina. In advanced stages the cancer may spread to adjacent organs or can travel through the lymphatic system and metastasize in the bone, liver, brain, or lungs.

Causative factors include a history of unprotected sexual intercourse with multiple partners, sexually transmitted diseases (especially HPV) and poor or neglected obstetric/gynecological health care, having more than one child, and beginning sexual intercourse at an early age. Chapter 11 has more information on STDs.

Radiation therapy may be used. For women who wish to have children, doctors will attempt to use methods that do not cause sterilization, but in some cases, a partial or complete hysterectomy may be indicated.

Colorectal Cancer (koh`·luh·rek´·tuhl kan´·suhr)

L. Colon; L. Straight; Gr. Crab

Description—Colorectal cancer consists of malignant tumors in the colon and rectum. Early symptoms include change in bowel habits, and dull, abdominal pain. Later symptoms include weight loss, fatigue, anemia, weakness, constipation, diarrhea, and blood in the stools (Figure 12-17). Colon cancer is most common in people over 40 years old, and affects both men and women. Diet is a major factor. Diets high in animal fat and low in fiber increase the risk of colorectal cancer. Complications of ulcerated colitis, family history of colorectal cancer, and a history of intestinal polyps also increase risk. A person who has or has had colorectal cancer may have a colostomy. Chapter 9 has more information on colostomies.

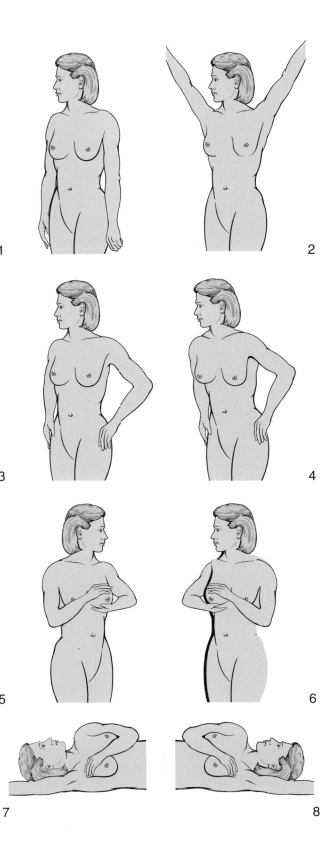

1

2

3

4

5

6

7

8

Figure 12-12. Breast self-examination. While in an upright position, the woman stands in front of a mirror and inspects her breasts in the normal position (1). The inspection should be repeated while she assumes three additional positions: raising her arms above her head (2), placing her hands on her hips (3), and flexing her shoulders forward (4). The breasts should then be palpated while in an upright position by holding the breast with one hand and by examining it with the fingers of the other hand (5 and 6). Palpation should be repeated while lying down with one hand extended above the head (7 and 8).

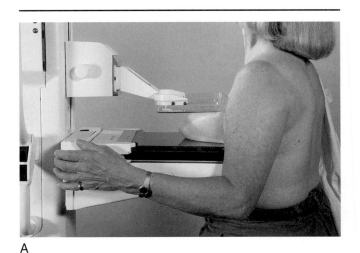

A

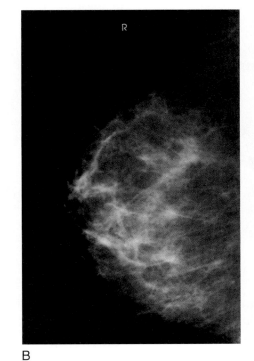

B

Figure 12-13. **A,** Clinical setting for mammograms. **B,** Normal mammogram.

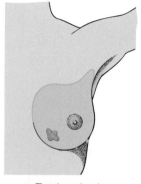

Total or simple
mastectomy

Modified radical
mastectomy

A

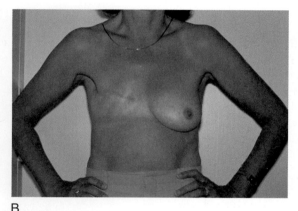

B

Figure 12-14.   Mastectomy. **A,** Diagram of mastectomy. **B,** Woman with mastectomy.

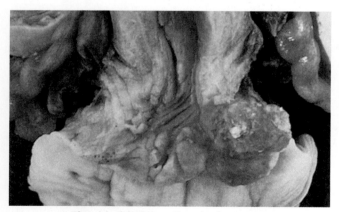

Figure 12-15.   Cervical cancer.

Endometrial Cancer (en`·doh·mee´·tree·uhl kan´·suhr)

Gr. Inward; Womb; Crab

 Description—Endometrial cancer is cancer of the endometrium (lining) of the uterus (Figure 12-18). It occurs most often in women in

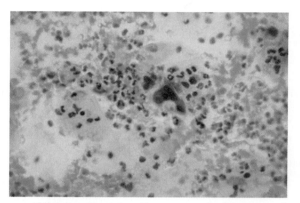

Figure 12-16.   Positive Pap smear indicative of cervical cancer.

Box **12-5**

Breast Massage

Breast massage is learned through special training and involves specific techniques that are mainly modified petrissage (kneading).

These techniques are geared toward increasing blood flow and lymphatic drainage and are most effective when nearby muscles, such as pectoralis major, have been relaxed first. It is also important to always obtain client consent first, and to never touch the nipple during the treatment. Some areas of the country may have regulations against touching the female breasts during massage, so therapists need to be very clear about the legalities of breast massage.

Indications for breast massage include congestion and swelling; discomforts of pregnancy, breastfeeding, and weaning; assistance with monitoring for lumps in the breast; premenstrual and postmenopausal tenderness; postsurgical symptoms (e.g., mastectomy), including loosening scar tissue; breast pain; and breast injuries.

their fifties and sixties. Factors associated with increased risk of this cancer include infertility, lack of ovulation, taking estrogen supplements, uterine polyps, diabetes, hypertension, and obesity. Symptoms include abnormal vaginal bleeding in postmenopausal women and abdominal and low back pain. The cancer is usually detected through uterine wall biopsies. The usual treatment is a hysterectomy followed by postoperative radiation therapy.

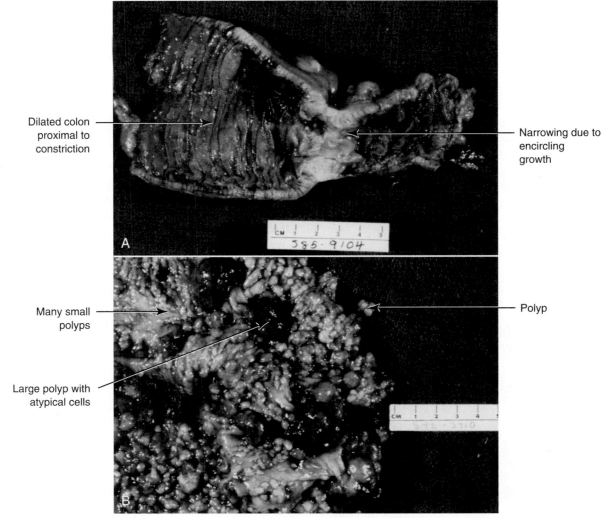

Dilated colon proximal to constriction

Narrowing due to encircling growth

Many small polyps

Large polyp with atypical cells

Polyp

Figure 12-17. Colorectal cancer. **A,** Circumferential malignant growth (cancer) obstructing flow of feces and causing proximal dilation of the colon. **B,** Polyposis and malignant changes.

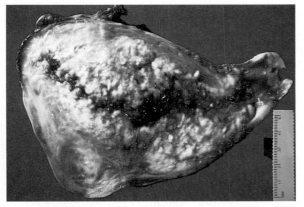

Figure 12-18. Endometrial cancer.

Laryngeal Cancer (luh·rin´·juhl kan´·suhr)

Gr. Larynx; Crab

Description—Laryngeal cancers are tumors in the structures of the larynx. They are 20 times more common in men than women, and usually occur between the ages of 50 and 70 years. Chronic alcoholism and heavy cigarette smoking increase the risk of developing laryngeal cancer. The first sign is persistent hoarseness. Later, symptoms of sore throat, painful breathing, painful swallowing, and enlarged cervical lymph nodes can develop. Radiation therapy is generally indicated for small tumors. A total laryngectomy, along with radiation, is the treatment for large tumors. After the procedure, speech production is impaired.

Speech production using the esophagus or an electrical device may be learned.

Leukemia (loo·kee´·mee·uh)

Gr. White; Blood

🚦 **Description**—Also called cancer of the blood, leukemia is a cancer characterized by elevated white blood cell count. There are many types of leukemia named for their dominant cell type (e.g., granulocytic, lymphocytic, myelogenous) and the severity of the disease (i.e., acute, chronic). Acute leukemia is a malignant disease of blood-forming tissues resulting in uncontrolled production and accumulation of immature leukocytes. Chronic leukemia results in an accumulation of mature leukocytes that do not die at the end of their life span (Figures 12-19 and 12-20). Complications include anemia and bleeding problems because the immature white blood cells crowd out functioning red blood cells and platelets. There can also be uncontrolled infection because of lack of mature or normal leukocytes.

Lymphoma (lim·foh´·muh)

L. Water; Gr. Tumor

🚦 **Description**—Lymphoma is a neoplasm (tumor) of lymphoid tissue that is usually malignant but, in rare cases, may be benign. Typically, lymphoma presents itself as enlarged lymph nodes. This is followed by weakness, fever, weight loss, and anemia. When the condition becomes widespread, the spleen and liver can enlarge, and gastrointestinal disturbances are noted. Bone lesions frequently develop. Men are more likely than women to develop lymphoid tumors. Treatments include radiation therapy and chemotherapy. There are many types of lymphoma. Two such types are Hodgkin's disease and malignant or non-Hodgkin's lymphoma.

Hodgkin's Disease

Thomas Hodgkin, British Physician; 1798-1866

Description—Hodgkin's disease is a cancer of the lymph nodes, evidenced by painless, progressive enlargement of lymph nodes that may spread to other areas (Figure 12-21). Other symptoms include fever, night sweats, weight loss, fatigue, itching, and anemia (Figures 12-22 and 12-23). The disease progresses in stages.

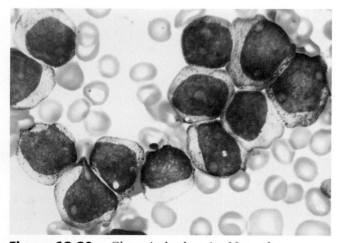

Figure 12-19. Acute leukemia. Note the accumulation of immature leukocytes.

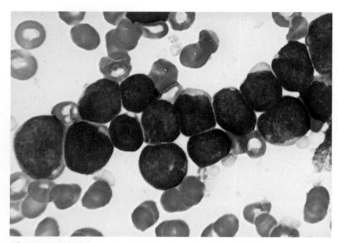

Figure 12-20. Chronic leukemia. Note the accumulation of mature leukocytes.

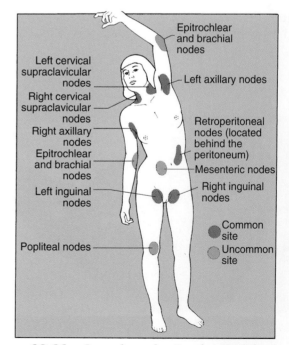

Figure 12-21. Lymph node sites for Hodgkin's disease.

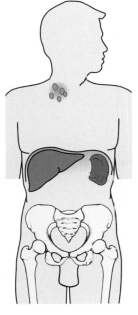 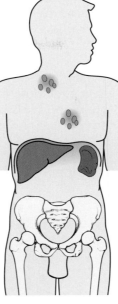 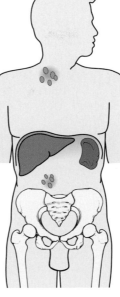 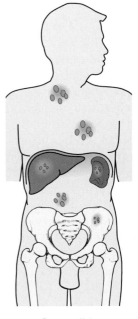

Stage I
Involvement of single
lymph node or group
of nodes

Stage II
Involvement of two
or more sites on same
side of diaphragm

Stage III
Disease on both sides
of diaphragm. May
include the spleen

Stage IV
Widespread extralymphatic
involvement (liver, bone
marrow, lung, skin)

Figure 12-22. Stages of Hodgkin's disease.

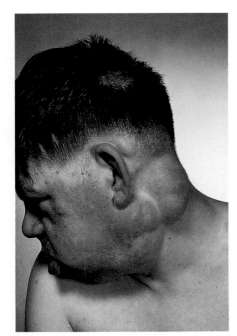

Figure 12-23. Enlargement of lymph nodes seen in Hodgkin's disease.

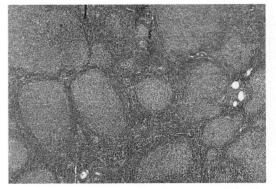

Figure 12-24. Cancer cells of non-Hodgkin's lymphoma.

Malignant Lymphomas (Non-Hodgkin's Lymphoma, Lymphosarcoma)
(lim`·foh·sahr·koh´·muh)

Gr. Of Bad Kind; L. Water; Gr. Tumor

Description—This is actually a group of malignant lymphomas, the only common feature being an absence of the giant Reed-Sternberg cells characteristic of Hodgkin's disease. These cells arise from the lymphoid tissue (Figure 12-24). The clinical picture is similar to that of Hodgkin's disease, except that the disease is initially more widespread, the most common manifestation being painless enlargement of lymph nodes.

Liver Cancer

A.S. Lifer; Gr. Crab

Description—Liver tumors can be primary cancers; however, cancers elsewhere in the body that have metastasized cause some liver tumors. In many cases, liver cancer is associated with cirrhosis of the liver. Other predisposing factors include hepatitis, nutritional deficiency, alcoholism, and exposure to carcinogens.

Symptoms include weakness, abdominal pain, abdominal swelling, mild jaundice, bloating, and liver tenderness and enlargement (Figure 12-25). Medical treatment consists primarily of surgical removal of the cancerous areas of the liver, depending on the severity of disease. Chemotherapy is sometimes used. Radiation treatment is more harmful to the liver than to the cancer and so is usually avoided.

Lung Cancer (Bronchogenic Carcinoma)

(brahn·koh·je´·nik kahr`·suh·noh´·muh)

A. S. Lung; Gr. Crab

Description—Lung cancer is caused by a long-term irritant such as air pollution, cigarette smoke, asbestos, or coal dust (Figure 12-26). Cigarette smoke is the main cause of lung cancer. Initially, there are usually no symptoms, and the cancer is usually not detected until the late stages when symptoms include chronic cough, difficulty breathing, chest pain, coughing up blood, weight loss, and fatigue (Figure 12-27).

Oral Cancer

L. Mouth; Gr. Crab

Description—Oral cancer is characterized by malignant tumors on the lip or within the oral cavity (Figure 12-28). This cancer type is eight times more common in men than in women. Influ-

ential factors are heavy alcohol and tobacco use, poor oral hygiene, syphilis, and overexposure to sun. Painless lesions that do not heal accompanied by enlarged cervical and axillary lymph nodes may be the initial signs of oral cancer (Figure 12-29). Small and medium-sized lesions are treated by excision or radiation. Large oral tumors are removed by more extensive surgery with removal of involved lymph nodes and postoperative radiation therapy.

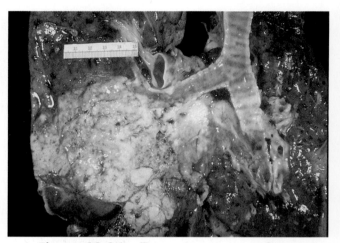

Figure 12-26.   Tumor in cancerous lung.

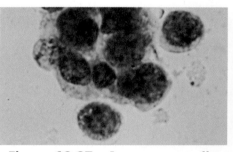

Figure 12-27.   Lung cancer cells.

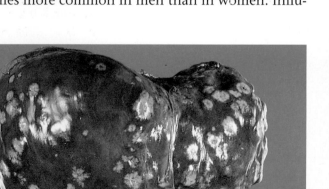

Figure 12-25.   Liver cancer.

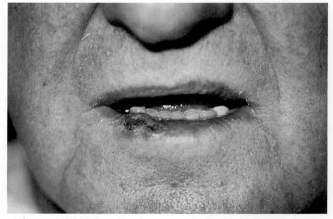

Figure 12-28.   Oral cancer lesion on lip surface.

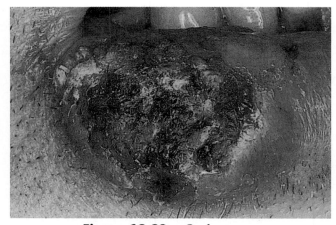

Figure 12-29. Oral cancer.

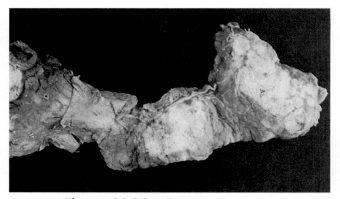

Figure 12-31. Pancreatic cancer.

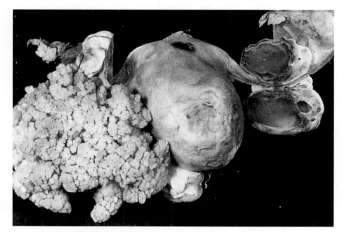

Figure 12-30. Ovarian cancer.

Ovarian Cancer

L. Egg; Gr. Crab

Description—Ovarian cancer is a malignant tumor of the ovaries, usually occurring in women in their fifties. The tumors may occur only on one side or they may appear bilaterally. In the early stages of tumor development, the woman is typically asymptomatic; thus diagnosis does not occur until the tumor has reached an advanced stage (Figure 12-30). Symptoms may include abnormal vaginal bleeding such as irregular menstrual cycles, excessive menstrual bleeding, or postmenopausal bleeding. Other signs of advanced stage ovarian cancer are abdominal swelling, abdominal pain, leg pain with edema, weight loss, constipation, and a palpable abdominal mass.

Ovarian tumor occurrence rates are increasing in the United States. Ovarian cancer rates are more likely in women with a history of repeated miscarriage, endometriosis, infertility, or those who have delayed childbearing. Other risk factors for the

disease include those who have had previous radiation treatments to the organs of the pelvis and exposure to carcinogens.

Treatment for ovarian cancer is usually a total hysterectomy. Surgery may be followed by chemotherapy, radiation, or both.

Pancreatic Cancer

Gr. Flesh; Gr. Crab

Description—Pancreatic cancer is a malignant tumor of the pancreas. Occurrences are higher in men than women. Besides gender, predisposing factors include heavy smokers, patients with diabetes mellitus, and exposure to carcinogenic compounds such as PCBs (polychlorinated biphenyl). Pancreatic cancer rates are higher in industrialized areas than in rural areas.

Symptoms include weakness, weight loss, anorexia, stomach pain, back pain, flatulence, itching, and in some patients, clay-colored stools. Another sign of pancreatic cancer is recent-onset diabetes. An abdominal mass is often palpable (Figure 12-31).

Medical treatment may include partial pancreatectomy and/or excision of the common bile duct, duodenum, and part of the stomach. Radiation or chemotherapy is sometimes used to buy the patient more time; however, prognosis is generally poor. Patients with pancreatic cancer seldom survive a year beyond diagnosis.

Prostate Cancer

Gr. Standing Before; Gr. Crab

Description—Prostate cancer progresses slowly, affecting an increasing proportion of male Caucasians after the age of 50 years. It is the third leading cause of deaths from cancer, with more than 120,000 new cases reported each year. The cause is unknown, but it is believed to be hormone-related. It often goes undetected, and then is suspected during diagnosis of identifying bladder or uretal obstruction, painful urination, or blood in the urine. Prostate cancer can be detected early by blood test measuring prostate-specific antigen (PSA). It may also be discovered by digital rectal examination followed by a needle biopsy. Treatment may include surgery, radiation and chemotherapy, and hormones, depending on the age of the patient and extent of the disease. Cancer may spread to the bones of the pelvis, spine, or ribs.

Skin Cancer

O. Norse Skin; Gr. Crab

Description—The three most common skin cancers are basal cell carcinoma, squamous cell carcinoma, and malignant melanoma and are discussed next. Ninety percent of all reported skin cancers can be abated through early detection and treatment. The best preventive measure anyone can take to reduce skin cancer is to avoid overexposure to the sun. This is more important for light-skinned people. Darker skinned people have fewer incidents of skin cancer because they have more pigment, or melanin, to protect their cells from ultraviolet radiation. Using a sunscreen lotion with a sun protection factor (SPF) of 15 or more is advisable.

Basal Cell Carcinoma

(bay´·zuhl sel´ kahr`·suh·noh´·muh)

L. Base; Cell; Gr. Cancer; Tumor

Description—Basal cell carcinoma accounts for about 75% of all cancers of the skin. This type of cancer is slow growing and is characterized by lesions that begin as small raised nodules that ulcerate (Figure 12-32). The primary cause of basal cell carcinoma is excessive exposure to sunlight. Basal cell carcinoma is the least dangerous skin cancer and rarely metastasizes.

Squamous Cell Carcinoma

(skwah·muhs sel´ kahr`·suh·noh´·muh)

L. Scalelike; Cell; Gr. Cancer; Tumor

Description—Squamous cell carcinoma is more aggressive than basal cell carcinoma and accounts for about 20% of all cases of skin cancer (Figure 12-33). Squamous cell carcinoma also arises from the epidermis, beginning as a scaly pigmented area that may develop into an ulcerated crater (Figure 12-34). This type of cancer is common on sun-exposed

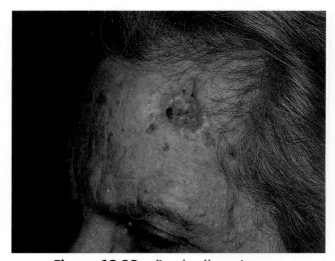

Figure 12-32. Basal cell carcinoma.

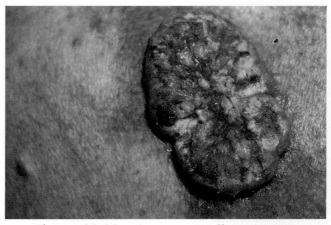

Figure 12-33. Squamous cell carcinoma.

areas or in the mouth (tobacco chewers) or on the lips (cigarette and cigar smokers).

Malignant Melanoma

(muh·lig´·nuhnt me`·luh·noh´·muh)

Gr. Of Bad Kind; Black; Tumor

Description—One of the most malignant and lethal skin cancer types, melanoma is a group of melanocytes that has mutated into cancer. Accounting for about 5% of all skin cancers, it often begins as a raised dark lesion with irregular borders and appears uneven in color (Figure 12-35). It typically occurs in light-skinned people who are exposed to ultraviolet radiation over many years. Melanoma is more likely to metastasize than any other form of cancer and can kill within months of diagnosis.

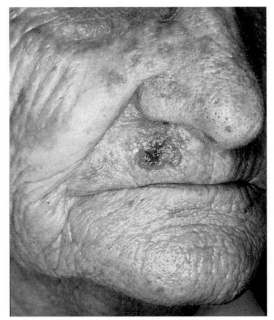

Figure 12-34. Squamous cell carcinoma on upper lip.

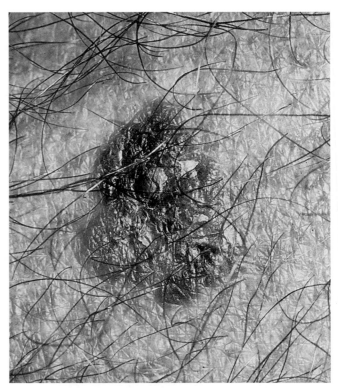

Figure 12-35. Malignant melanoma.

Stomach Cancer

Gr. Gullet; Gr. Crab

Description—Stomach cancer is the presence of neoplastic tumors in the lining of the stomach (Figure 12-36). In the early stages, symptoms may not be noticeable. As the cancer progresses, the patient may experience weight loss, anemia, fatigue, the presence of blood in the stool, and a range of digestive disorders. Stomach cancer has been associated with cases of gastritis (see Chapter 9). The cause of stomach cancer is unknown, and its incidence varies greatly. In the United States, it is only the seventh most common form of cancer, but in Japan it is the most common cancer.

Medical treatment may include surgery, radiation, chemotherapy, or any combination of the three. Prognosis is generally poor, because the cancer is usually not diagnosed until the later stages.

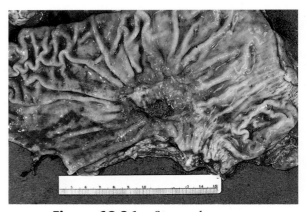

Figure 12-36. Stomach cancer.

SUMMARY

Cancer, or neoplasia, is any abnormal growth of new tissue and may be classified as benign or malignant. Benign means that the tumor is confined to one area of the body. Malignant means that the cancer spreads through the body by a process called metastasis. The method of travel is through the bloodstream or lymphatic system. Many malignant tumors are curable if they are detected at an early stage.

Although massage is not a treatment for cancer itself, it is often used to treat the symptoms of the cancer and the side effects of the cancer treatment. Massage has many benefits including lowering stress and fatigue, reducing edema, boosting immune function, improving sleep, and reducing pain. Medical consent needs to be obtained before performing massage on a patient with cancer, and special precautions are needed depending on the type of cancer and associated medical treatment. Cancer is treated one of three ways: surgery, chemotherapy, or radiation therapy. Bone marrow transplants are occasionally used.

The most common types of cancers are lung, breast, colon, uterus, oral, and bone cancer. Other cancers include bladder, brain, cervical, liver, ovarian, pancreatic, prostate, skin, and stomach cancer.

The incidence of different kinds of cancer varies greatly with age, ethnicity, gender, and geographic location. The definitive cause of cancer is not known, but cancer has been linked to exposure to certain chemicals, tobacco, ionizing radiation, ultraviolet rays, and some viruses. Studies suggest that genetics also plays an important role.

Resources

American Brain Tumor Association
2720 River Road, Suite 146
Des Plains, IL 60018

American Cancer Society
1599 Clifton Road NE
Atlanta, GA 30329
800-ACS-2345 (800-227-2345)

Antismoking Helpline
800-4-CANCER (800-524-1234)
800-638-6070 (in Alaska)
800-524-1234 (in Hawaii)

Cancer Care Counseling Line
800-813-HOPE (800-813-4673)
www.cancercareinc.org

Centers for Disease Control and Prevention
Building 1 South, Room SSB249
1600 Clifton Road NE
Atlanta, GA 30333
404-329-3492
www.cdc.gov

Leukemia Society of America
733 Third Avenue
New York, NY 10017
212-573-8484
www.leukemia.org

Melanoma Research Foundation
PO Box 747
San Leandro, CA 94577
800-MRF-1290
MRFI@melanoma.org

National Alliance of Breast Cancer Associations
9 East 37th Street, 10th Floor
New York, NY 10016
800-719-9154

National Cancer Institute
Building 31, Room 10A24
9000 Rockville Pike
Bethesda, MD 20892
800-4-CANCER (800-524-1234)
800-638-6070 (in Alaska)
800-524-1234 (in Hawaii)
www.nci.nih.gov

National Cervical Cancer Coalition
16501 Sherman Way, Suite 110
Van Nuys, CA 91406
800-685-5531

SELF-TEST

List the letter of the answer to the term or phrase that best describes it.

A. Benign tumor
B. Cancer
C. Carcinogens
D. Carcinomas
E. Malignant tumor
F. Melanomas
G. Metastasize
H. Neoplasm
I. Oncogenes
J. Oncology
K. Oncoviruses
L. Sarcomas

_____ 1. Viruses that cause cancer by stimulating cells to divide abnormally.
_____ 2. A cancerous tumor.
_____ 3. A word synonymous with tumor.
_____ 4. Cancers that grow from melanocytes.
_____ 5. Cancer-causing agents.
_____ 6. The study of tumors.
_____ 7. A disease characterized by uncontrollable growth of abnormal cells that form a tumor.
_____ 8. Cancer-causing genes.
_____ 9. When cancerous cells spread to other parts of the body.
_____ 10. Cancers that develop from muscle cells or connective tissue.
_____ 11. Cancers that arise from epithelial tissue.
_____ 12. A tumor that does not metastasize.

Use the index below as a convenient, quick, condensed reference. It is advised to go to the complete entry in the appropriate chapter for additional information.

Abortion: Avoid deep abdominal massage until client has completely healed.

Acne vulgaris: (ak´·nee vuhl·gar´·uhs) Local contraindication of infected area.

Acquired immunodeficiency syndrome: Adjust massage to client's stamina and vitality (i.e., slower, gentler, shorter duration, assist client on and off table).

Acrochordon: (a·kroh·kohr´·duhn) See entry under Skin tags.

Acromegaly: (a`·kroh·me´·guh·lee) Obtain physician clearance if symptoms are severe. Adjust massage if client is in pain.

Acute idiopathic polyneuritis: See entry under Guillain-Barré syndrome.

Addison's disease: Obtain physician clearance if symptoms are severe. Adjust massage to client's stamina and vitality (i.e., slower, gentler, shorter duration, assist client on and off table).

Adhesive capsulitis: (ad·hee´·siv kap`·soo·lai´·tis) Use techniques to increase ROM. Address shoulder girdle and rotator cuff muscles, biceps and triceps brachii, and deltoid.

Age spots: Massage is fine.

AIDS: See entry for Acquired immunodeficiency syndrome.

Albinism: (al´·buh·ni`·zuhm) Massage is fine.

Allergic dermatitis: See entry under Contact dermatitis.

Allergic rhinitis: See entry under Hay fever.

Allergies: Ascertain and avoid all known and suspected allergens (e.g., pet dander, nut oils). Ask client to review ingredient list of the massage lubricant.

Alzheimer's disease: (alz´·hai`·merz duh·zeez´) Use techniques to prevent joint stiffening and muscle contractures and to maintain mobility. Allow client to determine treatment length, but do not exceed 90 minutes.

Amenorrhea: (ah`·me`·nuh·ree´·uh) Massage is fine.

Amputation: Inquire about surgical procedure; use information to locate trigger points in affected muscles. Adjust massage if an area is sensitive or numb. Avoid chafing or friction wounds if prosthetics are worn.

Amyotrophic lateral sclerosis: (ay`·mai·uh·troh´·fik la´·tuh·ruhl skluh·roh´·sis) See entry under Lou Gehrig's disease.

Anemia: Adjust massage to client's stamina and vitality (i.e., slower, gentler, shorter duration, assist client on and off table). If anemia is due to a bleeding disorder, use lighter pressure.

Aneurysm: Obtain physician consent. If client has been diagnosed with an abdominal aortic aneurysm, abdominal massage is contraindicated.

Angina pectoris: Massage is fine. Keep client warm. Avoid using heat or cold packs. If client has an attack during treatment, assist the client in taking necessary medications (e.g., nitroglycerin). If nitroglycerin is taken by client while in the office, make sure the client sits or lies down for at least an hour.

Angioleukitis: (an`·jee·oh`·loo·kai´·tis) See entry under Lymphangitis.

Angiolymphitis: (an`·jee·oh`·lim·fai´·tis) See entry under Lymphangitis.

Ankylosing spondylitis: (an`·ki·loh´·sing spawn`·duh·lai´·tis) Position client for comfort. Use techniques to retain joint mobility, strengthen weak muscles, and stretch tight ones; do not force ankylosed joints into movement.

Anorexia nervosa: (a·nuh·rek´·see·uh nuhr·voh´·suh) Obtain physician clearance if symptoms are severe.

Anterior compartment syndrome: If symptoms are acute, seek medical attention. If chronic, elevate affected limb during treatment. Use heat and techniques that loosen fascia and relax muscles. End treatment with ice.

Anxiety disorders: Massage is fine. Obtain name and phone number of contact person and physician in case panic attack occurs during treatment.

Apnea: (ap´·nee·uh) Massage is fine. Position client for comfort.

Appendicitis: (uh·pen`·duh·sai´·tis) Massage is contraindicated.

Arteriosclerosis: (ahr·tee`·ree·oh·skluh·roh´·sis) Physician clearance is recommended. Avoid deep pressure massage.

Asthma: Position client for comfort. Ascertain and avoid all known and suspected allergens. If client uses a bronchodilator, have it handy. Focus treatment on primary and secondary muscles of respiration.

Atherosclerosis: (a`·thuh·roh`·skluh·roh´·sis) Physician clearance is recommended. A lighter massage is indicated.

Athlete's foot: Local contraindication of infected area.

Atopic dermatitis: See entry for Eczema.

Atrophy: (a´·truh·fee) Massage using strokes that are slow, superficial, and soothing with intermittent use of manual vibration and cross-fiber hacking percussion.

Baker's cyst: Local contraindication of involved area.

Basal cell carcinoma: (bay´·zuhl sel´ kahr`·suh·noh´·muh) See entry for Bladder cancer.

Bed sore: See entry under Decubitus ulcer.

Bell's palsy: Lighter pressure on face, directed upward.

Benign prostatic hyperplasia: (buh·nain´ pruh·sta´·tik hai`·puhr·play´·zhee·uh) See entry under Benign prostatic hypertrophy.

Benign prostatic hypertrophy: (buh·nain´ pruh·sta´·tik hai`·puhr·troh´·fee) Avoid abdomen if pressure causes pain. Position client for comfort.

Biliary calculus: (bi´·lee·er`·ee kal´·kyuh·luhs) See entry under Cholecystitis.

Bipolar disorder: Massage considerations are the same as for Anxiety disorders.

Birthmarks: Massage is fine.

Bladder cancer: Obtain physician consent. Once granted, adjust the massage to cancer type. Adjust massage according to cancer treatment client is undergoing (e.g., surgery, radiation therapy, chemotherapy). If client has a low platelet count, use lighter pressure. If the client is nauseated, avoid aromatherapy and pressure and speed that rock the client (e.g., joint mobilizations, stretches, jostling). Adjust massage to client's stamina and vitality (i.e., slower, gentler, shorter duration, assist client on and off table). Avoid massage over IVs, catheters, surgical wounds over known cancer and tumor sites, and radiation burns.

Bladder infection: See entry under Cystitis.

Blood blister: See entry under Hematoma.

Boil: See entry under Furuncle.

Bone cancer: See entry for Bladder cancer.

Brachial plexus injury: See entry under Thoracic outlet syndrome.

Brain tumors: See entry for Bladder cancer.

Breast cancer: See entry for Bladder cancer.

Bronchitis: (brahng·kai´·tis) Massage is contraindicated if client has acute bronchitis and fever. For chronic bronchitis, position client for comfort, including postural drainage. Percuss and vibrate ribcage for up to 5 minutes. Focus on the muscles of respiration.

Bronchogenic carcinoma: (brahn·koh·je´·nik kahr`·suh·noh´·muh) See entry under Bladder cancer.

Bruise: Local contraindication until bruise turns yellowish. Massage on bruise while it is bluish/purple is fine.

Buerger's disease: See entry under Thromboangiitis obliterans.

Bulimia: (buh·lee´·mee·uh) Massage is fine.

Bunion: Local contraindication if infected area is sensitive or if pressure causes pain.

Burns: Obtain physician clearance for recent but healed burns. Once granted, use lighter pressure (including healed skin graft) and techniques that help break up adhesions and increase mobility. All forms of thermotherapy (e.g., hot pack) are contraindicated. All forms of cryotherapy (e.g., cold pack) are contraindicated for third-degree burns.

Bursitis: Local contraindication of infected area if in acute stage. Cold packs can be applied to reduce swelling. If chronic, assess joint mobility and pain with movement, and, if indicated, joint mobilizations, stretches, and friction to maintain joint mobility. Ice after treatment.

Calcaneal spur: See entry under Plantar fasciitis.

Callus: (ka´·luhs) See entry under Corn.

Candidiasis vaginitis: (kan`·duh·dai´·uh·sis va`·ji·nai´·tis) See entry under Vaginal candidiasis.

Carbuncle: (kahr´buhn·kuhl) See entry under Furuncle.

Cardiac arrest: See entry for Myocardial infarction.

Cardiac murmur: See entry under Heart murmur.

Carpal tunnel syndrome: Local contraindication of inflamed area. If chronic, use techniques to reduce edema (e.g., elevating the limb, centripetal gliding strokes, lymphatic drainage). Use moist heat, cross-fiber friction, and passive movement of the elbow, wrist, and finger joints. Identify and avoid risk factors (e.g., improper arm-to-wrist angle, excessive wrist flexion).

Cataract: If visually impaired, explain everything that happens during the massage verbally.

Cellulitis: (sel`·yuh·lai´·tuhs) Local contraindication of infected area if contained to a small area. Otherwise, massage is contraindicated.

Cerebral palsy: Obtain physician clearance if symptoms are severe. Position client for comfort. If client uses a wheelchair, determine if treatment needs to be performed while client is in the chair. Do not force muscles into a stretch. If client is unable to speak, devise a code of communication.

Cerebrovascular accident: See entry under Stroke.

Cervical cancer: See entry for Bladder cancer.

Chickenpox: Massage is contraindicated.

Chlamydia: (kluh·mi´·dee·uh) Massage is contraindicated.

Chloasma: (khloh`·az´·muh) Massage is fine.

Cholecystitis: (koh`·luh·sis·tai´·tis) Massage is contraindicated during acute stage. For chronic cholecystitis, massage is fine if symptoms are not severe. Position client for comfort and avoid abdominal area.

Choledocholithiasis: (koh·luh·doh·kuh·luh·thai´·uh·sis) See entry under Cholecystitis.

Chondromalacia patellae: (kawn`·droh`·muh·lay´·shee·uh puh·te´·lay) Local contraindication of inflamed area.

Chronic chorea: See entry under Huntington's chorea.

Chronic fatigue syndrome: Treatment time should be of shorter duration if client is currently fatigued.

Chronic obstructive pulmonary disease: See entries for Asthma, Emphysema, Cystic fibrosis, Pneumoconiosis, and Chronic bronchitis.

Cirrhosis of the liver: (suh·roh·sis uhv thuh li·vuhr) Massage is contraindicated.

Clinical depression: See entry under Anxiety disorders.

Clubfoot: Use lighter pressure over the affected area.

Cluster headaches: See entry for Migraine headaches.

Cold sore: See entry under Herpes simplex.

Colitis: See entry under Ulcerative colitis.

Colorectal cancer: (koh`·luh·rek´·tuhl kan´·suhr) See entry for Bladder cancer.

Common cold: Massage is contraindicated for 2-3 days after cold symptoms start. Afterward, massage is fine if symptoms are not severe.

Concussion: Massage is contraindicated.

Condyloma acuminatum: See entry for Genital warts.

Congestive heart failure: Obtain physician clearance. Once granted, use lighter pressure; massage should be of shorter duration. If client has edema in extremities, lymphatic massage is contraindicated.

Conjunctivitis: (kuhn·junk´·tuh·vai`·tis) Massage is contraindicated.

Constipation: If not due to a contraindicated disease, massage is okay. Position client for comfort.

Contact dermatitis: Local contraindication of infected area if contained to a small area. Otherwise, massage is contraindicated.

Contracture: Use techniques to increase blood flow, reduce adhesions, stretch and release fascia, and elongate muscles.

Contusion: See entry for Bruise.

Contusion (head injury): Massage is contraindicated.

Corn: Avoid affected area if pressure causes pain.

Coronary artery disease: Physician clearance is recommended. Use lighter pressure and avoid deep pressure if client is prone to thrombosis.

Cradle cap: See entry under Seborrheic dermatitis.

Cretinism: (kree´·tuh·ni·zuhm) Obtain physician clearance. Once granted, use lighter pressure, avoiding neck/throat region.

Crohn's disease: Position client for comfort. Avoid abdomen if pressure causes pain.

Cubital tunnel syndrome: Local contraindication of inflamed area.

Cushing's disease: Obtain physician clearance if symptoms are severe.

Cystic fibrosis: (sis´·tik fai·broh´·sis) Obtain physician clearance if symptoms are severe. Position client for comfort and use postural drainage. Percuss and vibrate ribcage for up to 5 minutes. Focus on muscles of respiration.

Cystitis: (sis·tai´·tis) Position client for comfort and avoid abdomen if pressure causes pain.

Dandruff: See entry under Seborrheic dermatitis.

de Quervain's disease: See entry under de Quervain's tendonitis.

de Quervain's tendonitis: (duh·kwer´·vaynz ten`·duh·nai´·tis) Local contraindication of inflamed area.

Decubitus ulcer: (duh·kyoo´·buh·tuhs ul´·ser) Local contraindication of involved area.

Deep vein thrombosis: See entry under Thrombophlebitis.

Degenerative joint disease: See entry under Osteoarthritis.

Dementia: Obtain physician clearance. Once granted, see entry under Alzheimer's disease. Adjust massage to client's stamina and vitality (i.e., slower, gentler, shorter duration, assist client on and off table). If client is unable to speak for herself, get this information from client's caregiver.

Depression: See entry for Anxiety disorders.

Detached retina: Massage considerations are the same as for Cataracts.

Diabetes insipidus: (dai`·uh·bee´·teez in·si´·pi·duhs) Adjust massage to client's stamina and vitality (i.e., slower, gentler, shorter duration, assist client on and off table). Make sure client has necessary medication handy during treatment.

Diabetes mellitus: (dai`·uh·bee´·teez me´·luh·tuhs) Use lighter pressure. Avoid vigorous massage (e.g., percussion, vibration). Inform client of any bruises or breaks in the skin, especially the feet. If client is taking insulin, avoid injection site for at least 10 days on or around the injection site. Make sure client has necessary medications handy during treatment. Be prepared to make accommodations for client's medication administration or food intake during treatment.

Diarrhea: If not due to a contraindicated disease, massage is okay. Avoid abdomen if pressure causes pain.

Discoid lupus erythematosus: See entry under Lupus.

Dislocation: If recent, local contraindication of involved area. Once healed, use techniques to increase mobility. Avoid over-stretching and joint movements of affected joint.

Diverticulitis: (dai`·vuhr·tik`·yuh·lai´·tis) Massage is contraindicated if symptoms are severe. Position client for comfort and avoid abdomen if pressure causes pain.

Diverticulosis: (dai`·vuhr·ti`·kyuh·loh´·sis) Massage considerations are the same as for Diverticulitis.

Dupuytren's contracture: (doo´·pyuh·trenz` kuhn·trak´·chuhr) Use moist heat to soften fascia and techniques to increase circulation to affected area.

Dysmenorrhea: (dis`·men`·uh·ree´·uh) Massage is fine if symptoms are not severe. Position client for comfort. Avoid abdomen if pressure causes pain.

Ecchymosis: (e`·ki·moh´·suhs) See entry for Bruise.

Eczema: (eg´·zuh·muh) Avoid affected area if open and has a watery discharge or if pressure causes pain.

Edema: Massage is contraindicated if client has a history of heart or kidney disease or if due to a contraindicated disease. Otherwise, elevate area and use lymphatic drainage techniques. Work proximal areas first, then distal areas.

Embolism: Obtain physician clearance. Once granted, avoid deep, vigorous massage. If a client is taking anticoagulants, use lighter pressure.

Emphysema: (em`·fuh·zee´·muh) Position client for comfort. Focus on muscles of respiration. Adjust massage to client's stamina and vitality (i.e., slower, gentler, shorter duration, assist client on and off table).

Encephalitis: (en`·se`·fuh·lai´·tis) Massage is contraindicated.

Endocarditis: (en`·doh·kahr`·dai´·tuhs) Massage is contraindicated.

Endometrial cancer: (en`·doh·mee´·tree·uhl kan´·suhr) See entry for Bladder cancer.

Endometriosis: (en`·doh·mee`·tree·oh´·sis) Massage is fine. Position client for comfort.

Enterogastritis: (en`·tuh·roh·gas`·trai´·tis) See entry under Gastroenteritis.

Ephelis: (e´·fuh·lis) See entry under Freckle.

Epidermal cyst: (e·puh·der´·muhl sist´) See entry under Sebaceous cyst.

Epidermoid cyst: (e·puh·der´·moid sist´) See entry under Sebaceous cyst.

Epidural hematoma: Massage is contraindicated.

Epilepsy: (e´·puh·lep`·see) See entry under Seizure disorders.

Erb's palsy: Position client for comfort; may need to prop up and use lighter pressure on affected arm. Use techniques to increase muscle function, reduce swelling, and reduce contracture.

Fainting: See entry under Syncope.

Fever: Massage is contraindicated.

Fever blisters: See entry under Herpes simplex.

Fibrocystic breast disease: Massage is fine. Position client for comfort.

Fibroids: Massage is fine. Position client for comfort. Abdominal massage may be contraindicated if the pressure of massage causes pain.

Fibroid tumors: See entry under Fibroids.

Fibroma: See entry under Fibroids.

Fibromyalgia: Adjust massage to client's stamina and vitality (i.e., slower, gentler, shorter duration, assist client on and off table).

Fibrositis: See entry under Fibromyalgia.

Flaccid: (fla´·sid) Use techniques to increase muscle tone, increase blood flow, and assist in the removal of metabolic wastes.

Flu: See entry under Influenza.

Folliculitis: (fuh·lik`·yuh·lai´·tuhs) Local contraindication of infected area.

Fractures: While bone is immobilized, the involved area is a local contraindication, but massage can be performed close to the immobilized part using techniques to maintain circulation, joint mobility, muscle tone, reduce edema, decrease spasms, and reduce pain. Work proximal areas first, then distal areas. Once healed (physician determined), begin slowly for about a week, using techniques to help client regain joint mobility and increase tone in muscles that may have atrophied.

Freckle: Massage is fine.

Frozen shoulder: See entry for Adhesive capsulitis.

Furuncle/carbuncle: (fyur´·uhng·kuhl) Local contraindication of affected area. Avoid swollen lymph nodes.

Gallstones: Same as for Cholecystitis.

Ganglion cyst: Local contraindication of affected area.

Gastritis: Massage is contraindicated for acute gastritis. For chronic gastritis, massage is fine. Position client for comfort. Abdominal massage is contraindicated if pressure causes pain.

Gastroenteritis: (gas`·troh·en`·tuh·rai´·tis) If due to infectious agent, massage is contraindicated. If due to other factors, massage is fine. Position client for comfort. Abdominal massage is contraindicated if pressure causes pain.

Gastroesophageal reflux disease: (gas`·troh·uh·sah`·fuh·jee´·uhl ree´·fluhks duh·zeez´) Massage is fine if symptoms are not severe. Ask client not to eat a large meal prior to massage. Position client for comfort and avoid abdomen if pressure causes pain.

Genital herpes: Position client for comfort. Avoid abdomen if pressure causes pain.

Genital warts: Avoid abdomen if pressure causes pain.

German measles: Massage is contraindicated.

Glaucoma: (glah·koh´·muh) Massage considerations are the same as for Cataracts. Avoid pressure over eyes during facial massage. Position client for comfort; the face cradle may not be comfortable.

Glomerulonephritis: (gluh·mer`·yuh·loh`·ni·frai´·tis) Obtain physician clearance. Once granted, use lighter pressure. The massage should be of shorter duration. Do not use lymphatic massage to reduce edema.

Goiter: Adjust massage to client's stamina and vitality (i.e., slower, gentler, shorter duration, assist client on and off table). Avoid neck/throat region.

Gonorrhea: (gah`·nuh·ree´·uh) Massage is contraindicated.

Gout: Local contraindication of affected area during acute phase; this includes joint mobilizations.

Gouty arthritis: Local contraindication of affected area.

Graves' disease: Adjust massage to client's stamina and vitality (i.e., slower, gentler, shorter duration, assist client on and off table). Avoid neck/throat region and enlarged lymph nodes.

Guillain-Barré syndrome: (gee·lan´ bah·ray´ sin´·drohm) Obtain physician clearance. Once granted, use techniques to prevent muscle contractures, increase muscle tone of flaccid muscles, reduce adhesions, and improve mobility.

Hallux valgus: (ha´·luhks val´·guhs) See entry under Bunion.

Hammertoe: Use lighter pressure over the affected area.

Hay fever: Massage is contraindicated during acute allergic attack. Otherwise, massage is fine. Position the client for comfort (lying prone and/or using face cradle both cause nasal congestion). Ascertain and avoid all known and suspected allergens.

Head cold: See entry under Common cold.

Headaches: If not due to a contraindicated disease, massage is okay. If due to muscular contraction or tension, focus on muscles of the neck, shoulder, and back (e.g., trapezius, levator scapulae, splenius capitis and cervicis, suboccipitals, scalenes, sternocleidomastoid). Use moist heat.

Heart attack: See entry under Myocardial infarction.

Heart murmur: Obtain physician clearance if murmur is severe. Once granted, use lighter pressure.

Hemangioma: (hee·man·jee·oh´·muh)   Local contraindication of affected area.

Hematoma: Local contraindication of affected area.

Hemiplegia: See entry for Quadriplegia.

Hemophilia: (hee·moh·fee´·lee·uh) Massage is contraindicated for moderate to severe cases. For mild cases, obtain physician clearance. Once granted, lighter massage is indicated. Avoid stretches and joint mobilizations.

Hemorrhage: (he´·muh·rij) Massage is contraindicated.

Hemorrhoids: General massage is fine.

Hepatitis: Massage is contraindicated during acute phase. If client has chronic hepatitis, obtain physician clearance. Once granted, avoid abdominal massage.

Hernia: If client is in pain from the hernia, medical attention is needed. If not, position client for comfort and avoid herniated area. If client has a surgical mesh, use lighter pressure over mesh site, especially first 3 months after surgery. Deep pressure and myofascial release are contraindicated over mesh site.

Herniated disk: Obtain physician clearance. Once granted, use techniques to relieve pain. Focus on iliopsoas, paraspinals, and quadratus lumborum. Use heat if you follow treatment with ice. Avoid massage and traction of the involved area.

Herpes progenitalis: (her´·pees proh·je`·nuh·ta´·lis) See entry under genital herpes.

Herpes simplex: (her´·pees sim´·pleks) Local contraindication of infected area.

Herpes zoster: See entry under Shingles.

High blood pressure: See entry under Hypertension.

High cholesterol in the blood: See entry under Atherosclerosis.

Hives: During acute phase, massage is contraindicated. Otherwise, local contraindication where wheals are still visible, but not inflamed.

Hodgkin's disease: See entry for Bladder cancer.

Huntington's chorea: Obtain physician clearance. Once granted, position client for comfort. If client uses a wheelchair, determine if treatment needs to be performed while client is in the chair.

Hyaline membrane disease: See entry under Respiratory distress syndrome.

Hyperadrenalism: (hai·puhr·uh·dree´·nuh·li·zuhm) See entry under Cushing's disease.

Hypercholesterolemia: (hai`·puhr·kuh·les`·tuh·ruh·lee´·mee·uh) See entry under Atherosclerosis.

Hyperesthesia: (hai`·puhr·es·thee´·zhee·uh) Obtain physician clearance. If not due to a contraindicated disease, massage is okay.

Hyperparathyroidism: (hai`·puhr·pa`·ruh·thai´·roid·i`·zuhm) Obtain physician clearance if symptoms are severe. Avoid areas of bone fractures or areas where pressure causes pain. Carefully administer or avoid techniques such as stretches or mobilization and avoid vigorous massage in areas where bones are fragile.

Hyperpituitarism: (hai`·puhr·pi·too`·uh·tar´·ee·izm) Obtain physician clearance if symptoms are severe. Avoid areas where pressure causes pain. Carefully administer or avoid techniques such as stretches or mobilization and avoid vigorous massage.

Hypertension: If not controlled by diet, exercise, and/or medication, client should not receive massage. Otherwise, use stress reduction techniques to help lower blood pressure Client may need assistance to get up from table after the treatment.

Hyperthyroidism: (hai`·puhr·thai´·roid·i`·zuhm) Obtain physician clearance if symptoms are severe. Adjust massage to client's stamina and vitality (i.e., slower, gentler, shorter duration, assist client on and off table). Avoid neck/throat region.

Hypoadrenalism: (hai`·poh·uh·dree´·nuh·li·zuhm) See entry for Addison's disease.

Hypoglycemia: (hai`·poh·glai`·see´·mee·uh) Adjust massage to client's stamina and vitality (i.e., slower, gentler, shorter duration, assist client on and off table).

Hypoparathyroidism: (hi`·poh·pa`·ruh·thai´·roid·i`·zuhm) Obtain physician clearance if symptoms are severe. Adjust massage to client's stamina and vitality (i.e., slower, gentler, shorter duration, assist client on and off table). If client has tingling in the hands and/or feet, the pressure of massage over these areas needs to be lighter. Use techniques to maintain flexibility.

Hypopituitarism: (hai`·poh·pi·too`·uh·tar´·ee·izm) Obtain physician clearance if symptoms are severe. Adjust massage to client's stamina and vitality (i.e., slower, gentler, shorter duration, assist client on and off table, use of extra drape if client chills easily).

Hypotension: (hai`·poh·ten´·shuhn) Client may need assistance off table after massage. Clients with severe hypotension may need to be massaged in seated position.

Hypothyroidism: (hai`·poh·thai´·roid·i`·zuhm) Obtain physician clearance if symptoms are severe. Adjust massage to client's stamina and vitality (i.e., slower, gentler, shorter duration, assist client on and off table, use of extra drape if client chills easily). Avoid neck/throat region.

Ichthyosis vulgaris: (ik·thee·oh´·sis vuhl·ga´·ris) Avoid massage over areas that are inflamed or where pressure causes pain.

Icterus: See entry under Jaundice.

Impetigo: (im`·puh·tee´·goh) Massage is contraindicated.

Infectious rhinitis: (in·fek´·shuhs rai·nai´·tis) See entry under Common cold.

Influenza: (in·floo·en´·zuh) Massage is contraindicated.

Insomnia: Massage is fine, unless it is due to a condition that is a massage contraindication.

Intestinal obstruction: Massage is contraindicated.

Irritable bowel syndrome: Massage is fine if symptoms are not severe. Position client for comfort, avoiding abdomen if pressure causes pain.

Irritant dermatitis: See entry under Contact dermatitis.

Ischemic contracture: See entry under Dupuytren's contracture.

Ischemic heart disease: See entry under Coronary artery disease.

Jaundice: (jahn´·dis) Massage is contraindicated.

Jock itch: Avoid infected area unless infection is widespread, then massage is contraindicated.

Juvenile rheumatoid arthritis: See entry for Rheumatoid arthritis.

Kidney failure: Massage is contraindicated.

Kidney stones: Obtain physician clearance if client is taking medication for treatment of kidney stones. Once granted, massage only if symptoms are not severe. Position client for comfort.

Kyphosis: (kai·foh´·sis) Focus on involved muscles (pectoralis major/minor, serratus anterior, rhomboids major/minor), taking care not to over stretch the spine. If due to osteoporosis, use lighter pressure.

Laryngeal cancer: (luh·rin´·juhl kan´·suhr) See entry for Bladder cancer.

Laryngitis: (lar`·uhn·jai´·tis) If not due to a contraindicated disease, massage is okay.

Leukemia: (loo·kee´·mee·uh) See entry for Bladder cancer.

Leukoderma: (loo`·koh·der´·muh) See entry under Vitiligo.

Lice: Massage is contraindicated.

Liver cancer: See entry for Bladder cancer.

Liver spots: See entry for Age spots.

Lockjaw: See entry under Tetanus.

Lordosis: (lohr·doh´·sis) Focus on muscle of anterior and posterior pelvic tilt (e.g., abdominal muscles, quadratus lumborum, psoas major, erector spinae).

Lou Gehrig's disease: Obtain physician clearance. Once granted, position client for comfort. If client uses a wheelchair, determine if treatment needs to be performed while client is in the chair.

Low blood pressure: See entry under Hypotension.

Lung cancer: See entry for Bladder cancer.

Lupus: Massage is contraindicated during flare-ups. Otherwise, carefully administer stretches and mobilizations. Use lighter pressure if client is taking corticosteroids and antiinflammatory drugs. Avoid exposing client who is taking immunosuppressants to any form of infection.

Lyme arthritis: See entry under Lyme disease.

Lyme disease: Adjust massage to client's stamina and vitality (i.e., slower, gentler, shorter duration, assist client on and off table), using techniques to retain joint mobility. Massage is contraindicated if client is experiencing widespread inflammation.

Lymphangitis: (lim`·fuhn·jai´·tis) Massage is contraindicated.

Lymphedema: See entry under Edema.

Lymphoma: (lim·foh´·muh) See entry for Bladder cancer.

Lymphosarcoma: (lim`·foh·sahr·koh´·muh) See entry for Bladder cancer.

Macular degeneration: Massage is fine.

Malignant lymphoma: See entry for Bladder cancer.

Malignant melanoma: (muh·lig´·nuhnt me`·luh·noh´·muh) See entry for Bladder cancer.

Mask of pregnancy: See entry under Chloasma.

Mastitis: Avoid upper chest. Position client for comfort.

Measles: Massage is contraindicated.

Melasma: (muhl·az´·muh) See entry for Chloasma.

Meningitis: Massage is contraindicated.

Menopause: Massage is fine. Adjust room temperature for client comfort.

Menstruation: Avoid deep pressure on abdomen; instead, a moist hot pack may be used. Focus on low back (e.g., quadratus lumborum, erector spinae, latissimus dorsi) and gluteals.

Migraine headaches: Do not massage during a migraine headache. Otherwise, massage is fine between attacks.

Miscarriage: See entry for Abortion.

Mole: See entry under Birthmarks.

Mononucleosis: (mah`·noh·noo`·klee·oh´·sis) Massage is contraindicated.

Multiple sclerosis: Adjust massage to client's stamina and vitality (i.e., slower, gentler, shorter duration, assist client on and off table). Massage is contraindicated during flare-ups. Use techniques to relax client, decrease tone in rigid muscles, and prevent stiffness and contractures. Heat and cold therapies are contraindicated.

Mumps: Massage is contraindicated.

Muscle cramp: See entry under Muscle spasm.

Muscle spasm: Determine cause before treatment. If indicated, use techniques to increase local circulation and to mechanically lengthen and spread muscle fibers apart.

Muscular dystrophy: Use techniques to increase blood flow, to activate muscle spindles in weak muscles (if functional), and to increase peristaltic activity in the colon.

Muscular rheumatism: See entry under Fibromyalgia.

Myasthenia gravis: (mai`·uhs·thee´·nyuh gra´·vis) Obtain physician clearance if symptoms are severe. Use techniques to slow muscle atrophy and to maintain flexibility.

Myocardial infarction: (mai·oh·kahr´·dee·uhl in·fahrk´·shuhn) Massage is contraindicated if MI was recent and client is weak and debilitated. If client has a history of myocardial infarction, obtain physician clearance. Once granted, use lighter pressure of shorter duration. If client is further along in recovery and has regained most of his strength, use moderate pressure. If client has completely recovered and regained all of his strength, a more vigorous massage can be performed. Avoid using heat or cold packs. If an attack occurs during treatment, assist the client in taking necessary medications, then call EMS.

Myocarditis: (mai`·oh·kahr·dai´·tis) Massage is contraindicated.

Myofascial fibrocystitis: See entry under Fibromyalgia.

Myxedema: (mik`·suh·dee´·muh) See entry for Hypothyroidism.

Nephrotic syndrome: (nuh·frah´·tik sin´·drohm) Obtain physician clearance. Once granted, adjust massage to client's stamina and vitality (i.e., slower, gentler, shorter duration, assist client on and off table). Do not try to reduce edema with lymphatic massage.

Nerve compression: Obtain physician clearance. Once granted, focus on muscles in area of compression or muscles innervated by the nerve being compressed.

Nerve entrapment: Use techniques to reduce tension in involved muscles. Work deeply, but briefly.

Nerve impingement: See entry under Nerve compression.

Neuropathy: (nuh·rahp´·uh·thee) Obtain physician clearance. Once granted, either avoid massage of affected area or use lighter pressure. If not due to a contraindicated disease, massage is okay.

Nevi: (ne´·vee) See entry under Birthmarks.

Non-Hodgkin's lymphoma: See entry for Bladder cancer.

Obesity: Position client for comfort. Carefully apply pressure in areas containing large amounts of adipose tissue. If client is edematous due to inactivity, elevate legs during treatment and use lymphatic massage. If requested, use a sheet or an extra-large towel as a top drape. If needed, be prepared to massage client on the floor.

Obsessive compulsive disorder: Massage considerations are the same as for Anxiety disorders.

Onychomycosis: (ah`·nee·koh·mai·koh´·sis) Local contraindication of affected area.

Open wounds: Local contraindication of affected area.

Oral cancer: See entry for Bladder cancer.

Oral candidiasis: (ohr´·uhl kan`·duh·dai´·uh·sis) See entry under Thrush.

Osgood-Schlatter disease: (ahz´·guud-shla´·ter duh·zez´) Local massage is contraindicated during acute phase. Afterward, massage is fine. Focus treatment on reducing adhesion around knee and reducing tension in the quadriceps.

Osteitis deformans: (ays`·tee·ai´·tis duh·fohr´·muhnz) See entry under Paget's disease.

Osteoarthritis: (aws´·tee·oh·ahr·thrai´·tuhs) Deep pressure stretching and joint mobilizations are contraindicated. Use techniques to warm and loosen surrounding tissues.

Osteochondrosis: (ahs`·tee·oh·kuhn·droh´·sis) See entry under Osgood-Schlatter disease.

Osteomyelitis: (ahs`·tee·oh·mai·lai´·tis) Local contraindication of infectious wounds.

Osteoporosis: Use lighter pressure over bones. Limit or avoid joint mobilizations.

Ovarian cancer: See entry for Bladder cancer.

Ovarian cysts: Position client for comfort and avoid abdomen if pressure causes pain.

Paget's disease: Massage is fine.

Pancreatic cancer: See entry for Bladder cancer.

Pancreatitis: Massage is contraindicated if in acute stage. Otherwise, obtain physician clearance. Once granted, massage is fine if symptoms are not severe. Position client for comfort, avoiding abdomen if pressure causes pain.

Panic attack: See entry under Anxiety disorders.

Paraplegia: See entry for Quadriplegia.

Parkinson's disease: Obtain physician clearance if symptoms are severe. Use techniques to reduce rigidity.

Paronychia: (pa`·ruh·ni´·kee·uh) Local contraindication of affected area.

Parotitis: (par`·uh·tai´·tis) See entry under mumps.

Patellofemoral syndrome: See entry under Chondromalacia patellae.

Pediculosis capitis: (pi·di`·kyuh·loh´·sis ka´·pi·tis) See entry under Lice.

Pediculosis corpus: See entry under Lice.

Pediculosis palpebrarum: See entry under Lice.

Pediculosis pubis: (pi·di`·kyuh·loh´·sis pyoo´·bis) See entry under Lice.

Pelvic inflammatory disease: Massage is contraindicated.

Pericarditis: (pe`·ree·kahr·dai´·tis) Massage is contraindicated.

Peripheral vascular disease: Local contraindication if symptoms are severe (i.e., numbness, severe pain). Avoid or use lighter pressure in areas that are mildly numb or tingling.

Peritonitis: (pe`·ruh·tuh·nai´·tis) Obtain physician clearance. Once granted, avoid the abdomen. Adjust massage to client's stamina and vitality (i.e., slower, gentler, shorter duration, assist client on and off table). Do not massage if client is debilitated.

Petechiae: (puh·tee´·kee·ay) Local contraindication of affected area.

Pharyngitis: (far`·uhn·jai´·tis) If not due to a contraindicated disease, massage is okay.

Phlebitis: (fluh·bai´·tuhs) Local contraindication of affected area.

Phobias: See entry under Anxiety disorders.

Pinkeye: See entry under Conjunctivitis.

Plantar fasciitis: (plan´·tuhr fa`·shee·ai´·tis) Use techniques to reduce adhesions. Thoroughly massage leg muscles.

Pleurisy: (plur´·uh·see) Obtain physician clearance. If not due to a contraindicated disease, massage is okay, and treatment should focus on primary and secondary muscles of respiration.

Pleuritis: (plur´·ai·tis) See entry under Pleurisy.

Pneumoconiosis: (noo`·moh·koh`·nee·oh´·sis) Obtain physician clearance if symptoms are severe. Adjust massage to client's stamina and vitality (i.e., slower, gentler, shorter duration, assist client on and off table). Focus on primary and secondary muscles of respiration. Orient client with head lower than chest to induce positional drainage, then vibrate and percuss the ribcage.

Pneumonia: (nuh·moh´·nyuh) Massage is contraindicated during acute phase. Otherwise, obtain physician clearance. Once granted, percuss and vibrate the ribcage. Focus on the muscles of respiration.

Poliomyelitis: (poh`·lee·oh·mai`·lai´·tis) If in chronic, noninfective stage, use lighter pressure. Use techniques to reduce contractures, retain joint mobility, and loosen adhesions.

Polycystic kidney disease: Obtain physician clearance. Once granted, use lighter pressure, avoiding the abdomen.

Polycystic kidneys: See entry under Polycystic kidney disease.

Polyps: In the case of cancerous polyps, obtain physician clearance. Once granted, position client for comfort. Local massage of affected area is contraindicated if pressure causes pain.

Postherpetic neuralgia: (pohst`·her·pe´·tik nu·ral´·gee·uh) See entry under Shingles.

Postpartum depression: See entry under Anxiety disorders.

Postpoliomyelitis sequela: See entry under Poliomyelitis.

Postpoliomyelitis syndrome: See entry under Poliomyelitis.

Postpolio syndrome: Massage considerations are the same as for Poliomyelitis.

Posttraumatic stress disorders: See entry under Anxiety disorders.

Preeclampsia: Unless under strict physician supervision, massage is contraindicated. If authorized, avoid lymphatic massage.

Pregnancy: Position client for comfort and avoid deep abdominal massage. Massage is contraindicated in first trimester if client has a history of miscarriage. Avoid rocking movements if client is nauseated. Avoid prone and full supine position after eighteenth week of pregnancy. Use lighter pressure in medial thigh region and administer with an open, flat hand. Avoid heating blankets and hot packs. Elevate ankles, knees, and feet if edematous.

Pregnancy-induced hypertension: See entry under Preeclampsia.

Premenstrual syndrome: Massage is fine. Position client for comfort. Abdominal massage is contraindicated if pressure causes pain.

Pressure sore: See entry under Decubitus ulcer.

Prosopalgia: (prah`·suh·pal´·gee·uh) See entry under trigeminal neuralgia.

Prostatitis: (prah·stuh·tai´·tis) Position client for comfort and avoid abdomen if pressure causes pain.

Prostate cancer: See entry for Bladder cancer.

Psoriasis: (suh·rai´·uh·sis) Massage is fine. Avoid affected areas if pressure causes pain. Scales may dislodge during treatment.

Pulmonary edema: Massage is contraindicated if symptoms are severe or if due to congestive heart failure. Otherwise, obtain physician clearance. Once granted, position client for comfort and use lighter pressure of shorter duration.

Pulmonary embolism: Massage is contraindicated.

Pyelonephritis: (pai`·uh·loh`·ni·frai´·tis) Massage is contraindicated.

Quadriplegia: Position client for comfort and use lighter pressure in areas that lack sensation. Use techniques that increase circulation. Avoid electric vibrators, joint mobilizations, and stretches. If client uses a wheelchair, determine if treatment needs to be performed while client is in the chair.

Rabies: Massage is contraindicated.

Radiculopathy: (ruh·dik`·yuh·lah´·puh·thee) Obtain physician clearance. Once granted, use lighter pressure over affected area.

Raynaud's disease: See entry under Raynaud's syndrome.

Raynaud's syndrome: (ray·nohs´) Pressure is determined by client's pain level (lighter pressure if client is experiencing more pain; more pressure if client is experiencing less pain). Use techniques to increase local circulation, reduce stress, and relax smooth muscle. Heat and ice packs are contraindicated.

Reflex sympathetic dystrophy: Obtain physician clearance. Once granted, use lighter pressure and techniques to increase mobility, if symptoms are not severe.

Regional enteritis: (ree´·juh·nuhl en·tuh·rai´·tis) See entry under Crohn's disease.

Regional ileitis: (ree´·juh·nuhl i`·lee·ai´·tis) See entry under Crohn's disease.

Renal calculi: (ree´·nuhl kal´·kyuh·lee) See entry under Kidney stones.

Renal failure: See entry under Kidney failure.

Renal stones: See entry under Kidney stones.

Repetitive motion injury: See entries under Repetitive strain injury.

Repetitive strain injury: Tailor massage to type of RSI (see entries for carpal tunnel, thoracic outlet, etc.). Avoid area if inflamed.

Respiratory distress syndrome: Massage is contraindicated.

Rheumatoid arthritis: Massage is contraindicated during flare-ups. Otherwise, use techniques that reduce stress and increase joint mobility.

Ringworm: Massage is contraindicated.

Rosacea: (roh·zay´·shuh) Avoid hot immersion baths and use lighter pressure on affected areas.

Rubella: (roo·be´·luh) See entry under German measles.

Ruptured disk: See entry under Herniated disk.

Scabies: Massage is contraindicated.

Scars: Obtain physician clearance for recent but fully healed scars. Use cross-fiber and chucking friction and myofascial release directly on scar. Use techniques to increase muscle tone and strength, alleviate muscle spasms and tense spots, increase tissue flexibility, increase joint mobility, and counteract muscle weakness.

Sciatica: Modify treatment according to cause (e.g., herniated disk, tight piriformis muscle). Once determined, either avoid involved area or address involved musculature, using techniques to relax muscles, reduce atrophy, prevent spasms, and reduce edema.

Scleroderma: (skler`·uh·der´·muh) Obtain physician clearance. Once granted, massage is fine if symptoms are not severe. Use techniques to help reduce adhesions and increase local circulation. Passive and active stretches and joint mobilization help retain mobility.

Scoliosis: (skoh·lee·oh´·sis) If not due to a contraindicated condition, massage is okay. Position client for comfort. Focus on iliopsoas, quadratus lumborum, and paraspinal muscles. Avoid overstretching the spine.

Seasonal affective disorder: Adjust massage to client's stamina and vitality (i.e., slower, gentler, shorter duration, assist client on and off table).

Sebaceous cyst: (suh·bay´·shuhs sist´) Local contraindication of affected area.

Seborrheic dermatitis: (se·buh·ree´·ik der·muh·tai´·tis) Massage is fine, unless due to a contraindicated disease. If the latter is the case, local and possibly general massage may be contraindicated.

Seborrheic keratosis: (se`·buh·ree´·ik ka`·ruh·toh´·sis) Local contraindication of affected area.

Seizure disorders: Know and limit triggers for seizures. If seizure occurs during treatment, place client on side and provide light immobilization to prevent client from falling off table. Call 911 if seizure lasts more than 5 minutes.

Senile lentigo: (see´·nail len´·tah·goh) See entry under Age spots.

Separation: Position client for comfort. Avoid undue pressure over separated bones. Avoid joint mobilizations until client is completely healed.

Severe acute respiratory syndrome (SARS): Massage is contraindicated.

Shingles: Local contraindication of infected area. General massage is fine if client feels up to it.

Shin splints: Local contraindication if condition is acute. If chronic, massage tibialis anterior and posterior. Use RICE (rest, ice, compression, elevation) on both acute and chronic cases.

Shock: Massage is contraindicated.

Sickle cell anemia: See entry under Sickle cell disease.

Sickle cell disease: Obtain physician clearance. Once granted, avoid massage during flare-ups. If in remission, adjust massage to client's stamina and vitality (i.e., slower, gentler, shorter duration, assist client on and off table).

Sinusitis: If client has fever, massage is contraindicated. Otherwise, massage is fine. Position client for comfort; lying prone and/or using the face cradle since increases sinus congestion. Moist heat, deep ischemic pressure over the frontal and sphenoidal sinuses, and steam inhalation may help relieve congestion.

Skin cancer: See entry for Bladder cancer.

Skin tags: If area is sensitive, adjust pressure. Take care not to pull skin tags during treatment.

Slipped disk: See entry under Herniated disk.

Sore throat: See entry under Pharyngitis.

Spastic colon: See entry under Irritable bowel syndrome.

Spasticity: Obtain physician clearance if symptoms are severe. Adjust massage if sensations are impaired. Avoid joint mobilizations. Use techniques to prevent adhesions and contractures.

Spider capillaries: See entry under Telangiectasia.

Spina bifida: Obtain physician clearance if symptoms are severe. Position client for comfort. If client uses a wheelchair, determine if treatment needs to be performed while client is in the chair. Avoid lumbosacral area and forcing muscles into stretch. Use techniques to prevent contractures, prevent pressure ulcers, reduce spasticity, and reduce any edema in the legs.

Spinal cord injury: See entry for Quadriplegia.

Spondylolisthesis: (spahn`·duh·loh·lis´·thuh·sis) Massage is fine if symptoms are not severe. Use strokes to loosen tight erector spinae muscles and latissimus dorsi. Tight muscles in the area can be stretched but should not be forced.

Spondylosis: (spahn·duh·loh´·sis) Position client for comfort.

Sprain: Obtain physician clearance. Once granted, use RICE (rest, ice, compression, elevation) for the first 72 hours. Avoid stretching the injured area.

Squamous cell carcinoma: (skwah·muhs sel´ kahr`·suh·noh´·muh) See entry for Bladder cancer.

Still's disease: See entry under Rheumatoid arthritis.

Stomach cancer: See entry for Bladder cancer.

Strain: Obtain physician clearance. Once granted, use RICE (rest, ice, compression, elevation) for the first 72 hours. Then, treatment times should be of short duration and become longer as the injury heals. Avoid stretching of injured area and massage done distal to injury site. Use techniques to maintain range of motion and to prevent adhesion formation.

Stretch marks: Avoid affected areas if pressure causes pain. Use lighter pressure over affected areas.

Striae: (stri´·e) See entry under Stretch marks.

Stroke: Obtain physician clearance. Once granted, use techniques to prevent joint stiffness, decrease muscle spasticity, and address postural changes. Carefully administer joint mobilizations. Adjust massage to client's stamina and vitality (i.e., slower, gentler, shorter duration, assist client on and off table). Treatments can be gradually increased to 1 hour. Deep pressure is contraindicated.

Subdural hematoma: Massage is contraindicated.

Substance abuse: Avoid deep pressure during early stages of withdrawal.

Syncope: (sing´·kuh·pee) Massage is contraindicated.

Syphilis: Massage is contraindicated.

Systemic lupus erythematosus: See entry under Lupus.

Systemic sclerosis: See entry under Scleroderma.

Telangiectasia: (te`·lan`·jee·ek·tay´·zhee·uh) Use lighter pressure over affected area.

Temporomandibular joint dysfunction: (tem`·puh·roh·man·dib´·yuh·luhr joint´ dis·funk´·shuhn) Treat involved muscles (i.e., masseter, temporalis, medial and lateral pterygoids, trapezius, rhomboids, levator scapula, scalenes, splenius muscles, suboccipitals).

Tendinitis: Local contraindication for 72 hours if due to injury. Otherwise, use appropriate techniques on involved tendons. End session with ice.

Tetanus: Massage is contraindicated.

Thoracic outlet syndrome: Treat involved muscles (i.e., pectoralis minor, scalenes, muscles of the entire shoulder girdle and arm).

Thromboangiitis obliterans: (thrahm`·boh·an·jee·ai´·tis uh·bli´·tuh·ranz) Local contraindication of affected area if client has possibility of blood clot formation. Deep pressure is contraindicated because skin may be thin and/or painful. Heat and cold packs are contraindicated.

Thrombophlebitis: (thrahm`·boh·fluh·bai´·tis) Local massage of affected area is contraindicated. Avoid deep pressure in the inner thigh area.

Thrombosis: See entry under Thrombophlebitis.

Thrush: Massage may be contraindicated, depending on the cause. If not due to a contraindicated disease, massage is okay.

Tic douloureux: (tik´ doh´·luh·roo) See entry under Trigeminal neuralgia.

Tinea corporis: See entry under Ringworm.

Tinea cruris: (ti·nee´·uh krur´·uhs) See entry under Jock itch.

Tinea pedis: (ti·nee´·uh pee´·dis) See entry under Athlete's foot.

Tinea unguium: (ti·nee´·uh un´·gwee·uhm) See entry under Onychomycosis.

Tonsillitis: (tahn`·suh·lai´·tis) Massage is contraindicated.

Torticollis: (tohr·tuh·koh´·luhs) Focus on sternocleidomastoid, trapezius, scalenes, and the splenius muscles. Use moist heat.

Toxemia: See entry under Preeclampsia.

Transient ischemic attack: Obtain physician clearance. Once granted, use lighter pressure if client is on anticoagulant therapy. Refer to a physician if client experiences tingling, numbness, or loss of movement during or immediately after the massage session.

Trichomoniasis: (tri`·kuh·muh·nai´·uh·sis) Massage is contraindicated.

Trigeminal neuralgia: (trai·je´·muh·nuhl nu·ral´·gee·uh) Obtain physician clearance if symptoms are severe. Avoid affected area if pressure causes pain.

Tuberculosis: (tu`·buhr·kyuh·loh´·suhs) Massage is contraindicated until client is no longer infectious (physician determined). Adjust massage to client's stamina and vitality (i.e., slower, gentler, shorter duration, assist client on and off table).

Ulcerative colitis: Position client for comfort. Abdominal massage is contraindicated if pressure causes pain.

Ulcers: Position client for comfort. Abdominal massage is contraindicated if pressure causes pain.

Unipolar disorder: See entry under Anxiety disorders.

Upper respiratory infection: See entry under Common cold.

Uremia: Obtain physician clearance. Once granted, adjust massage to client's stamina and vitality (i.e., slower, gentler, shorter duration, assist client on and off table). If client bruises easily, use lighter pressure and of short duration.

Urethritis: (yuh·ri·thrai´·tis) Massage is contraindicated.

Urinary incontinence: Massage is okay. Abdominal massage is contraindicated if client is uncomfortable.

Urinary tract infection: Massage is fine, unless symptoms are severe. Abdominal massage is contraindicated if pressure causes pain.

Urticaria: (uhr·tuh·kar´·ee·uh) See entry under Hives.

Vaginal candidiasis: (va´·ji·nuhl kan`·duh·dai´·uh·sis) Massage is contraindicated during acute systemic candidiasis.

Varicella: (vahr`·uh·se´·luh) See entry under Chickenpox.

Varicose veins: Local contraindications if blood clots or inflammation is present. Otherwise, massage is fine. Elevate the legs during treatment.

Venereal warts: See entry under Genital warts.

Venous thrombosis: See entry under Thrombophlebitis.

Verruca: (vuh·roo´·kuh) See entry under Wart.

Vertigo: Obtain physician clearance. If not due to a contraindicated condition, massage is okay.

Vitiligo: (vi·tuh·lai´·goh) Massage is fine.

Volkmann's contracture: (vohlk´·muhnz` kuhn·trak´·chuhr) See entry under Dupuytren's contracture.

Wart: Local contraindication of affected area.

Whiplash: Obtain physician clearance. Once granted, rule out other prevailing disorders (i.e., vertebral luxation). Local contraindication for 72 hours after initial injury. For anterior/posterior whiplash, focus on longus colli, scalenes, splenius muscles, sternocleidomastoid, levator scapula, and upper trapezius. For lateral whiplash, focus on scalenes and sternocleidomastoid. End session with ice.

Wryneck: See entry under Torticollis.

Xerosis: (zuh·roh´·sis) Massage is fine.

This section includes a listing of the documented effects of massage. Although every effort has been made to cite reliable sources, there are varying degrees of the quality of research. Literature in massage therapy tends to lack the rigorous application of empirical research methods and oftentimes is anecdotal in nature. The reference section at the end of this book has a complete list of works cited. If you have any concerns about a particular claim, obtain the actual research and peruse the study.

Indications of Massage for Specific Conditions and for Specific Individuals

Alzheimer's disease: Massage decreased physical expressions of agitation (e.g., pacing, wandering) and improved sleep patterns.

Anemia: An increase in red blood cells and an increase in oxygen saturation in the blood suggest that massage is beneficial for individuals with anemia.

Asthma: Massage improved pulmonary functions and reduced the occurrence of asthma attacks. Peak airflows increased on average 57%. Forced vital capacity increased 24%, forced expiratory volume increased 27%, and peak expiratory flow rate increased 30%. Parents of asthmatic children reported reduced anxiety when they massaged their children.

Attention deficit hyperactivity disorder: Individuals diagnosed with attention deficit hyperactivity disorder (ADHD) who receive massage were less fidgety and hyperactive and spent more time completing assigned tasks.

Autism: Massaged autistic children spent less time in solitary play and had an increase in attention to sounds and their social relatedness to their teachers. Teachers reported that these children spent more time on task behaviors and exhibited less stereotypical behavior such as touch aversion.

Burn victims: Burn victims who were massaged experienced a decrease in pain and itching as well as reduced anxiety before débridement. Massage also lowered feelings of depression and anger.

Cancer and oncology patients: A reduction of edema, pain, anxiety, and feelings of anger and depression were reported with an improved quality of life when cancer patients had routine massages. Increased parasympathetic activity may be the underlying mechanism for these changes. The pressure stimulation associated with touch increases vagal activity, which in turn lowers sympathetic arousal and stress hormone levels. The pressure is critical because light stroking is generally aversive (much like a tickle stimulus) and does not produce these effects. Decrease in stress hormones in turn leads to enhanced immune functions. This is evidenced by an increase in lymphocyte and natural killer cell (NK) counts along with an increase of cytotoxicity of NK cells. Furthermore, massage used with antiemetic medication was more cost-effective in controlling high-dose chemotherapy-induced nausea and vomiting. Nausea and vomiting are some of the most dreaded side effects of chemotherapy. Massage proves to be beneficial in improving patient participation and compliance in high-dose chemotherapy, which offers hope for a potential cure or at least a partial remission from cancer.

Cerebral palsy: Massage promotes circulation of blood and lymph and relieves muscular tension in individuals with cerebral palsy. Increases in flexibility were also reported.

Chronic fatigue syndrome: Clients with chronic fatigue syndrome (CFS) experience reduced feelings of depression and anxiety, as well as fewer somatic symptoms such as pain and fatigue. Massage clients with CFS also reported an increase in the hours of sleep. CFS affected muscle strength; improved grip strength was also documented for clients receiving massages.

Constipation: Elimination problems were relieved through abdominal massage.

Cystic fibrosis: Children with cystic fibrosis experienced a reduction in anxiety, improved mood, decreased depression, and increased peak airflow readings when massaged.

Dementia: A decrease in the episodes of dysfunctional behavior was found in patients with dementia. Hand massage and calming music are effective interventions to reduce the level of agitation in agitated nursing home residents with dementia. Decreasing a hand massage from 10 minutes to 5 minutes resulted in less consistently observed reductions in agitation, suggesting that a 5-minute intervention is not sufficient.

Diabetes: Blood glucose levels decreased, and anxiety and depression were reduced with massage. An increase in dietary compliance was also reported.

Eating disorders: Patients with anorexia nervosa and bulimia reported a reduction of depression and anxiety, as well as improved eating habits. These individuals also reported improved mood and an increase in positive body image with regular massage treatments.

Elderly: Benefits were reported in both the persons giving and receiving massages. Individuals who gave the massages reported an improved affect; decreased anxiety, stress, and depression; and an improved lifestyle. Individuals who received massages stated that they experienced an improved mood and a decrease in anxiety, stress, and depression.

Employees: An experimental group of corporate employees exhibited improved cognitive functions as evidenced by decreased anxiety and depression, as well as increased emotional control and overall well-being. In addition, participants reported a decrease in general sleep disturbances.

Fibromyalgia: Not only were stress, anxiety, and feelings of depression reduced with massage, but decreases in pain, stiffness, fatigue, and insomnia were also documented in individuals with fibromyalgia. Massage was rated more effective than standard physical therapy or prescriptive drugs.

Headaches: Most headaches (muscular, cluster, eye strain, mental fatigue, sinus, etc.) were relieved with massage. Subjects also reported more headache-free days and less analgesic use as a result of pain reduction. In individuals with migraine headaches, the hours slept at night increased, and the amount of night wakings decreased.

High blood pressure: Massage decreased blood pressure (both systolic and diastolic readings) and helped to promote healthy lifestyle habits in patients with hypertension.

HIV positive: Both the number of natural killer cells and their ability to fight pathogens increased (cytotoxicity) after massage. This finding suggests that patients with HIV who receive regular massage will probably experience fewer opportunistic infections, such as pneumonia and other viruses that often kill them. Massage also helped individuals with HIV relax and helped to decrease their anxiety and depression.

Hospitalized and hospice patients: Postoperative pain was reduced and patients had a decline in heart rate and blood pressure, indicating decreased stress and anxiety. Hospice patients experienced the same effects.

Infants: Preterm, cocaine-exposed, HIV-exposed, and full-term infants all benefited from massage. They experienced less colic, less repetitive crying, and improved feeding habits, and gained more weight than nonmassaged infants in the same categories. Massage (tactile and kinesthetic stimulation) is safe for preterm infants and improved their hospital course. Passive forms of touch therapy have been shown to soothe young and sick infants residing in the NICU (neonatal intensive care unit). For infants who have left the NICU and have been transferred to a grower nursery, massage facilitated further weight gain and appeared to enhance neurobehavioral maturation. Massage was more effective than rocking for inducing infant sleep. Improvement in temperament, including social ability, was also observed.

Injuries: Massage speeds the healing of overuse injuries, sprains, and strains.

Insomnia: Insomnia is alleviated by inducing relaxation.

Juvenile rheumatoid arthritis: Massage reduces anxiety, stress, pain (both muscle and joint pain), and morning stiffness in children with juvenile rheumatoid arthritis.

Low back pain: Low back pain is decreased by addressing trigger points. Medical costs were reduced by about 40% along with reduced analgesic use. Massage increased range of motion and promoted relaxation. Patients reported that massage made them feel cared for, happy, physically relaxed, less anxious, calm, and restful, and gave them a feeling of closeness with the individuals who gave massages. Massage was rated more effective than standard physical therapy or prescriptive drugs.

Lung disease: For clients with chronic obstructive lung disease, massage strengthened respiratory muscles, reduced heart rate, increased oxygen saturation in blood, decreased shortness of breath, and improved pulmonary functions. Respiratory drainage is encouraged through cupping tapotement and vibration on ribcage.

Lymphedema: Swelling resulting from lymphedema was reduced with massage if it was not a result of inflammation or heart or kidney disease. Edema resulting from traumatic inflammation may be aided with techniques such as manual lymphatic drainage.

Multiple sclerosis: Individuals with multiple sclerosis who received massages experienced reduced anxiety and depression, improved self-esteem, and positive body image; they implemented changes to their lifestyle that promoted health such as exercising and stretching.

Nerve entrapment: Conditions of nerve entrapment that occur when soft tissues constrict the nerve, such as carpal tunnel syndrome, thoracic outlet syndrome, and sciatica, were relieved by release of the myofascial component.

Poor circulation: Massage improved blood circulation.

Pregnancy and postpartum: Massaged pregnant women reported fewer obstetric and postpartum complications, reduced prematurity rates, shorter and less painful labors, and fewer days in hospital after labor and delivery. When nurses, midwives, or partners massaged the pregnant or laboring women's perineal area, injury such as tearing during fetal delivery was reduced. Feelings of postpartum depression declined with massage. Depressed adolescent mothers reported less stress, anxiety, and depression. These reports were supported by a reduction in stress hormones in the blood.

Premenstrual syndrome: Massage reduced swelling, reduced pain and anxiety, and improved the mood of women experiencing premenstrual syndrome.

Psychiatric patients: Child, adolescent, and adult psychiatric patients were observed to be better adapted to a group, and the medical staff reported better clinical progress with massage treatments. A decrease in depression and anxiety was noted with reduced cortisol levels and norepinephrine blood levels and increased dopamine levels. In many individuals, decreased self-destructive behavior and improved mental health status were reported in subjects of the massaged group. With child and adolescent patients, the percentage of time in bed for which sleep occurred increased, and nighttime wakefulness decreased correspondingly.

Rheumatoid arthritis: Massage reduced trigger point formation, pain, anxiety, and morning stiffness in individuals with adult and juvenile rheumatoid arthritis (see prior entry for more information on juvenile RA).

Skin conditions: Skin problems such as mild dryness and itching were alleviated by massage as a result of the increase of sebum production and blood circulation. In children with atopic dermatitis (eczema), there was a reduction in redness and scaling.

Spinal cord injuries: Individuals with spinal cord injuries reported shorter lengths of stay in rehabilitation programs or hospital settings, improved wound healing, fewer respiratory illnesses, fewer urinary tract infections, and swifter transition to productive work. Massage also fostered a reduction in sympathetic tone through its influence on the central nervous system, allowing for a greater impact of subsequent treatments.

Stress and anxiety: Stress and anxiety are reduced by activation of the parasympathetic nervous system and promotion of the relaxation response (including individuals with posttraumatic stress syndrome).

Temporomandibular joint dysfunction: The muscular component of temporomandibular joint dysfunction (TMJD) was addressed with massage, resulting in reduced pain and dysfunction.

Effects of Massage on the Cardiovascular System

Dilates blood vessels: The body responds to massage by reflexively dilating the blood vessels. This, in turn, aids in improving blood circulation and lowering blood pressure (discussed later).

Improves blood circulation: Deep stroking improves blood circulation by mechanically assisting venous blood flow back to the heart. The increase of blood flow is comparable to that of exercise. It has been documented that local circulation increases during massage up to three times more than circulation at rest.

Creates hyperemia: Increased blood flow creates a hyperemic effect, which is often visible on the surface of the skin.

Stimulates release of acetylcholine and histamine for sustained vasodilation: These two substances are released as a result of vasomotor activity, helping to prolong vasodilation.

Replenishes nutritive materials: Another benefit of increased circulation is that products such as nutrients and oxygen are transported to the cells and tissues more efficiently.

Promotes rapid removal of waste products: Not only are nutrients brought to cells and tissues, but metabolic waste products are removed more rapidly through massage. It is often said that massage "dilutes the poisons."

Reduces ischemia: Massage reduces ischemia and ischemic-related pain. Ischemia is also related to trigger point formation and their associated pain referral patterns.

Decreases blood pressure: Blood pressure is decreased by dilation of blood vessels. Both diastolic and systolic readings decline and last approximately 40 minutes after the massage session.

Reduces heart rate: Massage decreases heart rate through activation of the relaxation response.

Lowers pulse rate: As one would expect, a reduced heart rate lowers pulse rate.

Increases stroke volume: Stroke volume is the amount of blood ejected from the left ventricle during each contraction. As the heart rate decreases, there is more time for the cardiac ventricles to fill with blood. The result is a larger volume of blood pushed through the heart with each ventricular contraction, thereby increasing stroke volume.

Increases red blood cell count: The number of functioning red blood cells (RBCs) and their oxygen-carrying capacity are increased. It is speculated that this effect is achieved by (1) promoting the spleen's discharge of RBCs, (2) recruiting excess blood from engorged internal organs into general circulation, and (3) stimulating stagnant capillary beds and returning this blood into general circulation. All three events would increase RBC count.

Increases oxygen saturation in blood: When red blood cell count rises, there is greater oxygen saturation in the blood.

Increases white blood cell count: The presence of white blood cells (WBCs) increases after massage. The body may perceive massage as a stressor (an event that the body must adapt to) and recruits additional WBCs. The increase in WBC count enables the body to more effectively protect itself against disease.

Enhances the adhesion of migrating white blood cells: The surfaces of white blood cells become more "sticky" after a massage, increasing their effectiveness.

Increases platelet count: Gentle but firm massage strokes increase the number of platelets in the blood.

Effects of Massage on the Lymphatic/Immune Systems

Promotes lymph circulation: Lymph is a fluid that moves slowly within its own system of vessels. Lymphatic circulation depends entirely on pressure from muscle contraction, from pressure changes in the thorax and abdomen during breathing, or pressure from a massage.

Reduces edema: Massage reduces edema (swelling) by promoting lymph circulation, which helps remove waste from the system more effectively than either passive range of motion or electrical muscle stimulation.

Decreases the circumference of an area affected with edema: When an area swells, there is an increase in diameter. When the swelling subsides, circumference decreases.

Decreases weight in patients with edema: Fluid retention adds weight to a patient. When edema is addressed with massage, weight is consequently reduced.

Increases lymphocyte count: Lymphocytes are types of white blood cells. This indicates that massage supports immune functions.

Increases the number and function (or cytotoxicity) of natural killer cells: Natural killer cells are also types of white blood cells. This further suggests that massage strengthens immune functions and might help individuals with immune disorders.

Effects of Massage on the Skin and Related Structures

Increases skin temperature: Warming of the skin indicates a reduction of stress and other benefits outlined below.

Improves skin condition: As superficial blood vessels dilate and circulation increases, the skin appears hyperemic. This brings added nutrients to the skin, improving the skin's condition, texture, and tone. Clinical observations have determined that massage also improves the appearance (e.g., color and texture) of the skin.

Stimulates sebaceous glands: Stimulation of the sebaceous (oil) glands causes an increase in sebum production. This added sebum improves the skin's condition.

Stimulates sudoriferous glands: Sudoriferous (sweat) gland stimulation increases insensible perspiration. Insensible perspiration is the constant evaporative cooling that occurs as microscopic beads of perspiration evaporate from the skin's surface.

Improves skin pathologies: Unless there is a condition that contraindicates massage, skin pathologies may improve by decreasing redness, reducing thickening/hardening of the skin, increasing healing of skin abrasions, and reducing itching.

Reduces superficial keloid formation: Massage applied to scar tissue helps to reduce the formation of superficial keloids in the skin and excessive scar formation in the soft tissues beneath the site of massage application.

Effects of Massage on the Nervous and Endocrine Systems

Reduces stress: Stress is reduced by activation of the parasympathetic nervous system.

Reduces anxiety: Of interest, a reduction in anxiety is noted in both the persons who received the massage and the persons who gave the massage.

Promotes relaxation: General relaxation is promoted through activation of the relaxation response. Relaxation also has a diminishing effect on pain.

Decreases beta wave activity: Associated with relaxation, a decrease in beta brainwave activity occurred during and after the massage (EEG determined).

Increases delta wave activity: Increases in delta brainwave activity are linked to sleep and to relaxation; both are promoted with massage (EEG determined).

Increase in alpha waves: Confirmed by an EEG, an increase in alpha brainwave during massage indicates relaxation.

Increases dopamine levels: Increased levels of dopamine are linked to decreased stress levels and reduced depression.

Increases serotonin levels: Increased levels of serotonin suggest a reduction of both stress and depression. It is believed that serotonin inhibits transmission of noxious signals to the brain, indicating that increased levels of serotonin may also reduce pain.

Reduces cortisol levels: Massage reduces cortisol levels by activating the relaxation response. Elevated levels of cortisol not only represent heightened stress but also inhibit immune functions.

Reduces norepinephrine levels: Massage has been proven to reduce norepinephrine, a stress hormone, which is linked to the relaxation response.

Reduces epinephrine levels: Another stress hormone, epinephrine levels are reduced with massage.

Reduces feelings of depression: Both chemical and electrophysiological changes from a negative to a positive mood were noted and may underlie the decrease in depression after massage therapy.

Decreases pain: Massage relieves local and referred pain caused by hypersensitive trigger points, presumably by increasing circulation, thereby reducing ischemia. Massage also stimulates the release of endorphins (endogenous morphine), enkephalins, and other pain-reducing neurochemicals. General relaxation brought on by massage therapy also has a diminishing effect on pain. The pressure of a massage interferes with pain information entering the spinal cord by stimulating pressure receptors, further reducing pain (gate theory). Massage interrupts the pain cycle by relieving muscular spasms, increasing circulation, and promoting rapid disposal of waste products. Massage also improves sleep patterns. During deep sleep, a substance called somatostatin is normally released. Without this substance, pain is experienced.

Reduces analgesic use: Because pain is reduced with massage, the need for pain medication is also reduced.

Activates sensory receptors: Depending on factors such as stroke choice, direction, speed, and pressure, massage can stimulate different sensory receptors and have an impact on the massage outcome. For example, cross-fiber tapotement stimulates muscle spindles, which activates muscular contraction, whereas a slow passive stretch activates Golgi tendon organs, which inhibits muscular contraction. Activation of sensory pressure receptors reduces pain.

Faster and more elaborate development of the hippocampal region of the brain: The hippocampal region is part of the limbic system and its development is related to superior memory performance.

Increases vagal activity: Increased activity of the vagal nerve lowers physiological arousal and stress hormones. A decrease in stress hormones leads to enhanced immune functions. One of the branches of the vagus nerve found to be stimulated during massage is the nucleus-ambiguus branch (i.e., "smart" branch). Stimulation of this nerve branch increases facial expression and vocalization, which reduces feelings of depression.

Right frontal EEG activation shifted to left frontal EEG activation: Right frontal EEG activation is associated with a sad affect, and left frontal EEG activation is associated with a happy affect. This implies that the client experienced an improvement of mood during the massage.

Decreases H-amplitude levels during massage: A decrease of 60% to 80% was noted. This reduction is crucial for the comfort of patients with spinal cord injuries, as it signifies a decrease of muscle cramps and spasm activity.

Effects of Massage on Muscles

Relieves muscular tension: Massage relieves muscular restrictions, tightness, stiffness, and spasms. These effects are achieved by direct pressure and by increasing circulation, resulting in more flexible, supple, and resilient muscle tissues.

Relaxes muscles: Muscles relax as massage reduces excitability in the sympathetic nervous system.

Reduces muscle soreness and fatigue: Massage enhances blood circulation, thus increasing the amount of oxygen and nutrients available to the muscles. Increased oxygen and nutrients reduce muscle fatigue and postexercise soreness. Massage promotes rapid disposal of waste products, further reducing muscle fatigue and soreness. A fatigued muscle recuperates 20% after 5 minutes of rest and 100% after 5 minutes of massage. A reduction in postexercise recovery time was indicated by a decline in pulse rate and an increase in muscle "work" capacity.

Reduces trigger point formation: Trigger point formation is greatly reduced by the pressure applied to tissues during a massage, affecting trigger points in both muscle and fascia.

Manually separates muscle fibers: Compressive strokes and cross-fiber friction strokes separate muscle fibers, reducing muscle spasms.

Increases range of motion: When muscular tension is reduced, range of motion is improved. The freedom of the joints is dictated by the freedom of the muscles.

Improves performance (balance and posture): Many postural distortions are removed when trigger points are released and muscle tension is reduced. Range of motion increases, gait becomes more efficient, and the posture is more aligned and balanced, all of which improve performance.

Improves motor skills: Massage enhances motor skills.

Lengthens muscles: Massage mechanically stretches and broadens tissue, especially when combined with joint mobilizations and stretches. These changes are detected by Golgi tendon organs, which inhibit a contraction signal, further lengthening muscles. Massage retrains the tissue *from* a contracted state *to* an elongated state, increasing resting length.

Increases flexibility: By lengthening muscles and promoting muscular relaxation, massage has also been shown to increase muscle flexibility.

Tones weak muscles: Muscle spindle activity is increased during massage strokes (e.g., tapotement, vibration). An increase in muscle spindle activity creates muscle contractions, helping tone weak muscles. This effect is particularly beneficial in cases of prolonged bed rest, flaccidity, and atrophy.

Reduces the creatine kinase activity in the blood: Creatine kinase is an enzyme that helps ensure that enough adenotriphosphate is available for muscle contraction. By reducing the activity of creatine kinase in the blood, massage indirectly helps decrease muscle contraction, thereby increasing muscle relaxation.

Improves muscular nutrition: As a result of an increase in blood-transported nutrients, massage improves muscular nutrition. This hastens muscle recovery and enables muscles to function at maximum capacity.

Decreases electromyography (EMG) readings: This signifies a decrease in neuromuscular activity and a reduction of neuromuscular complaints.

Effects of Massage on Connective Tissues

Reduces keloid formation: Massage applied to scar tissue helps to reduce keloid formation in scar tissue.

Reduces excessive scar formation: Deep massage reduces excessive scar formation, helping to create an appropriate scar that is strong yet does not interfere with the muscle's ability to broaden as it contracts.

Decreases adhesion formation: The displacement of scar tissue during massage helps to reduce formation of adhesions. This, in turn, facilitates normal, pain-free motion of the affected muscles and joints.

Releases fascial restrictions: Pressure, and the heat it produces, converts fascia from a gel-state to a sol state (thixotropy), reducing hyperplasia. Fascia loosens and melts, becoming more flexible and elastic. Softening of the fascia surrounding muscles allows them to be stretched to their fullest resting length, increasing joint range of motion.

Increases mineral retention in bone: Massage increases the retention of nutrients such as nitrogen, sulfur, and phosphorus in bones.

Promotes fracture healing: When a bone is fractured, the body forms a network of new blood vessels at the break site. Massage increases circulation around the fracture, promoting fracture healing. Increased circulation around a fracture leads to increased deposition of callus to the bone. Callus is formed between and around the broken ends of a fractured bone during healing and is ultimately replaced by compact bone.

Improves connective tissue healing: Occurring only with deep pressure massage, proliferation and activation of fibroblasts were noted. Fibroblasts stimulate the production of connective tissue, which promotes tissue healing by increasing collagen production and increasing the tensile strength of healed tissue.

Reduces surface dimpling of cellulite: Massage flattens out adipose globules located under the skin and makes the skin seem smoother. Cellulite, a type of adipose tissue, appears as groups of small dimples or depressions under the skin, caused by an uneven separation of fat globules below the skin's surface, which are displaced by manual manipulation. Massage does not reduce the amount of cellulite below the skin; instead, it temporarily alters the shape and appearance of cellulite.

Effects of Massage on the Respiratory System

Reduces respiration rate: Massage slows down the rate of respiration because of activation of the relaxation response.

Strengthens respiratory muscles: The muscles of respiration have a greater capacity to contract, helping to improve pulmonary functions.

Decreases the sensation of dyspnea: Dyspnea is shortness of breath or difficult breathing and is lessened as a result of massage.

Decreases asthma attacks: Through increased relaxation and improved pulmonary functions, the client experiences fewer asthma attacks.

Reduces laryngeal tension: Laryngeal tension may occur as a result of excessive public speaking or singing. Massage reduces the tension on the muscles of the throat.

Increases fluid discharge from the lungs: The mechanical loosening and discharge of phlegm in the respiratory tract increase with rhythmic alternating pressures. Tapotement (cupping) and vibration on the rib cage are often used to enhance this effect. Phlegm loosening and discharge are further enhanced when combined with postural drainage (promoting fluid drainage of the respiratory tract through certain body positions) and when the client is encouraged to cough.

Improves pulmonary functions: Relaxation plays a significant role in how massage improves pulmonary function, but massage also loosens tight respiratory muscles and fascia. The affected pulmonary functions are:

- ***Increased vital capacity:*** This is the amount of air that can be expelled at the normal rate of exhalation after a maximum inhalation, representing the greatest possible breathing capacity.
- ***Increased forced vital capacity:*** This is the amount of air that can be forcibly expelled after a forced inhalation.
- ***Increased forced expiratory volume:*** This is the volume of air that can be forcibly expelled after a full exhalation.
- ***Increased forced expiratory flow:*** This is the volume of air that can be forcibly expelled after a full inhalation.
- ***Improved peak expiratory flow:*** This is the greatest rate of airflow that can be achieved during forced expiration beginning with the lungs fully inflated.

Effects of Massage on the Digestive System

Promotes evacuation of the colon: By increasing peristaltic activity in the colon through abdominal massage, bowel contents move toward the anus for elimination.

Relieves constipation: Because evacuation of the colon is promoted, constipation is relieved.

Relieves colic and intestinal gas: Increased peristaltic activity also helps relieve colic and intestinal gas.

Stimulates digestion: Massage also promotes activation of the parasympathetic nervous system, which stimulates digestion.

Effects of Massage on the Urinary System

Increases urine output: Massage activates dormant capillary beds and recovers lymphatic fluids for filtration by the kidney. This, in turn, increases the frequency of urination and amount of urine produced. Massage is also relaxing. This promotes general homeostasis and increases urine output.

Promotes the excretion of nitrogen, inorganic phosphorus, and sodium chloride in urine: Levels of these metabolic wastes are elevated in urine after massage.

Miscellaneous Effects of Massage

In various research studies, the following effects were noted:

Reduces fatigue and increases vigor: Many clients experienced a sense of renewed energy after massage by taking a break from the stresses of the day.

Improves sleep patterns: When clients went to sleep, they reported a deeper sleep and felt more rested on waking.

Reduces job related and posttraumatic stress: Massage reduces many types of stress. In particular, job-related stress and posttraumatic stress decreased after massage.

Improves mood: The mental health status and mood improved in the subjects of the massaged group.

Decreases feelings of anger: Clients reported a decrease in aggression and feelings of anger with massage.

Improves body image: Massage improved body image in clients who stated having a poor body image before the massage session.

Improves self-esteem: Individuals who received and who gave massages reported enhanced self-esteem.

Promotes communication and expression: Individuals who received and gave massages reported an increase in the quantity and quality of their social interactions. They talked more freely and openly and enjoyed themselves more during these social interactions. Massage can also assist the ease of emotional expression through relaxation.

Improves lifestyle habits: After massage, clients reported improved lifestyle habits such as increased activities of daily living, fewer cups of coffee, fewer somatic symptoms, fewer doctor visits, and increased levels of exercising (walking).

Increases physical well-being: Massage enhances well-being through stress reduction and subsequent relaxation.

Reduces touch aversion and touch sensitivity: Massage given to victims of rape and spousal abuse reported a reduction in touch aversion. Hypersensitivity to touch reduced in other individuals.

Increases academic performance: A decrease in math computation time and an increase in math accuracy were noted in massage studies.

Increases mental alertness: Massage increases mental alertness by relaxing the body/mind and by removing unwanted stress.

Satisfies emotional needs: Clients reported using the therapeutic relationship to satisfy their emotional needs for attention, acceptance, caring, and nurturing touch, which were not being met through their other relationships.

Endangerment sites are areas of the body that contain superficial delicate anatomical structures that are relatively unprotected and are therefore prone to injury. These sites merit caution during treatment. Endangerment sites include such structures as nerves, blood vessels, organs, and small or prominent bony projections. The areas that these structures lie in may be treated, and often are, during a massage session. However, caution must be exercised, and the massage therapist should work slowly, lightly, and carefully when in or around these sites. Exceptions to this rule would be energy work and techniques where little or no pressure is used.

Nerves: When nerves are compressed during massage, the client may experience numbness, tingling, burning, or shooting pain. It is doubtful that this compression will damage the nerve, but it may alarm the client or make the client feel uncomfortable. If the pressure is prolonged, the client may experience a temporary loss of motor control.

Blood vessels: Pressure applied to superficial blood vessels may cause a temporary reduction in blood flow and may possibly affect blood pressure. Arteries and veins lie in proximity to each other, and caution of one generally reflects caution of the other. The massage therapist should note that many of these endangerment sites are common pulse point locations.

When massaging an area where there is a known or suspected artery, the massage therapist should apply light pressure and feel for a pulse. If a pulse is felt, prolonged pressure on the specific pulse location should be avoided.

Bony structures: Compression of certain small, fragile, or prominent bony areas may cause pain, bruising of surface tissues, and, in some cases, fracture of the bony projection.

Organs/glands: Pressure or striking movements such as percussion to the kidney or eye area may cause bruising, sharp pain, nausea, or temporary dysfunction. Swollen lymph nodes are local contraindications.

Anomalies: Any abnormal findings, such as suspicious lumps, masses, or moles are endangerment sites. Massage over these sites is a local contraindication, and the massage therapist needs to point these areas out to the client.

The following are specific areas of each type of endangerment site. All endangerment sites are bilaterally symmetrical, with the exception of those located on the midline of the body. It is important for the massage therapist to remember that he or she can and should work these areas, but to be mindful of these anatomical structures.

- **Abdomen:** The structures to be aware of regarding pressure in the abdomen are the:
  - abdominal and descending aorta
  - liver
  - linea alba
  - lumbar plexus
  - vagus nerve
  - xiphoid process
- **Axilla:** The axillary region contains several nerves and blood vessels that can become compressed during massage such as the:
  - axillary arteries
  - axillary nerves
  - brachial arteries
  - brachial plexus
  - median nerves
  - musculocutaneous nerves
  - radial nerves
  - ulnar nerves
- **Elbow:** The areas of endangerment of the elbow are the:
  - brachial arteries (antecubital)
  - cubital veins (antecubital)
  - median nerves (antecubital)
  - radial arteries (antecubital)
  - radial nerves (lateral epicondyles of the humerus)
  - ulnar arteries (antecubital)
  - ulnar nerves (medial epicondyles of the humerus—ulnar notch)

- **Face:** Direct pressure should be avoided on the:
  - eyeball
  - facial arteries (alongside the upper and lower jaw)
  - transverse facial arteries (anterior to the ear)
- **Femoral Triangle/Medial Thigh:** The borders of the femoral triangle are the gracilis, the sartorius, and the inguinal ligament. This area contains the:
  - femoral arteries
  - femoral nerves
  - great saphenous veins
  - obturator nerves
- **Low Back:** Percussion and electrical massagers should be used cautiously on the low back. Two structural areas that can be damaged are:
  - floating ribs
  - kidneys
- **Popliteal:** Located behind the knee are the:
  - common peroneal nerves
  - popliteal arteries
  - tibial nerves
- **Throat:** The throat region contains two triangular regions: the anterior and the posterior cervical triangles. The *anterior cervical triangle*, whose defining borders are the trachea, base of the mandible, and the sternocleidomastoid, contains six endangerment sites, which are the:
  - common carotid arteries
  - external carotid arteries
  - hyoid bone
  - internal jugular veins
  - thyroid gland
  - trachea
  - vagus nerves

The *posterior cervical triangle*, which has the clavicle, the sternocleidomastoid, and the trapezius as its defining borders, contains several endangerment sites. They are the:

- brachial plexus
- external jugular veins
- facial nerve (just posterior to the mandibular ramus)
- subclavian artery
- styloid processes of the temporal bone (located anterior to insertion of the sternocleidomastoid and posterior to the angle of the mandible)

Hydrotherapy is a common component of massage therapy. Hydrotherapy is used not only during treatment but also as home care for the client. Below is a list of contraindications for both the use of heat and the use of cold.

Contraindications of Heat

Acute injury
Autoimmune conditions
Clients who have an aversion to heat
Over a fresh bruise or any hemorrhage under the skin
Recent burns, including sunburn
Cardiac impairment
Cerebrovascular accident (CVA) or stroke survivor
Edematous conditions
Directly over the eyes
Fever
Hypertension or hypotension
Over injection sites that are less than 10 days old
Immediately after an injury (because of the possibility of internal bleeding, wait 72 hours)
Inflammation
Over joint prosthetics
Malignant or chronic illness
Significant obesity
Open wounds, blisters, or abrasion burns
Pectoralis angina
Phlebitis (or thrombophlebitis)
Over implanted devices such as a pacemaker
Pregnancy, with the exception of paraffin baths on hands, elbows, knees, and feet
Rosacea
Sensory impairments, individuals who cannot report subjective reactions (e.g., infants or some older people), or when the client has the inability to react appropriately to excessive temperature changes (e.g., infants or older people, people with diabetes, mentally handicapped clients, clients who have multiple sclerosis or Raynaud's syndrome)
Skin infections or rashes
Thromboangiitis obliterans
Over a tumor or cyst
Clients who are weak or debilitated

Contraindications of Cold

Arthritis
Clients who have an aversion to cold
Cerebrovascular accident (CVA) or stroke survivor
Cold or plastic allergies
Over injection sites that are less than 3 days old
Open wounds
Hypertension (cold application may cause a transient increase in blood pressure)
Over implanted devices such as a pacemaker
Pectoralis angina
Rheumatoid conditions
Sensory impairments, individuals who cannot report subjective reactions (e.g., infants or older people), or when the client has the inability to react appropriately to excessive temperature changes (e.g., infants, older people, people with diabetes, those who are mentally handicapped, clients who have multiple sclerosis or Raynaud's syndrome)
Skin infections or rashes
Thromboangiitis obliterans

Common abbreviations, symbols, prescriptive directions, medical terminology, pathologies, modalities, and findings are listed here.

Symbols or Abbreviations	Meaning
#	number
>	greater than
@	at
+	positive, plus, present, and
<	less than, minus, negative, absent
≈	approximately
↑	increase, above
2°	secondary, due to, as a result of
A&P	anterior & posterior, anatomy & physiology
a; pre	before
AAS	active assisted stretching
Abd, ABD	abduction (abdomen, abdominal)
Abs	abdomen, abdominal
Abr	abrasion
AC	acromioclavicular
ACL	anterior cruciate ligament
Add, ADD	adduction
Adh	adhesion, fibrosis
ADL	activities of daily living
AI	accidental injury
AIDS	acquired immunodeficiency syndrome
AK	above knee
ALS	amyotrophic lateral sclerosis, Lou Gehrig's disease
ANT	anterior
AOB	alcohol on breath
AROM	active ROM
aroma	aromatherapy
ASAP	as soon as possible
ASIS	anterior superior iliac spine
ASP	abnormal spine posture
BA	backache
bi	biceps
bid	twice a day
BIL	bilateral
BP	blood pressure

Symbols or Abbreviations	Meaning
BPH	benign prostatic hypertrophy
BS	bowel sounds, breathing sounds
c̄	with
c/o	complains of
C1->7	cervical vertebrae, spine
CAD	coronary artery disease
CAUD	caudal
CC	chief complaint
CEPH	cephalic
CFS	chronic fatigue syndrome
CHD	congenital heart disease, coronary heart disease, childhood disease
CHF	congestive heart failure
CNT	could not test
CON	congested
COPD	chronic obstructive pulmonary disease
CP	cerebral palsy
crep	crepitus
CST	craniosacral therapy
CSTx	continue same treatment
CTS	carpal tunnel syndrome
CV	cardiovascular
CVA	cerebrovascular accident
D/C	discontinue
DDD	degenerative disc disease
DEV	deviation
DH	dominant hand
dist.	distal
DJD	degenerative joint disease
DKA	did not keep
DM	diabetes mellitus
DOB	date of birth
DOE	dyspnea (shortness of breath) on exertion
DOI	date of injury
DP	direct pressure
DVT	deep vein thrombosis
Dx	diagnosis
ed	edema
EENT	eye, ear, nose, throat
ENT	ear, nose, throat
ES	erector spinae group

Symbols or Abbreviations	Meaning	Symbols or Abbreviations	Meaning
Eval	evaluate	LBP	low back pain
ever	eversion	LE	lower extremities
EXT	external, extension	LEV	levator scapulae
ext. rot.	external rotation	LLQ	left lower quadrant (abdomen)
FB	foreign body	LMD	local medical doctor
FH	family history	LN	lymph node
Fl up	flare up	LOC	loss of consciousness, level of consciousness
Flat	flatulence		
FLEX	flexion	lord	lordosis
FOOSH	fell on outstretched hand	LS	lumbosacral
FROM	full range of motion	LUQ	left upper quadrant (abdomen)
FT	fibrous tissue	M	murmur
ft	foot	MAEW	moves all extremities well
Fx	fracture	mas	massage
gastroc	gastrocnemius	max	maximum
GERD	gastroesophageal reflux disease	MET	muscle energy technique
GBS	Guillain Barré syndrome	MFR	myofascial release
GI	gastrointestinal	MFW	myofascial web, continuous fascial planes
GYN	gynecologic, gynecological		
HA	headache	MGF	maternal grandfather
HBP	high blood pressure	MGM	maternal grandmother
HEENT	head, eyes, ears, nose, throat	MI	myocardial infarction (heart attack)
HIV+	human immunodeficiency virus, positive		
		min	minimum
HOH	hard of hearing	MLD	manual lymphatic drainage
HPI	history of present illness	Ms	muscle, musculoskeletal
hs	at bedtime	MS	multiple sclerosis
HT	hypertonus, tension, tight muscles	MVA	motor vehicle accident
		N & V	nausea and vomiting
HTR	hypertrophy	NA	nonapplicable, no answer
Hx	history	NKA	no known allergies
ICS	intercostal space	NMT	neuromuscular therapy
IF	iliofemoral	NT	nose and throat
IHD	ischemic heart disease	O–<	recumbent
IM	intramuscular	OA	osteoarthritis
INF	inferior	OCD	obsessive compulsive disorder
INFLAM	inflammation	OTC	over-the-counter Rx
INT	internal	P & B	pain and burning
int. rot.	internal rotation	p̄; post	after
inver	inversion	PAROM	passive-assisted ROM
IP	iliopsoas	Pas Ex	passive exercise
IT	ischial tuberosity	PB	paraffin bath
ITB	iliotibial band	PE	physical examination
IV	intravenous	pecs	pectoralis major and minor
KUB	kidneys, ureters, bladder	per, /	through or by
kyph	kyphosis	PGF	paternal grandfather
L	left	PGM	paternal grandmother
L1->5	lumbar vertebrae, spine	PKD	polycystic kidney disease
Lat	lateral, left anterior thigh	PI	present illness
lats	latissimus dorsi	PID	pelvic inflammatory disease
LB	low back	PMH	past medical history

Symbols or Abbreviations	Meaning
PMS	premenstrual syndrome
PNF	proprioceptive neuromuscular facilitation
POM	pain on motion
prn	as needed, as necessary
PROM	passive ROM
PROX	proximal
PSNS	parasympathetic nervous system
Pt	patient
PT	physical therapy
PTSD	posttraumatic stress disorder
Px	prognosis, physical examination
q	every
qd	every day
qh	every hour
QL	quadratus lumborum
qod	every other day
qwk	once a week
R	right
RA	rheumatoid arthritis
RLQ	right lower quadrant (abdomen)
ROM	range of motion
ROS	review of symptoms/systems
RSD	reflex sympathetic dystrophy
RSI	repetitive strain injury
RUQ	right upper quadrant (abdomen)
Rx	prescription, drug, or medication
s̄; w/o	without
S1->5	sacral vertebrae, sacrum
SCM	sternocleidomastoid
SCS	strain, counterstrain
SFLE	stress from life experience
SFT	soft-tissue mobilization

Symbols or Abbreviations	Meaning
SI	sacroiliac
SLE	systemic lupus erythematosus
SNS	sympathetic nervous system
SOB	shortness of breath
SOBOE	shortness of breath on exercise
SP	spasm
spr	sprain
SQ	subcutaneous
st	stiffness
stat	immediately
STI	soft tissue injury
str	strain
SUP	superior, supination
SwM	Swedish massage
Sx	symptoms
T1->12	thoracic vertebrae, spine
TeP	tender point
TFL	tensor fascia lata
Ther-X	therapeutic exercise or procedure
TIA	transient ischemic attack
TMJ	temporal mandibular joint
TMJD	temporomandibular joint dysfunction
TOS	thoracic outlet syndrome
TP	trigger point
TPR	temperature, pulse, and respiration
traps	trapezius
Tx	treatment, therapy
UE	upper extremity
URI	upper respiratory infection (common cold)
UTI	urinary tract infection
VV	varicose vein
WNL	within normal limits
x	times
XFF	cross-fiber friction

Abdenour J: *TN Magazine*, Mountvale, NJ, 1999, Medical Economics Company.

American Massage Therapy Association: *Code of Ethics*, Evanston, Ill, 1994.

Applegate EJ: *The anatomy and physiology learning system*, ed 2, Philadelphia, 2000, WB Saunders.

Barnes L: Cryotherapy—putting injury on ice, *Physician Sportsmed* 7:130-136, 1979.

Barr JS, Taslitz N: Influence of back massage on autonomic functions, *Phys Ther* 50:1679-1691, 1970.

Barstow C: *Tending body and spirit: massage and counseling with elders*, Boulder, Co, 1985, Author.

Bass E, Davis L: *The courage to heal*, Philadelphia, 1988, Harper & Row.

Beeken JE et al: The effectiveness of neuromuscular release massage therapy in five individuals with chronic obstructive lung disease, *Clin Nurs Res* 7:309-325, 1998.

Bell AJ: Massage and the physiotherapist, *Physiotherapy*. JCSP, 1964.

Bernal GR: How to calm children through massage, *Childhood Educ* 74: 34-42, 1997.

Bodian M: Use of massage following lid surgery, *Eye, Ear, Nose, Throat Monthly*: 542-547, 1969.

Boltn R: *People skills*, New York, 1979, Simon & Schuster, Inc.

Bonica JJ: The management of myofascial pain syndromes, *Phys Ther Rev* 39: 1959.

Burch S: *Holistic pathology for body-centered therapies*, Lawrence, Kans, 2002, Health Positive! Publishing.

Burch S: *Recognizing health and illness: pathophysiology for massage therapy and bodyworks*, ed 2, Lawrence, Kans, 2002, Health Positive! Publishing.

Burley-Allen M: *Listening: the forgotten skill*, New York, 1995, John Wiley & Sons.

Cady SH, Jones GR: Massage therapy as a workplace intervention for reduction of stress, *Percept Mot Skills* 84:157-158, 1997.

Chaitow L: *Palpation skills: assessment and diagnosis through touch*, New York, 2000, Churchill Livingstone.

Chaitow L: *Soft tissue manipulation*, Rochester, Vermont, 1988, Healing Arts Press.

Chaitow L, DeLany JW: *Clinical application of neuromuscular techniques*, vols 1 and 2, New York, 2001, Churchill Livingstone.

Charting made incredibly easy! Springhouse, Pa, 1998, Springhouse Corp.

Cherkin DC et al: Randomized trial comparing traditional Chinese medical acupuncture, therapeutic massage, and self-care education for chronic low back pain, *Arch Intern Med* 161:1081-1088, 2001.

Consumer Reports: The mainstreaming of alternative medicine, *Consumer Reports Magazine* 2000.

Coward DD: Lymphedema prevention and management knowledge in women treated for breast cancer, *Oncol Nurs Forum* 26:1047-1053, 1999.

Cox N, Lawrence C: *Diagnostic problems in dermatology*, St Louis, 1998, Mosby.

Curties D: *Breast massage*, Moncton, New Brunswick, Canada, 1999, Curties-Overzet Publications, Inc.

Curties D: *Massage therapy and cancer*, Moncton, New Brunswick, Canada, 1999, Curties-Overzet Publications, Inc.

Cuthbertson DP: Effects of massage on metabolism: a survey, *Glasgow Med J* 131:1933.

Cyriax J: Treatment by manipulation, massage, and injection. In *Textbook of orthopedic medicine*, vol 2, ed 11, London, 1984, Bailliere-Tindall.

D'Ambrogio KJ, Roth GB: *Positional release therapy: assessment & treatment of musculoskeletal dysfunction*, Philadelphia, 1997, Mosby.

Damjanov I: *Pathophysiology for the health-related professions*, ed 2, Philadelphia, 2000, WB Saunders.

Davis NM: *Medical abbreviations: 7000 conveniences at the expense of communications and safety*, ed 5, Huntington Valley, Pa, 1990, Neil M. Davis Associates.

De Domenico G, Wood E: *Beard's massage*, Philadelphia, 1997, WB Saunders.

Dennis W, Pergrouhi N: Infant development under environmental handicap, *Psychol Monogr General and Applied* 71: 1957.

Despard LL: *Textbook of massage and remedial gymnastics*, ed 3, New York, 1932, Oxford University Press.

Diego M et al: Massage therapy effects on immune function in adolescents with HIV, *Int J Neurosci* 106: 2001.

Diego M et al: Spinal cord injury benefits from massage therapy, Manuscript submitted for publication, 1998.

Dolan DW: *Objective structural findings in massage therapy: key to insurance reimbursement & specialty physician referrals*, Jacksonville, Fla, 1995, Advanced Therapeutics America.

Dorland's electronic medical dictionary, ed 29, Philadelphia, 2000, WB Saunders.

Drez D: *Therapeutic modalities for sports injuries*, St Louis, 1986, Times Mirror/Mosby College Publishing.

Eisenberg DM, et al: Trends in alternative medicine use in the United States, 1990-1997: results of a follow-up national survey, *JAMA* 280:1569-1575, 1998.

Escalona A, Field T, Cullen C: Behavior problem preschool children benefit from massage therapy, *Early Child Development and Care*, In Review, 2001.

Evans P: The healing process at a cellular level: a review, *Physiotherapy* JCSP, 66: 1980.

Expert 10-minute physical examination, St Louis, 1997, Mosby.

Falconer J: Being of service, *Massage and Bodywork: Nurturing Body, Mind, and Spirit* Feb/Mar:132-137, 2002.

Fassbender HG: *Pathology of rheumatic diseases,* New York, 1975, Springer-Verlag.

Ferell-Torry AT, Glick OJ: The use of therapeutic massage as a nursing intervention to modify anxiety and the perception of cancer pain, *Cancer Nurs* 16:93-101, 1993.

Field T: *Touch in early development,* Hillsdale, NJ, 1995, Erlbaum.

Field T: *Touch therapy,* St Louis, 2000, Churchill Livingstone.

Field T, Grizzle N, Scafidi F, Schanberg S: Massage and relaxation therapies' effects on depressed adolescent mothers, *Adolescence* 31:903-911, 1996.

Field T et al: Massage therapy for infants of depressed mothers, *Infant Behavior and Development* 19: 1996.

Field T et al: Children with asthma have improved pulmonary functions after massage therapy, *J Pediatr* 132: 1998.

Field T et al: Sexual abuse effects are lessened by massage therapy, *J Bodywork Movement Ther* 1:607-617, 1997.

Field T et al: Pregnant women benefit from massage therapy, *J Psychosom Obstet Gynecol* 19:31-38, 1999.

Field T et al: Massage therapy lowers glucose levels in children with diabetes mellitus, *Diabetes Spectrum* 10: 237-239, 1997.

Field T, Hernandez-Reif M, Seligman S: Juvenile rheumatoid arthritis: benefits from massage therapy, *J Pediatr Psychol* 22:607-617, 1997.

Field T et al: Labor pain is reduced by massage therapy, *J Psychosom Obstet Gynecol* 18:286-291, 1997.

Field T et al: Elder retired volunteers benefit from giving massage therapy to infants, *J Appl Gerontol* 17: 1998.

Field T et al: Massage therapy reduces anxiety and enhances EEG pattern of alertness and math computations, *Int J Neurosci* 86:197-205, 1996.

Field T et al: Autistic children's attentiveness and responsively improved after touch therapy, *J Autism Dev Disord* 27:333-338, 1997.

Field T et al: Massage reduces anxiety in child and adolescent psychiatric patients, *J Am Acad Child Adolesc Psychiatry* 31:125-131, 1992.

Field T et al: Postburn itching, pain, and psychological symptoms are reduced with massage therapy, *J Burn Care Rehabil* 21: 2000.

Field T et al: Burn injuries benefit from massage therapy, *J Burn Care Rehabil* 19:241-244, 1998.

Field T et al: Job stress reduction therapies, *Altern Ther Health Med* 3:54-56, 1997.

Field T, Quintino O, Hernandez-Rief M, Koslovsky G: Adolescents with attention deficit hyperactivity disorder benefit from massage therapy, *Adolescence* 33:103-108, 1998.

Field T et al: Bulimic adolescents benefit from massage therapy, *Adolescence* 33:555-563, 1998.

Field T, Seligman S, Scafidi F: Alleviating posttraumatic stress in children following Hurricane Andrew, *J Appl Dev Psychol* 17: 1996.

Field T et al: Chronic fatigue syndrome: massage therapy effects on depression and somatic symptoms in chronic fatigue, *J Chronic Fatigue Syndr* 3:43-51, 1997.

Fraser J, Kerr JR: Psychophysiological effects of back massage on elderly institutionalized patients, *J Adv Nurs* 18:238-245, 1993.

Frazier MS, Drzymkowski JW: *Essentials of human diseases and conditions,* ed 2, Philadelphia, 2000, WB Saunders.

Garner DM, Olmsted MP, Polivy J: *Anorexia nervosa: recent developments in research,* New York, 1983, Alan R. Liss.

Gehlsen GM, Ganion LR, Helfst R: Fibroblast responses to variation in soft tissue mobilization pressure, *Med SciSports Exerc* 31:531-535, 1999.

Goldberg J, Seaborne D, Sullivan S: The effects of therapeutic massage on H–reflex amplitude in persons with a spinal cord injury, *Phys Ther* 74:728-737, 1994.

Goodman C, Boissommault W, Fuller K: *Pathology: implications for the physical therapist,* ed 2, Philadelphia, 2003, WB Saunders.

Gould BE: *Pathophysiology for the health-related professionals,* ed 2, Philadelphia, 2002, WB Saunders.

Grafelman T: *Graf's anatomy and physiology guide for the massage therapist,* Aurora, Co, 1998, D.G. Publishing.

Habif T, Campbell J, Quitadamo M, Zug K: *Skin disease: diagnosis and treatment,* St Louis, 2001, Mosby.

Hammer WI: The use of transverse friction massage in the management of chronic bursitis of the shoulder and hip, *J Manipulative Physiol Med* 69:107-111, 1993.

Hart S et al: Anorexia nervosa symptoms are reduced by massage therapy, *J Treatment Prevention* 9: 2001.

Helm K, Marks J Jr: *Atlas of differential diagnosis in dermatology,* New York, 1998, Churchill Livingstone.

Herlihy B, Maebius N: *The human body in health and illness,* ed 2, Philadelphia, 2003, WB Saunders.

Hernandez-Reif M et al: Cystic fibrosis symptoms are reduced with massage therapy intervention, *J Pediatr Psychol* 151:183-199, 1999.

Hernandez-Reif M et al: High blood pressure and associated symptoms were reduced by massage therapy, *J Bodywork Movement Ther* 4: 2000.

Hernandez-Reif M et al: Low back pain is reduced and range of motion improved after massage therapy, *Int J Neurosci* 106: 2001.

Hernandez-Reif M et al: Massage therapy for breast cancer, Manuscript submitted for publication, 1998.

Hernandez-Reif M et al: Migraine headaches are reduced by massage therapy, *Int J Neurosci* 96:1-11, 1998.

Hernandez-Reif M et al: Multiple sclerosis patients benefit from massage therapy, *J Bodywork Movement Ther* 2:168-174, 1998.

Hernandez-Reif M et al: Premenstrual syndrome symptoms are relieved by massage therapy, *J Psychosom Obstet Gynecol* 21: 2000.

Hillard D: Massage for the seriously mentally ill, *J Psychosoc Nurs* 33:29-30, 1995.

Holland B, Pokorny M: Slow stroke back massage: its effect on patients in a rehabilitation setting, *Rehabil Nurs* 26:182-186, 2001.

Honeyman U: *Pathophysiology for massage technicians: a companion to the Merck manual,* Corvallis, Oregon, 1995, Author.

Hoppenfeld S: *Physical examination of the spine and extremities,* Norwalk, Conn, 1976, Appleton-Century-Crofts.

Hovind H, Nielsen SL: Effect of massage on blood flow in skeletal muscle, *Scand J Rehabil Med* 6:74-77, 1974.

Hulme J, Waterman H, Hillier VF: The effect of foot massage on patients' perception of care following laparoscopic sterilization as day case patients, *J Adv Nurs* 30:460-468, 1999.

Ignatiavicius DD, Bayne MV: *Medical-surgical nursing: a nursing process approach,* Philadelphia, 1991, WB Saunders.

Ironson G et al: Massage therapy is associated with enhancement of the immune system's cytotoxic capacity, *Int J Neurosci* 84:205-218, 1996.

Jacob S, Francone C: *Elements of anatomy and physiology,* Philadelphia, 1989, WB Saunders.

Jacobs M: Massage for the relief of pain: anatomical and physiological considerations, *Phys Ther Rev* 40: 1960.

Jancin B: Massage effective in treating chronic low back pain, *Family Practice News* 29: 1999.

Johnson R: Perineal massage for the prevention of perineal trauma in childbirth, *Lancet* 355:250-251, 2000.

Jones NA, Field T: Massage and music therapies attenuate frontal EEG asymmetry in depressed adolescents, *Adolescence* 34:529-534, 1999.

Juhan D: *Job's body, a handbook for bodyworkers,* Barrington, NY, 1987, Station Hill Press.

Kendall FP, McCreary E, Provance PG: *Muscle testing and function,* ed 4, Baltimore, 1993, Williams and Wilkins.

Kim EJ, Buschmann MT: The effect of expressive physical touch on patients with dementia, *Int J Nurs Stud* 36:235-243, 1999.

Klafs C, Arnheim DD: *Modern principles of athletic training,* St Louis, 1981, Mosby.

Knight K: *Cryotherapy: theory, technique and physiology,* Chattanooga, 1985, Chattanooga Corporation.

Kresge CA: Massage and sports. In *Sports medicine, fitness, training, injuries,* Baltimore, 1987, Urban and Schwarzenberg.

Krieger D: Therapeutic touch: the imprimatur of nursing, *Am J Nurs* 5:784-787, 1975.

Krusen FH: *Physical medicine,* Philadelphia, 1941, WB Saunders.

Larson E, Mayur T, Laughon BA: Influence of two hand washing frequencies on reduction in colonizing flora with three products used by health care personnel, *Am J Infect Control* 1989.

Leibold G: *Practical hydrotherapy,* Wellingborough, England, 1980, Thorson Publishers Limited.

Leivadi S, Hernandez-Reif M, Field T: Massage therapy and relaxation effects on university dance students, *J Dance Sci* 3:108-112, 1999.

Lindrea KB, Stainton MC: A case study of infant massage outcomes, *Am J Matern/Child Nurs* 25:95-99, 2000.

Little L, Porche DJ: Manual lymph drainage, *J Assoc Nurses AIDS Care* 9:78-81, 1998.

Louisiana State Department of Social Services: *Uniform federal accessibility standards accessibility checklist,* United States Architectural and Transportation Barriers Compliance Board, 1995.

Loving J: *Massage therapy: theory and practice,* Stanford, Conn, 1998, Appleton & Lange.

Lowe WW: *Functional assessment in massage therapy,* Corvallis, Oregon, 1995, Pacific Orthopedic Massage.

Lucia SP, Richard JF: Effects of massage on blood platelet production, *Proc Soc Exp Biol Med* 1933.

Lundeberg T: Long-term results of vibratory stimulation as a pain relieving measure for chronic pain, *Pain* 20:153-158, 1984.

Lundeberg T et al: Effect of vibratory stimulation on experimental and clinical pain, *Scand J Rehabil Med* 19:153-158, 1988.

Lundeberg T et al: Vibratory stimulation compared to placebo in alleviation of pain, *Scand J Rehabil Med* 19: 1987.

MacDonald G: Easing the chemotherapy experience with massage, *Massage Magazine* 84:85-91, 2000.

MacDonald G: *Medicine hands: massage therapy for people with cancer,* Tallahassee, 1999, Findhorn Press.

Mackey B: Massage therapy and reflexology awareness, *Nurs Clin North Am* 36:159-170, 2001.

Mathias M: Personal communication, 1998.

McConnellogue K: The courage to touch: massage and cancer, *Massage Bodywork: Nurturing Body, Mind, and Spirit,* 12-20, 2000.

McKay M, Davis M, Fanning P: *Messages: the communication skills book,* Oakland, Calif, 1987, New Harbinger Publications.

McKechnie A et al: Anxiety states: a preliminary report on the value of connective tissue massage, *J Psychosom Res* 27:125-129, 1983.

Meek S: Effects of slow stroke back massage on relaxation in hospice clients, *IMAGE: Journal of Nursing Scholarship* 25:17-21, 1993.

Mellion MB: *Sportsmedicine secrets,* Philadelphia, 1994, Hanley and Belfus, Inc.

Mennell JB: *Physical treatment,* ed 5, Philadelphia, 1945, Blakiston.

The Merck manual of diagnosis and therapy, Whitehouse Station, NJ, 1999, Merck Research Laboratories.

Mitchell JK: *Massage and exercise in system of physiological therapeutics,* Philadelphia, 1904, Blakiston.

Mock HE: Massage in surgical cases. *American Medical Association handbook of physical medicine,* Chicago, 1945, Council of Physical Medicine.

Modi N, Glover J: Massage therapy for preterm infants, Research paper presented at a Touch Research Symposium, April 1995.

Morelli M, Seaborne DE, Sullivan J: Changes in H reflex amplitude during massage of triceps surae in healthy subjects, *J Orthop Sports Phys Ther* 12:55-59, 1990.

Morelli M, Seaborne DE, Sullivan J: H-reflex modulation during manual muscle massage of human triceps surae, *Arch Phys Med Rehabil* 72:915-919, 1991.

Mosby's guide to physical examination, ed 54, St Louis, 2003, Mosby.

Mosby's medical, nursing, and allied health dictionary, ed 4, St Louis, 1994, Mosby.

Mosby's medical, nursing, and allied health dictionary, ed 6, St Louis, 2002, Mosby.

Myers TW: *Anatomy trains: myofascial meridians for manual and movement therapists,* New York, 2001, Churchill Livingstone.

National Association for Nurse Massage Therapists: *Standards of Practice,* February 16, 1992.

National Certification Board of Massage Therapy: *Code of Ethics,* McLean, Va, 1995.

Netter FH: *Atlas of human anatomy,* ed 2, Teterboro, NJ, 2000, ICON Learning Systems.

Newton D: *Pathology for massage therapists,* ed 2, Portland, 2001, Simran Publications.

Nikola RJ: *Creatures of water,* Salt Lake City, 1997, Europa Therapeutic.

Nishiyama S, Inoue S, Ueki H, Monk B: *Atlas of regional dermatology: diagnosis and treatment,* St Louis, 2001, Mosby.

Nixon N et al: Expanding the nursing repertory: the effectiveness of massage in postoperative pain, *Aust J Adv Nurs* 14:21-26, 1997.

Nordschow M, Bierman W: Influence of manual massage on muscle relaxation: effects on trunk flexion, *Phys Ther* 42:653-657, 1962.

Ogg S: Lafayette General Hospital, Lafayette, Louisiana, 1997, personal communication.

Ottoson D, Ekblom AT, Hansson P: Vibratory stimulation for the relief of pain of dental origin, *Pain* 10:37-45, 1981.

Pemberton R: Physiology of massage. In *American Medical Association handbook of physical therapy,* ed 3, Chicago, 1939, Council of Physical Therapy.

Persad RS: *Massage therapy and medication: general treatment principles,* Toronto, 2002, Toronto Press.

Premkumar K: *Anatomy and physiology: the massage connection,* ed 2, Baltimore, 2004, Lippincott Williams & Wilkins.

Premkumar K: *Pathology A to Z: a handbook for massage therapists,* Calgary, Canada, 2002, VanPub Books.

Preyde M: Effectiveness of massage therapy for subacute low-back pain: a randomized controlled trial, *Can Medl Assoc J* 162:1815-1820, 2000.

Prudden B: *Pain erasure,* New York, 1980, Random House.

Puustjarvi K, Pontinen PJ: The effects of massage in patients with chronic tension headaches, *Acupunct Electrother Res Int J* 15: 1990.

Reed B, Held JM: Effects of sequential connective tissue massage on autonomic nervous system of middle-aged and elderly adults, *Physical Therapy* 68:1231-1234, 1988.

Reese NB: *Muscle and sensory testing,* Philadelphia, 1999, WB Saunders.

Rich GJ: *Massage therapy: the evidence for practice,* St Louis, 2002, Mosby.

Richards A: Hands on help, *Nursing Times* 94: 1998.

Rodenburg JB et al: Warm-up, stretching, and massage diminish harmful effects of eccentric exercise, *Int J Sports Med* 15: 1994.

Rogeness GA, Javors MA, Pliszka SR: Neurochemistry and child/adolescent psychiatry, *Am Acad Child Adolesc Psychiatry* 31: 1992.

Rounseville C: Phantom limb pain: the ghost that haunts the amputee, *Orthop Nurs* 11(2):67-71, 1992.

Rowe M, Alfred D: The effectiveness of slow stroke massage in diffusing agitated behaviors in individuals with Alzheimer's disease, *J Gerontol Nurs* 25(6):22-34, 1999.

Rubino J: *Been there done that,* Charlottesville, VA, 1997, Upline Press.

St. John P: *St. John Neuromuscular Therapy Seminars, Manual I.* Largo, Fla, 1995.

Salvo S: *Massage therapy: principles and practice,* ed 2, Philadelphia, 2003, WB Saunders.

Samples P: Does sports massage have a role in sports medicine? *The Physician and Sportsmedicine* 15: 1987.

Sansone P, Schmitt L: Providing tender touch massage to elderly nursing home residents: a demonstration project, *Geriatr Nurs* 21:303-308, 2000.

Schachner L et al: Atopic dermatitis symptoms decrease in children following massage therapy, *Pediatc Dermatol* 15: 1998.

Schanberg S: Genetic basis for touch effects. In *Touch in early development,* Hillsdale, NJ, 1994, Erlbaum.

Scott D et al: The antiemetic effect of clinical relaxation: report of an exploratory pilot study, *J Psychosoc Oncol* 1:71-83, 1983.

Scull CW: Massage: physiological basis, *Arch Phys Med* 1945.

Shealy NC: *Alternative medicine: the complete family guide,* Versailles, Ky, 1996, Rand McNally.

Simons DG, Travell JG, Simons LS: *Myofascial pain and dysfunction, the trigger point manual,* vols 1 and 2, ed 2, Philadelphia, 1999, Lippincott Williams and Wilkins.

Smith L et al: The effects of athletic massage on delayed onset muscle soreness, creatine kinase, and neutrophil count: a preliminary report, *J Orthop Sports Phys Ther* 19(2):93-99, 1994.

Sohen-Moe C: Taking care of business: the ultimate client interview. *Massage Therapy J* 133-136, 1996.

Starlanyl D, Copeland ME: *Fibromyalgia & chronic myofascial pain: a survival manual,* ed 2, Oakland, Calif, 2001, New Harbinger Publications, Inc.

Stewart K: Massage for children with cerebral palsy, *Nursing Times* 2(50), 2000.

Strong J, Unruh AM, Wright A, Baxter GD: *Pain: a textbook for therapists,* New York, 2002, Churchill Livingstone.

Successful business handbook, Evergreen, Col, 2001, Associated Bodywork & Massage.

Sullivan SJ: Does massage decrease laryngeal tension in a subject with complete tetraplegia? *Percept Mot Skills* 84:169-170, 1997.

Sullivan SJ et al: Effects of massage on alpha motoneuron excitability, *Phys Ther* 71:555-560, 1991.

Sunshine W et al: Fibromyalgia benefits from massage therapy and transcutaneous electrical stimulation, *J Clin Rheumatol* 2:18-22, 1997.

Taber's cyclopedic medical dictionary, ed 13, Philadelphia, 1977, FA Davis.

Tappan FM, Benjamin PJ: *Tappan's handbook of healing massage techniques*, Lahore, NJ, 1998, Appleton and Lange.

Tepperman PS, Devilin M: Therapeutic heat and cold: a practitioner's guide, *Postgrad Med* 73:69-76, 1983.

Thibodeau G, Patton K: *Structure and function of the body*, ed 11, St Louis, 2000, Mosby.

Thibodeau G, Patton K: *The human body in health and disease*, ed 2, St Louis, 1977, Mosby.

Thompson DL: *Hands heal: documentation for massage therapy*, ed 2, Seattle, 2001, Lippincott Williams & Wilkins.

Torres LS: *Basic medical techniques and patient care for radiologic technologies*, Philadelphia, 1993, JB Lippincott.

Tortora GJ: *Introduction to the human body: the essentials of anatomy and physiology*, ed 3, New York, 1994, HarperCollins.

Tortora GJ, Grabowski SR: *Principles of anatomy and physiology*, ed 10, New York, 2003, John Wiley and Sons.

Touch training manual, Evergreen, Col, 1988, Associated Bodywork and Massage.

Travel J: Referred pain from skeletal muscles, *NY State J Med* 55: 1955.

Travell JG, Simons D: *Myofasical pain and dysfunction, the trigger point manual*, Baltimore, 1983, Williams & Wilkins.

Van Der Riet P: Effects of therapeutic massage on preoperative anxiety in a rural hospital: Part 1 and Part 2, *Aust J Rural Health* 1:17-21, 1993.

Vickers A, Zollman C: Massage therapies, *Br Med J* 319:7219, 1999.

Voss DE, Ionta MK, Myers BJ: *Proprioceptive neuromuscular facilitation*, Philadelphia, 1985, Harper & Row.

Wakim KG: *Manipulation, traction and massage*, New York, 1976, Robert E. Krieger.

Wakim KG et al: The effects of massage on the circulation in normal and paralyzed extremities, *Arch Phys Med* 30:135-144, 1949.

Wall PD, Melzack R: Pain mechanisms: a new theory, *Science* 150:971-979, 1965.

Walton T: Clinical thinking and cancer, *Massage Therapy J* Fall:133-137, 2000.

Weeks VD, Travel J: Postural vertigo due to trigger areas in the sternocleidomastoid muscle, *J Pediatr* 47: 1955.

Weidner N: Personal communication, 2003.

Werner R: *A massage therapist's guide to pathology*, ed 2, Philadelphia, 2002, Lippincott Williams and Wilkins.

Williams D: Touching cancer patients, *Massage Magazine* 84:74-79, 2000.

Williams RE: *The road to radiant health*, College Place, Wash, 1977, Color Press.

Zeitlin D et al: Immunological effects of massage therapy during academic stress, *Psychosom Med* 62:83-84, 2000.

CHAPTER 1

Baran R, Dawber RPR, Levene GM: *Color atlas of the hair, scalp, and nails,* London, 1992, Mosby-Wolfe. *1-8*

Centers for Disease Control and Prevention. *1-1, 1-2*

Copstead LC, Banasik JL: *Pathophysiology: biological and behavioral perspectives,* ed 2, Philadelphia, 2000, WB Saunders. *1-12*

Cox NH, Lawrence CM: *Diagnostic problems in dermatology,* St Louis, 1998, Mosby. *1-7, 1-9, 1-13, 1-14, 1-15, 1-16*

Hart CA, Broadhead RL: *Color atlas of pediatric infectious diseases,* London, 1992, Mosby-Wolfe. *1-6*

Kamal A, Brockelhurst JC: *Color atlas of geriatric medicine,* ed 2, 1991, Mosby. *1-3 (Courtesy Dr. RH MacDonald.)*

McLaren DS: *Color atlas and text of diet-related disorders,* London, 1992, Mosby-Wolfe. *1-4, 1-5*

Salvo S: *Massage therapy: principles and practice,* ed 2, Philadelphia, 2003, WB Saunders. *1-17, 1-18*

Stoy WA: *Mosby's first responder textbook,* St Louis, 1997, Mosby. *Table 1-2*

Zitelli BJ, Davis HW: *Atlas of pediatric physical diagnosis,* ed 4, St Louis, 2002, Mosby. *1-10*

Zitelli BJ, Davis HW: *Atlas of pediatric physical diagnosis,* ed 3, St Louis, 1997, Mosby. *1-11 (Courtesy Dr. Ellen Wald, Children's Hospital of Pittsburgh.)*

CHAPTER 2

Bloom A, Ireland J: *Color atlas of diabetes,* ed 2, London, 1992, Mosby-Wolfe. *2-11*

Canobbio MM: *Cardiovascular disorders,* St Louis, 1990, Mosby. *2-12*

Cox NH, Lawrence CM: *Diagnostic problems in dermatology,* St Louis, 1998, Mosby. *2-7*

Dockery GL: *Cutaneous disorders of the lower extremity,* Philadelphia, 1997, WB Saunders. *2-13*

du Vivier A: *Atlas of clinical dermatology,* ed 2, London, 1993, Gower Medical Publishing. *2-9*

Frazier MS, Drzymkowski JW: *Essentials of human diseases and conditions,* ed 2, Philadelphia, 2000, WB Saunders. *2-19*

Herlihy B, Maebius N: *The human body in health and illness,* ed 2, Philadelphia, 2003, WB Saunders. *2-16, 2-17*

Kamal A, Brockelhurst JC: *Color atlas of geriatric medicine,* ed 2, St Louis, 1991, Mosby. *2-8*

Lawrence CM, Cox NH: *Physical signs in dermatology: color atlas and text,* St Louis, 1993, Mosby. *2-14*

Lemmi FO, Lemmi CAE: *Physical assessment findings CD-ROM,* Philadelphia, 2000, WB Saunders. *2-32*

Salvo S: *Massage therapy: principles and practice,* ed 2, Philadelphia, 2003, WB Saunders. *2-2, 2-3, 2-5, 2-6, 2-20, 2-21, 2-25, 2-26*

Seidel H: *Mosby's guide to physical examination,* ed 5, St Louis, 2003, Mosby. *2-23, 2-27, 2-28, 2-29, 2-30, 2-31*

Seidel H: *Mosby's guide to physical examination,* ed 4, St Louis, 1999, Mosby. *2-18*

Zitelli BJ, Davis HW: *Atlas of pediatric physical diagnosis,* ed 4, St Louis, 2002, Mosby. *2-10*

Zitelli BJ, Davis HW: *Atlas of pediatric physical diagnosis,* ed 3, St Louis, 1997, Mosby. *2-15, 2-24*

CHAPTER 3

Baran R, Dawher RPR, Levene GM: *Color atlas of the hair, scalp, and nails,* London, 1991, Mosby-Wolfe. *Box 3-2 (fine scaling), 3-53*

Callen J et al: *Color atlas of dermatology,* ed 2, Philadelphia, 2000, WB Saunders. *3-5, 3-8, 3-25, 3-32, 3-36, 3-43, 3-49, 3-52, 3-54, 3-56, 3-59, 3-60, 3-62, 3-67*

Callen J et al: *Color atlas of dermatology,* Philadelphia, 1993, WB Saunders. *3-20, 3-23, 3-37 A, 3-66 A, 3-71 A*

Cerio R, Jackson WF: *A colour atlas of allergic skin disorders,* London, 1992, Mosby-Wolfe. *3-22*

Cohen BA: *Atlas of pediatric dermatology,* St Louis, 1993, Mosby. *Box 3-2 (erosion)*

Cotran RS, Kumar V, Collins T: *Robbins pathologic basis of disease,* ed 6, Philadelphia, 1999, WB Saunders. *3-37 B, 3-47*

Cox NH, Lawrence CM: *Diagnostic problems in dermatology,* St Louis, 1998, Mosby. *3-14 B, 3-16, 3-17*

Damjanov I: *Pathology for the health-related professions,* ed 2, Philadelphia, 2000, WB Saunders. *3-63*

Dockery GL: *Cutaneous disorders of the lower extremity,* Philadelphia, 1997, WB Saunders. *3-41*

Farrar WE et al: *Infectious diseases,* ed 2, London, 1992, Gower Medical Publishing. *Box 3-2 (wheal, vesicles caused by varicella)*

Frazier MS, Drzymkowski JW: *Essentials of human diseases and conditions,* ed 2, Philadelphia, 2000, WB Saunders. *3-9, 3-40 A, 3-40 C, 3-40 E, 3-40 G*

Goldman MP, Fitzpatrick RE: *Cutaneous laser surgery: the art and science of selective photothermolysis,* St Louis, 1994, Mosby. *Box 3-2 (hypertrophic nodule, hypertrophic scar, abrasion from tree branch)*

Gould B: *Pathophysiology for the health professions,* ed 2, Philadelphia, 2002, WB Saunders. *3-15 (Courtesy Dr. M McKenzie, Toronto.)*

Habif T, Campbell J, Quitadamo M, Zug K: *Skin disease: diagnosis and treatment,* St Louis, 2001, Mosby. *3-6, 3-7, 3-13, 3-14 A, 3-18, 3-24, 3-27, 3-29, 3-30, 3-31, 3-33, 3-34, 3-35, 3-42, 3-44, 3-46, 3-48, 3-50, 3-51, 3-55, 3-58, 3-68, 3-69*

Habif T: *Clinical dermatology: a color guide to diagnosis and therapy,* ed 4, St Louis, 2004, Mosby. *3-19*

Habif T: *Clinical dermatology: a color guide to diagnosis and therapy,* ed 3, St Louis, 1996, Mosby. *Box 3-2 (measles, plaque, statis ulcer), 3-64*

Habif T: *Clinical dermatology: A color guide to diagnosis and therapy,* ed 2, St Louis, 1990, Mosby. *3-61*

Henry MC, Stapleton ER: *EMT prehospital care,* ed 2, Philadelphia, 1997, WB Saunders. *3-40 B, 3-40 D, 3-40 F (Courtesy SL Wiener and J Barrett.), 3-40 H*

Jarvis C: *Physical examination and health assessment,* ed 4, Philadelphia, 2004, WB Saunders. *3-71 B*

Judd RL, Ponsell PP: *Mosby's first responder,* ed 2, St Louis, 1988, Mosby. *3-10, 3-11, 3-12*

Lemmi FO, Lemmi CAE: *Physical assessment findings CD-ROM,* Philadelphia, 2000, WB Saunders. *Box 3-2 (lipoma, telangiectasia, lichenification, scaling and fissures of athlete's foot)*

Lookingbill D, Marks J: *Principles of dermatology,* ed 3, Philadelphia, 2000, WB Saunders. *3-21, 3-39*

Lookingbill D, Marks J: *Principles of dermatology,* ed 2, Philadelphia, 1993, WB Saunders. *3-66 B, 3-66 C*

Salvo S: *Massage therapy: principles and practice,* ed 2, Philadelphia, 2003, WB Saunders. *3-1, Box 3-3, 3-4, 3-57*

Seidel H: *Mosby's guide to physical examination,* ed 5, St Louis, 2003, Mosby. *Box 3-2 (scab, striae)*

Weston WL, Lane AT, Morrelli JG: *Color textbook of pediatric dermatology,* ed 2, St Louis, 1996, Mosby. *Box 3-2 (lichen planus, acne, sebaceous cyst, keloid), 3-70*

Weston WL, Lane AT, Morrelli JG: *Color textbook of pediatric dermatology,* St Louis, 1991, Mosby. *Box 3-2 (vitiligo)*

White GM: *Color atlas of regional dermatology,* St Louis, 1994, Mosby. *Box 3-2 (blister)*

Zitelli BJ, Davis HW: *Atlas of pediatric physical diagnosis,* ed 4, St Louis, 2002, Mosby. *3-65*

Zitelli BJ, Davis HW: *Atlas of pediatric physical diagnosis,* ed 3, St Louis, 1997, Mosby. *3-2, 3-3 (Courtesy Dr. Mary Jelks.), 3-26 (Courtesy Dr. Michael Sherlock.), 3-28 (Courtesy Dr. Donald Kress, Children's Hospital of Pittsburgh.), 3-38 (Courtesy Dr. Michael Sherlock.), 3-45*

CHAPTER 4

American College of Rheumatology, reprinted from the Clinical Slide Collection of the Rheumatic Diseases, 1991, 1995, 1997. *4-21, 4-37*

Ashwill J, Droske S: *Nursing care of children: principles and practice,* Philadelphia, 1997, WB Saunders. *4-44*

Beare PG, Myers JL: *Adult health nursing,* ed 3, St Louis, 1998, Mosby. *4-15*

Black JM, Hawks JH, Keene AM: *Medical-surgical nursing: clinical management for positive outcomes,* ed 6, Philadelphia, 2001, WB Saunders. *4-17*

Black JM, Matassarin-Jacobs E: *Luckmann and Sorensen's medical-surgical nursing,* ed 4, Philadelphia, 1993, WB Saunders. *4-39*

Callen J et al: *Color atlas of dermatology,* ed 2, Philadelphia, 2000, WB Saunders. *4-45*

Callen J et al: *Color atlas of dermatology,* Philadelphia, 1993, WB Saunders. *4-35 B*

Damjanov I: *Pathology for the health-related professions,* ed 2, Philadelphia, 2000, WB Saunders. *4-36 (modified), 4-52, 4-53, 4-54, 4-55, 4-59, 4-60, 4-61*

Forbes CD, Jackson WF: *A color atlas and text of clinical medicine,* ed 2, St Louis, 1997, Mosby. *4-50, 4-56*

Forbes CD, Jackson WF: *A color atlas and text of clinical medicine,* London, 1993, Mosby Europe. *4-29*

Frazier MS, Drzymkowski JW: *Essentials of human diseases and conditions,* ed 2, Philadelphia, 2000, WB Saunders. *4-20, 4-33, 4-34, 4-38 A, 4-46, 4-57, 4-65*

Gould B: *Pathophysiology for the health professions,* ed 2, Philadelphia, 2002, WB Saunders. *4-32*

Herlihy B, Maebius N: *The human body in health and illness,* ed 2, Philadelphia, 2003, WB Saunders. *4-62*

Hoppenfeld S: *Physical examination of the spine and extremities,* Upper Saddle River, NJ, 1976, Pearson Education. *4-22, 4-23, 4-24, 4-25, 4-26, 4-27, 4-35 A, 4-49*

Jarvis C: *Physical examination and health assessment,* ed 4, Philadelphia, 2004, WB Saunders. *4-28 (Courtesy AE Chudley, MD.), 4-58*

Kamal A, Brockelhurst JC: *Color atlas of geriatric medicine,* ed 2, St Louis, 1991, Mosby. *4-18, 4-30, 4-51*

Miller-Keane, O'Toole M: *Miller-Keane encyclopedia and dictionary of medicine, nursing, and allied health,* ed 7, Philadelphia, 2003, WB Saunders. *4-14*

Monahan FD, Neighbors M: *Medical-surgical nursing: foundations for clinical practice,* ed 2, Philadelphia, 1998, WB Saunders. *4-13 (Courtesy Otto Bock Orthopedic Industry, Inc., Minneapolis.)*

Perkin GD: *Mosby's color atlas and text of neurology,* London, 1998, Times Mirror International Publishers. *4-48*

Phipps WJ, Sands J, Marek JF: *Medical-surgical nursing: concepts and clinical practice,* ed 5, St Louis, 1999, Mosby. *4-31*

Salvo S: *Massage therapy: principles and practice,* ed 2, Philadelphia, 2003, WB Saunders. *4-1, 4-2, 4-3 (modified), 4-4 (modified), 4-5 (modified), 4-6, 4-7 (modified), 4-8, 4-9, 4-10, 4-11, 4-12, 4-47, 4-66*

Seeley R, Stephens T, Tate P: *Anatomy and physiology,* ed 2, New York, 1992, McGraw-Hill. *4-40*

Seidel H: *Mosby's guide to physical examination,* ed 4, St Louis, 1999, Mosby. *4-38 B (Courtesy Charles W Bradley, DPM, MPA, and Caroline Harvey, DPM, California College of Podiatric Medicine.)*

Shipley M: *A colour atlas of rheumatology,* ed 3, London, 1993, Mosby Year Book Europe. *4-16*

Zitelli BJ, Davis HW: *Atlas of pediatric physical diagnosis,* ed 4, St Louis, 2002, Mosby. *4-19 (Courtesy Dr. M Sherlock.), 4-43, 4-64, 4-67*

Zitelli BJ, Davis HW: *Atlas of pediatric physical diagnosis,* ed 3, St Louis, 1997, Mosby. *4-41, 4-42, 4-63*

CHAPTER 5

American College of Rheumatology, reprinted from the Clinical Slide Collection of the Rheumatic Diseases, 1991, 1995, 1997. *5-10*

Apple DJ, Rabb MF: *Ocular pathology,* ed 4, St Louis, 1996, Mosby. *5-18 B*

Ballinger P, Frank E: *Merrill's atlas of radiographic positions and radiologic procedures,* vol 3, ed 10, St Louis, 2003, Mosby. *5-19*

Beare PG, Myers JL: *Adult health nursing,* ed 3, St Louis, 1998, Mosby. *5-9*

Black JM, Hawks JH, Keene AM: *Medical-surgical nursing: clinical management for positive outcomes,* ed 6, Philadelphia, 2001, WB Saunders. *5-16 (Courtesy University of Michigan WK Kellogg Eye Center.)*

Cotran RS, Kumar V, Collins T: *Robbins pathologic basis of disease,* ed 6, Philadelphia, 1999, WB Saunders. *5-34*

Crossman AR, Neary D: *Neuroanatomy: an illustrated color text,* Edinburgh, 1995, Churchill Livingstone. *5-35*

Forbes CD, Jackson WF: *A color atlas and text of clinical medicine,* London, 1993, Mosby Europe. *5-33*

Frazier MS, Drzymkowski JW: *Essentials of human diseases and conditions,* ed 2, Philadelphia, 2000, WB Saunders. *5-8 (Courtesy ARO Tool Products/Ingersoll-Rand Professional Tools.), 5-30*

Goodman C, Snyder T: *Differential diagnosis in physical therapy,* ed 3, Philadelphia, 2000, WB Saunders. *5-31, 5-32*

Hoppenfeld S: *Physical examination of the spine and extremities,* Upper Saddle River, NJ, 1976, Pearson Education. *5-29*

Kamal A, Brockelhurst JC: *Color atlas of geriatric medicine,* ed 2, St Louis, 1991, Mosby. *5-15*

Kanski J: *Clinical ophthalmology: a systematic approach,* ed 5, 2003, Butterworth-Heinemann. *5-14*

Kanski J, Nischal KK: *Ophthalmology: clinical signs and differential diagnosis,* London, 1999, Mosby International. *5-21*

Kumar V, Cotran RS, Robbins SL: *Basic pathology,* ed 6, Philadelphia, 1997, WB Saunders. *5-7 A, 5-7 B (Courtesy Eileen Bigio, MD, Department of Pathology, University of Texas Southwestern Medical Center.)*

Monahan FD, Neighbors M: *Medical-surgical nursing: foundations for clinical practice,* ed 2, Philadelphia, 1998, WB Saunders. *5-25*

Okazaki H, Scheithauer BW: *Atlas of neuropathology,* London, 1988, Gower Medical Publishing. *5-17 (Courtesy Mayo Clinic.), 5-23 (Courtesy Mayo Clinic.)*

Perkin GD: *Mosby's color atlas and text of neurology,* London, 1998, Times Mirror International Publishers. *5-20, 5-36*

Perkin GD, Hochberg FH, Miller DC: *Atlas of clinical neurology,* ed 2, London, 1993, Gower Medical Publishing. *5-26*

Phipps WJ, Sands J, Marek JF: *Medical-surgical nursing: concepts and clinical practice,* ed 5, St Louis, 1999, Mosby. *5-24*

Salvo S: *Massage therapy: principles and practice,* ed 2, Philadelphia, 2003, WB Saunders. *5-1, Box 5-1, 5-2, 5-3, 5-4, 5-5, 5-6, 5-11, 5-12, 5-13*

Swartz M: *Textbook of physical diagnosis: history and examination,* ed 4, Philadelphia, 2002, WB Saunders. *5-27*

Zitelli BJ, Davis HW: *Atlas of pediatric physical diagnosis,* ed 3, St Louis, 1997, Mosby. *5-18 A, 5-22, 5-28*

CHAPTER 6

Bryant RA: *Acute and chronic wounds: nursing management,* St Louis, 1992, Mosby. *6-9 (Courtesy Abbott Northwestern Hospital, Minneapolis.)*

Damjanov I: *Pathology for the health-related professions,* ed 2, Philadelphia, 2000, WB Saunders. *6-5 (modified), 6-10, 6-14 (modified)*

Damjanov I: *Pathology for the health-related professions,* Philadelphia, 1996, WB Saunders. *6-2*

Forbes CD, Jackson WF: *A color atlas and text of clinical medicine,* ed 2, St Louis, 1997, Mosby. *6-3, 6-4*

Frazier MS, Drzymkowski JW: *Essentials of human diseases and conditions,* ed 2, Philadelphia, 2000, WB Saunders. *6-15*

Potter PA, Perry AG: *Fundamentals of nursing,* ed 4, St Louis, 1997, Mosby. *6-8*

Salvo S: *Massage therapy: principles and practice,* ed 2, Philadelphia, 2003, WB Saunders. *6-1*

Seidel H: *Mosby's guide to physical examination,* ed 5, St Louis, 2003, Mosby. *6-7, 6-16*

Seidel H: *Mosby's guide to physical examination,* ed 4, St Louis, 1999, Mosby. *6-12*

Swartz M: *Textbook of physical diagnosis: history and examination,* ed 4, Philadelphia, 2002, WB Saunders. *6-11*

Thibodeau GA: *Anatomy and physiology,* St Louis, 1987, Mosby College Publishing. *6-13 (Courtesy Dr. Edmund Beard.)*

Zitelli BJ, Davis HW: *Atlas of pediatric physical diagnosis,* ed 3, St Louis, 1997, Mosby. *6-6 (Courtesy Dr. TP Foley, Jr.)*

CHAPTER 7

Barkauskas VH et al: *Health and physical assessment,* ed 2, St Louis, 1998, Mosby. *7-32*

Bingham BJG, Hawke M, Kwok P: *Atlas of clinical otolaryngology,* St Louis, 1992, Mosby. *7-27*

Callen J et al: *Color atlas of dermatology,* ed 2, Philadelphia, 2000, WB Saunders. *7-36, 7-44*

Chabner DA: *The language of medicine,* ed 6, Philadelphia, 2001, WB Saunders. *Box 7-1*

Copstead LC, Banasik JL: *Pathophysiology: biological and behavioral perspectives,* ed 2, Philadelphia, 2000, WB Saunders. *7-34 (Courtesy Beth Paine, Sacred Heart Medical Center.)*

Cotran RS, Kumar V, Collins T: *Robbins pathologic basis of disease,* ed 6, Philadelphia, 1999, WB Saunders. *7-25 (Courtesy William Edwards, MD.), 7-31*

Cox NH, Lawrence CM: *Diagnostic problems in dermatology,* St Louis, 1998, Mosby. *7-43*

Damjanov I, Linder J: *Pathology: a color atlas,* St Louis, 2000, Mosby. *7-13, 7-18, 7-21, 7-29*

Damjanov I: *Pathology for the health-related professions,* ed 2, Philadelphia, 2000, WB Saunders. *Box 7-4 (Kaposi's*

sarcoma), *7-19 (inset only), 7-23, 7-28, 7-33 (modified),
7-37*

Damjanov I: *Pathology for the health-related professions,*
Philadelphia, 1996, WB Saunders. *Box 7-4 (diseases
common in persons with AIDS)*

Dockery GL: *Cutaneous disorders of the lower extremity,*
Philadelphia, 1997, WB Saunders. *7-38*

Frazier MS, Drzymkowski JW: *Essentials of human diseases
and conditions,* ed 2, Philadelphia, 2000, WB Saunders.
7-14, 7-20

Goodman C, Boissonnault W, Fuller K: *Pathology: implications for the physical therapist,* ed 2, Philadelphia,
2003, WB Saunders. *7-15*

Goodman C, Snyder T: *Differential diagnosis in physical
therapy,* ed 3, Philadelphia, 2000, WB Saunders. *7-30*

Gould B: *Pathophysiology for the health professions,* ed 2,
Philadelphia, 2002, WB Saunders. *7-16, 7-19, 7-22,
7-39*

Habif T: *Clinical dermatology: a color guide to diagnosis and
therapy,* ed 4, St Louis, 2004, Mosby. *7-35, 7-45*

Habif T, Campbell J, Quitadamo M, Zug K: *Skin disease:
diagnosis and treatment,* St Louis, 2001, Mosby. *7-42*

Kumar V, Cotran RS, Robbins SL: *Basic pathology,* ed 6,
Philadelphia, 1997, WB Saunders. *7-17 (Courtesy Tom
Rogers, MD, University of Texas Southwestern Medical
School.), 7-24 (Courtesy Department of Pathology, Univer-
sity of Texas Southwestern Medical School.), 7-40*

Lewis SM, Heitkemper MM, Dirksen SR: *Medical-surgical
nursing: assessment and management of clinical problems,*
ed 5, St Louis, 2000, Mosby. *Box 7-2*

Potter PA, Perry AG: *Fundamentals of nursing,* ed 5, St
Louis, 2001, Mosby. *Box 7-3 (Courtesy Rolin Graphics.)*

Salvo S: *Massage therapy: principles and practice,* ed 2,
Philadelphia, 2003, WB Saunders. *7-1 (modified), 7-2
(modified), 7-3, 7-4, 7-5, 7-6, 7-7, 7-8, 7-9, 7-10*

Stone DR, Gorbach SL: *Atlas of infectious diseases,*
Philadelphia, 2000, WB Saunders. *7-46*

Swartz M: *Textbook of physical diagnosis: history and
examination,* ed 4, Philadelphia, 2002, WB Saunders.
7-41

Thibodeau GA, Patton, KT: *Anatomy and physiology,* ed 4,
St Louis, 1999, Mosby. *7-11*

Zitelli BJ, Davis HW: *Atlas of pediatric physical diagnosis,* ed 4, St Louis, 2002, Mosby. *7-12 (Courtesy JR
Zuberbuhler, MD.)*

Zitelli BJ, Davis HW: *Atlas of pediatric physical diagnosis,*
ed 3, St Louis, 1997, Mosby. *7-26, 7-47 (Courtesy Dr. M
Sherlock.)*

CHAPTER 8

Cotran RS, Kumar V, Collins T: *Robbins pathologic basis of
disease,* ed 6, Philadelphia, WB Saunders, 1999. *8-10
(Courtesy Dr. Eduardo Unis, Children's Hospital of
Pittsburgh.), 8-12, 8-25 A*

Damjanov I, Linder J: *Pathology: a color atlas,* St Louis,
2000, Mosby. *8-15, 8-16*

Damjanov I: *Pathology for the health-related professions,* ed
2, Philadelphia, 2000, WB Saunders. *8-9, 8-13*

Fletcher CDM, McKee PH: *An atlas of gross pathology,*
London, 1987, Gower Medical Publishing. *8-18*

Frazier MS, Drzymkowski JW: *Essentials of human diseases
and conditions,* ed 2, Philadelphia, 2000, WB Saunders.
8-6, 8-22

Gould B: *Pathophysiology for the health professions,* ed 2,
Philadelphia, 2002, WB Saunders. *8-20, 8-21 B (Courtesy RW Shaw, MD, North York General Hospital), 8-25 B
(modified)*

Huether SE, McCance KL: *Understanding pathophysiology,*
ed 2, St Louis, 2000, Mosby. *8-8*

Ignatavicius DD, Workman ML, Mishler MA: *Medical-
surgical nursing across the health care continuum,* ed 3,
Philadelphia, 1999, WB Saunders. *8-5*

Kumar V, Cotran RS, Robbins SL: *Basic pathology,* ed 6,
Philadelphia, 1997, WB Saunders. *8-17*

Salvo S: *Massage therapy: principles and practice,* ed 2,
Philadelphia, 2003, WB Saunders. *8-1, 8-2, 8-3, 8-14,
8-19, 8-23*

Thibodeau GA, Patton, KT: *Anatomy and physiology,* ed 4,
St Louis, 1999, Mosby. *8-7 (Courtesy Rolin Graphics.)*

Zitelli BJ, Davis HW: *Atlas of pediatric physical diagnosis,*
ed 3, St Louis, 1997, Mosby. *8-4 (Courtesy Dr. Meyer B
Marks.), 8-11, 8-24 (Courtesy Dr. Ellen Wald, Children's
Hospital of Pittsburgh.)*

CHAPTER 9

Cotran RS, Kumar V, Collins T: *Robbins pathologic basis
of disease,* ed 6, Philadelphia, 1999, WB Saunders.
9-43

Damjanov I, Linder J: *Pathology: a color atlas,* St Louis,
2000, Mosby. *9-16, 9-17, 9-18, 9-21, 9-22*

Damjanov I: *Pathology for the health-related professions,* ed
2, Philadelphia, 2000, WB Saunders. *9-11, 9-12, 9-35,
9-36, 9-40*

Efron G: Sinai Hospital of Baltimore. *9-19*

Fletcher CDM, McKee PH: *An atlas of gross pathology,*
London, 1987, Gower Medical Publishing. *9-9, 9-42*

Forbes CD, Jackson WF: *A color atlas and text of clinical
medicine,* London, 1993, Mosby Europe. *9-7, 9-39*

Frazier MS, Drzymkowski JW: *Essentials of human diseases
and conditions,* ed 2, Philadelphia, 2000, WB Saunders.
*Box 9-1 (colostomy), 9-10 (modified), 9-23, 9-24, 9-27,
9-37*

Gould B: *Pathophysiology for the health professions,* ed 2,
Philadelphia, 2002, WB Saunders. *9-31*

Kumar V, Cotran RS, Robbins SL: *Basic pathology,* ed 6,
Philadelphia, 1997, WB Saunders. *9-14*

Lemmi FO, Lemmi CAE: *Physical assessment findings
CD-ROM,* Philadelphia, 2000, WB Saunders. *9-34*

Lewis SM, Heitkemper MM, Dirksen SR: *Medical-surgical
nursing: assessment and management of clinical problems,*
ed 5, St Louis, 2000, Mosby. *9-20*

Miesiewicz JJ et al: *Atlas of clinical gastroenterology,* ed 2,
London, 1994, Gower Medical Publishing. *9-41*

Potter PA, Perry AG: *Basic nursing,* ed 4, St Louis, 1999, Mosby. *9-29*

Reschke E: Muskegon, Michigan, reprinted with permission. *Box 9-2 (adipose tissue)*

Salvo S: *Massage therapy: principles and practice,* ed 2, Philadelphia, 2003, WB Saunders. *9-1, 9-2, 9-3, 9-4, 9-5*

Seeley R, Stephens T, Tate P: *Anatomy and physiology,* ed 3, New York, 1995, McGraw-Hill. *9-15*

Seidel H: *Mosby's guide to physical examination,* ed 5, St Louis, 2003, Mosby. *9-26*

Swartz M: *Textbook of physical diagnosis: history and examination,* ed 4, Philadelphia, 2002, WB Saunders. *9-32*

Thibodeau GA, Patton KT: *Anatomy and physiology,* ed 4, St Louis, 1999, Mosby. *Box 9-2 (somatotypes)*

Wardlaw GM, Insel PM: *Perspectives in nutrition,* ed 3, St Louis, 1996, The McGraw-Hill Companies. *9-13*

Wilson SF, Giddens JF: *Health assessment for nursing practice,* ed 2, St Louis, 2001, Mosby. *9-6*

Winawer SJ: *Management of gastrointestinal diseases,* London, 1992, Gower Medical Publishing. *Box 9-1 (ileostomy)*

Zitelli BJ, Davis HW: *Atlas of pediatric physical diagnosis,* ed 3, St Louis, 1997, Mosby. *9-8, 9-25, 9-28, 9-33 (Courtesy Dr. GDW McKendrik.), 9-38*

CHAPTER 10

Damjanov I: *Pathology for the health-related professions,* ed 2, Philadelphia, 2000, WB Saunders. *10-9, 10-10*

Damjanov I: *Pathology for the health-related professions,* Philadelphia, 1996, WB Saunders. *10-3, 10-4*

Fletcher CDM, McKee PH: *An atlas of gross pathology,* London, 1987, Gower Medical Publishing. *10-5*

Forbes CD, Jackson WF: *A color atlas and text of clinical medicine,* ed 2, St Louis, 1997, Mosby. *Box 10-1 (patient undergoing hemodialysis)*

Gould B: *Pathophysiology for the health professions,* ed 2, Philadelphia, 2002, WB Saunders. *10-6 (modified)*

Lewis SM, Heitkemper MM, Dirksen SR: *Medical-surgical nursing: assessment and management of clinical problems,* ed 5, St Louis, 2000, Mosby. *Box 10-1 (hemodialysis figure)*

Phipps WJ, Sands J, Marek JF: *Medical-surgical nursing: concepts and clinical practice,* ed 5, St Louis, 1999, Mosby. *10-7*

Salvo S: *Massage therapy: principles and practice,* ed 2, Philadelphia, 2003, WB Saunders. *10-1, 10-2*

Zitelli BJ, Davis HW: *Atlas of pediatric physical diagnosis,* ed 2, London, 1992, Gower Medical Publishing. *10-8*

CHAPTER 11

Applegate E: *The anatomy and physiology learning system,* ed 2, Philadelphia, 2000, WB Saunders. *11-1, 11-2, 11-3, 11-4, 11-5, 11-6, 11-7, 11-8*

Behrman RE, Kliegman RM, Arvin AM: Slide set, *Nelson textbook of pediatrics,* ed 15, Philadelphia, WB Saunders, 1996. *11-15, 11-16*

Callen J et al: *Color atlas of dermatology,* ed 2, Philadelphia, 2000, WB Saunders. *11-18*

Chessel GSJ, Jamieson MJ, Morton RA, Petrie TC, Towler HMA: *Diagnostic tests in clinical medicine,* London, 1985, Wolfe Medical Publishing. *11-17*

Cotran RS, Kumar V, Collins T: *Robbins pathologic basis of disease,* ed 6, Philadelphia, 1999, WB Saunders. *11-30*

Damjanov I, Linder J: *Pathology: a color atlas,* St Louis, 2000, Mosby. *11-9, 11-22*

Damjanov I: *Pathology for the health-related professions,* Philadelphia, 1996, WB Saunders. *11-12, 11-14, 11-21*

Epstein O et al: *Clinical examination,* London, 1992, Gower Medical Publishing. *11-29*

Fletcher CDM, McKee PH: *An atlas of gross pathology,* London, 1987, Gower Medical Publishing. *11-13, 11-25*

Forbes CD, Jackson WF: *A color atlas and text of clinical medicine,* ed 2, St Louis, 1997, Mosby. *11-20*

Frazier MS, Drzymkowski JW: *Essentials of human diseases and conditions,* ed 2, Philadelphia, 2000, WB Saunders. *11-24*

Gould B: *Pathophysiology for the health professions,* ed 2, Philadelphia, 2002, WB Saunders. *11-23*

Greenberger NJ, Hinthorn DR: *History taking and physical examination: essentials and clinical correlates,* St Louis, 1993, Mosby. *11-27 (Courtesy US Public Health Service.)*

Lewis SM, Heitkemper MM, Dirksen SR: *Medical-surgical nursing: assessment and management of clinical problems,* ed 5, St Louis, 2000, Mosby. *11-11*

Monahan FD, Neighbors M: *Medical-surgical nursing: foundations for clinical practice,* ed 2, Philadelphia, 1998, WB Saunders. *11-31 (Courtesy Leonard Wolf, MD.)*

Morse SA, Moreland A, Holmes K: *Atlas of sexually transmitted diseases and AIDS,* ed 2, London, 1996, Gower Medical Publishing. *11-28*

Salvo S: *Massage therapy: principles and practice,* ed 2, Philadelphia, 2003, WB Saunders. *Box 11-2, 11-26*

Swartz M: *Textbook of physical diagnosis: history and examination,* ed 4, Philadelphia, 2002, WB Saunders. *11-19*

Tilton RC, Ballows A, Hohnadel DC: *Clinical laboratory medicine,* St Louis, 1992, Mosby. *11-10*

CHAPTER 12

American Cancer Society. *12-3 (data only), 12-4 (data only), 12-5 (data only)*

Ballinger PW: *Merrill's atlas of radiographic positions and radiologic procedures,* vol 2, ed 10, St Louis, 2003, Mosby. *12-13 A*

Ballinger PW: *Merrill's atlas of radiographic positions and radiologic procedures,* ed 9, St Louis, 1999, Mosby. *12-10*

Beare PG, Myers JL: *Adult health nursing,* ed 3, St Louis, 1998, Mosby. *12-14 A*

Belcher AE: *Cancer nursing,* St Louis, 1992, Mosby. *12-1*

Callen J et al: *Color atlas of dermatology,* Philadelphia, 1993, WB Saunders. *12-33*

Cawson RA, Eveson JW: *Oral pathology and diagnosis,* London, 1987, Heinemann Medical Books/Gower Medical Publishing. *12-29*

Chabner DA: *The language of medicine,* ed 6, Philadelphia, 2001, WB Saunders. *12-14 B*

Christiansen JL, Grzybowski JM: *Biology of aging,* St Louis, 1993, Mosby. *12-16*

Cotran RS, Kumar V, Collins T: *Robbins pathologic basis of disease,* ed 6, Philadelphia, 1999, WB Saunders. *12-26*

Damjanov I: *Pathology for the health-related professions,* ed 2, Philadelphia, 2000, WB Saunders. *12-2 (modified), 12-7, 12-8, 12-12, 12-22, 12-25, 12-28, 12-34*

Fletcher CDM, McKee PH: *An atlas of gross pathology,* London, 1987, Gower Medical Publishing. *12-15, 12-31*

Forbes CD, Jackson WF: *A color atlas and text of clinical medicine,* ed 2, St Louis, 1997, Mosby. *12-23*

Frazier MS, Drzymkowski JW: *Essentials of human diseases and conditions,* ed 2, Philadelphia, 2000, WB Saunders. *12-9*

Gould B: *Pathophysiology for the health professions,* ed 2, Philadelphia, 2002, WB Saunders. *12-17 (Courtesy RW Shaw, MD, North York General Hospital.), 12-35 (Courtesy Dr. M McKenzie.)*

Huether SE, McCance KL: *Understanding pathophysiology,* ed 2, St Louis, 2000, Mosby. *12-21*

Kumar V, Cotran RS, Robbins SL: *Basic pathology,* ed 6, Philadelphia, 1997, WB Saunders. *12-11, 12-18 (Courtesy Dr. Kyle Molberg, University of Texas Southwestern Medical Center.), 12-19, 12-20, 12-24 (Courtesy Dr. Robert McKenna, University of Texas Southwestern Medical Center.), 12-36*

McCance KL, Huether SE: *Pathophysiology: The biological basis for disease in adults and children,* ed 3, St Louis, 1998, Mosby. *12-27*

Salvo S: *Massage therapy: principles and practice,* ed 2, Philadelphia, 2003, WB Saunders. *12-6*

Swartz M: *Textbook of physical diagnosis: history and examination,* ed 4, Philadelphia, 2002, WB Saunders. *12-32*

Turk JL, Fletcher CDM: *Atlas of surgical pathology,* London, 1991, Gower Medical Publishing. *12-30*

Index

Page numbers followed by "b" indicate
box, "f" indicate figure, and "t" indicate
table.